A P P L I E D

Pharmaceutics

IN CONTEMPORARY

COMPOUNDING

SECOND EDITION

Robert Shrewsbury

University of North Carolina

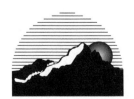

Morton Publishing Company

925 W. Kenyon Avenue, Unit 12

Englewood, CO 80110

http://www.morton-pub.com

BOOK TEAM

Publisher: Douglas Morton
Project Manager: Dona Mendoza
Copy Editor: Carolyn Acheson
Cover & Interior Design: Bob Schram, Bookends
Composition: Ash Street Typecrafters, Inc.

ISBN 10: 0-89582-744-1
ISBN 13: 978-089582-744-9

Printed in the United States of America

10   9   8   7   6   5   4   3   2

Preface

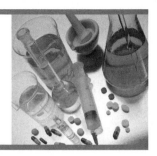

*P*HARMACEUTICS AND COMPOUNDING ARE INTIMATELY related and mutually inclusive. Pharmaceutics addresses the scientific considerations and methodologies needed to prepare and use pharmaceutical dosage forms on a large scale. Compounding is the extemporaneous preparation of the same type of dosage forms to meet an individual patient's need. This book is designed to convey a fundamental understanding of the principles and practices involved in both the development and the production of compounded dosage forms by applying pharmaceutical principles.

The first edition concentrated on the art of compounding and grew out of the author's personal experiences in conducting pharmaceutics and compounding laboratories at the University of North Carolina School of Pharmacy. These laboratories are part of a five-semester Pharmaceutical Care Laboratory sequence that has been in place at the school for more than a decade (*International Journal of Pharmaceutical Compounding* 10:353–358, 2006).

This second edition brings a balance of material between pharmaceutics and compounding and adds a dozen new chapters. Many of the previous chapters have been expanded significantly to strengthen the applicable pharmaceutics information and have been updated to reflect the state-of-the-art of compounding. Relevant principles of both compounding and pharmaceutics are organizationally presented in a similar order so the material in the later chapters builds on content from the earlier chapters. The book is illustrated extensively, and the illustrations are placed as close as possible to the corresponding text, as an aid to the reader.

Also, this second edition has the enhanced feature of Internet-based material, which supplements and expands even further the materials in the book. The online resource (http://pharmlabs.unc.edu) is an open website designed to enhance the presentation of material and increase students' preparation and learning. The site has been designated a Basic Resource for Pharmaceutical Education by the American Association of Colleges of Pharmacy (AACP) since 1999. Additional materials available on the website include: (1) laboratory exercises that can be adapted for either pharmaceutics or compounding; (2) formulation records of compounds

developed and used at the University of North Carolina School of Pharmacy; (3) instructional videos (all of the photo series in the book have a video clip counterpart); (4) instructional videos not found in the book; and (5) an interactive question bank for students to self-assess their own learning and understanding.

Three major organizational features are as follows: The first chapters (1–7) address the legal and operational basis of pharmaceutical compounding. These chapters cover the elements of a prescription to compound; legal requirements for the compounder in terms of training, equipment, and facilities; and stability considerations of the final formulation. Beginning with Chapter 8, the order of the chapters is based on the physical state of the formulation and progresses from solution dosage forms through the dispersed systems and powder based formulations, and ends with the modified release formulations. The last group of chapters (24–30) deals with the compounding and administration of sterile formulations in inpatient, outpatient, and home health care settings.

A search for relevant materials in any health science library will reveal that volumes of books have been written for each chapter covered in this work. Therefore, this book is not a complete and exhaustive treatise of the disciplines of pharmaceutics and compounding. It includes a consolidation of these materials plus the original materials of the author in a format that is easily accessible and understandable. The book was developed for four audiences: pharmacists, pharmacy educators, pharmacy students, and pharmacy technicians. Pharmacists and pharmacy technicians most likely will use the book as a stand-alone resource with some reliance on the additional support available at the website. Pharmacy educators and students, however, are more likely to use the book in conjunction with the website because detailed pharmaceutics laboratory procedures and accompanying learning aids are available online.

The author sincerely thanks Alexandra Gunn for producing many of the illustrations in this work. Alexandra is a graphic artist and web based multimedia designer who holds BFA and BA degrees from the School of the Art Institute of Chicago and North Carolina State University College of Design.

About the Author

Dr. Shrewsbury received his B.S. in Pharmacy from the University of Oklahoma in 1972 and his Ph.D. in Pharmaceutical Sciences from the University of Kentucky in 1977. He joined the University of North Carolina School of Pharmacy faculty in 1980 and is currently an Associate Professor in the Division of Pharmacy Practice and Experiential Education. His background training is in basic and applied biopharmaceutics and pharmacokinetics, and drug interaction mechanisms. More recently, his research interest have focused on classroom and laboratory instructional methodologies utilizing web based or technology based formats. He has authored books in pharmacy and pharmacology, and has written a number of online pharmacy courses and study guides.

For Laura, who has always been there.

CREDITS

Special Photo Credits — Copyright © — Reprinted with Permission

Chapter 1 – Professional Compounding Centers of America, Inc., Houston, TX, p. 1.

Chapter 2 – National Association of Boards of Pharmacy, Park Ridge, IL, pgs. 7, 11.

Chapter 3 – National Association of Boards of Pharmacy, Park Ridge, IL, p. 25.

Chapter 4 – National Association of Boards of Pharmacy, Park Ridge, IL, pgs. 27, 29, 33, 35.

Chapter 4 – Professional Compounding Centers of America, Inc., Houston, TX, pgs. 30, 32.

Chapter 4 – Perspective Press, p. 35.

Chapter 6 – International Journal of Pharmaceutical Compounding, Inc., Edmond, OK, p. 51.

Chapter 7 – Perspective Press, pgs. 55, 60, 61.

Chapter 7 – Professional Compounding Centers of America, Inc., Houston, TX, p. 57.

Chapter 13 – Professional Compounding Centers of America, Inc., Houston, TX, p. 108.

Chapter 15 – Perspective Press, p. 117.

Chapter 15 – Professional Compounding Centers of America, Inc., Houston, TX, p. 121.

Chapter 17 – Michigan Pharmacists Association Patient Education Program, Lansing, MI, p. 132.

Chapter 18 – Professional Compounding Centers of America, Inc., Houston, TX, p. 148.

Chapter 18 – American Pharmaceutical Association, Washington, DC, p. 154.

Chapter 19 – Capsugel, Inc., Peapack, NJ, pgs. 155, 156.

Chapter 20 – Professional Compounding Centers of America, Inc., Houston, TX, p. 170.

Chapter 24 – Perspective Press, pgs. 209, 210, 211, 215.

Chapter 24 – Morton Publishing Company, Englewood, CO, p. 217.

Chapter 25 – Perspective Press, pgs. 226, 228, 229.

Chapter 26 – National Institute of Diabetes and Digestive and Kidney Diseases, National Institute of Health, p. 244

Contents

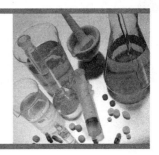

CHAPTER ONE

What Is Compounding and Why Do It?

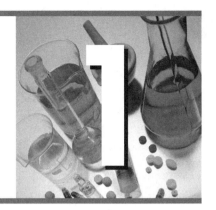

COMPOUNDING HAS ALWAYS BEEN A BASIC COMPONENT in the practice of pharmacy. There is an art, a *secundum artem*, to begin with only raw ingredients and formulate (or compound) a drug product that will meet the unique need of a patient. This art, this knowledge and skill, is unique to the profession of pharmacy.

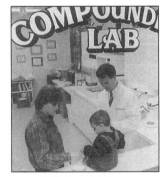

Clearly, the practice of pharmacy has undergone significant changes over the past three decades. In the 1980s and 1990s the number of compounded prescriptions began to increase as a result of the emergence of home health care, hospice care, pain management, and total parenteral nutrition, which requires that preparations be compounded. At the same time, many pharmaceutical manufacturers reduced the number of available dosage forms as a cost-saving measure. Also, most drugs did not have a pediatric indication and were not available in liquid dosage forms.

During the same time period, pharmacists assumed responsibility for patients' outcomes through the principles of pharmaceutical care and established themselves as problem solvers in their relationships with physicians, patients, and other health-care providers. Many pharmacists have chosen the ability to compound as the primary means to provide pharmaceutical care for their patients. Some have practice sites dedicated exclusively to compounding. Others do compounding as part of their practice. In either case, the contribution of compounding provides a means to resolve individual patients' problems. In 1995, the percentage of compounded prescriptions represented approximately 11% of all prescriptions dispensed.[1] Today, approximately 30 to 40 million compounded formulations are dispensed yearly in the United States.[2]

Definitions

Chapter <1075> Good Compounding Practices in the United States Pharmacopeia—National Formulary (USP/NF) defines *compounding* as

the preparation, mixing, assembling, packaging, or labeling of a drug or device in accordance with a licensed practitioner's prescription under an initiative based on the practitioner/patient/pharmacist/compounder relationship in the course of professional practice.

Compounding includes the following:

- Preparation of drugs or devices in anticipation of prescription drug orders based on routine, regularly observed prescribing patterns.

- Reconstitution or manipulation of commercial products that may require the addition of one or more ingredients as a result of a licensed practitioner's prescription drug order.

- Preparation of drugs or devices for the purposes of, or as an incident to, research, teaching, or chemical analysis.[3]

Compounding is not manufacturing in the legal sense. *Manufacturing* is defined in the same USP/NF chapter as

the production, propagation, conversion, or processing of a drug or device, either directly or indirectly, by extraction of the drug from substances of natural origin or by means of chemical or biological synthesis. Manufacturing also includes (1) any packaging or repackaging of the substance(s) or labeling or relabeling of containers for the promotion and marketing of such drugs or devices; (2) any preparation of a drug or device that is given or sold for resale by pharmacies, practitioners, or other persons; (3) the distribution of inordinate amounts of compounded preparations or the copying of commercially available drug products; and (4) the preparation of any quantity of a drug product without a licensed prescriber/patient/licensed pharmacist/compounder relationship.

Various Facets of Compounding

Compounding has different facets. Some compounding involves reconstituting a lyophilized powder to form a simple solution. More complex compounding operations include formulation of a suspension, an ointment, lozenges, suppositories, and sustained release capsules. In most hospitals, compounding involves the preparation of intravenous (IV) admixtures, parenteral nutrition solutions, and radiopharmaceuticals. For home health care settings, compounding requires the preparation of cassettes, syringes, and other devices for home-infusion administration. Table 1.1 outlines several categories of compounding:

TABLE 1.1: CATEGORIES OF COMPOUNDING

Category	Compounding Activity
1	Nonsterile – Simple Mixing of two or more commercial products.
2	Nonsterile – Complex Compounding with the bulk drug substance or when calculations are required.
3	Sterile – Risk Level I See Chapter <797> Pharmaceutical Compounding – Sterile Preparations.
4	Sterile – Risk Level II See Chapter <797> Pharmaceutical Compounding – Sterile Preparations.
5	Sterile – Risk Level III See Chapter <797> Pharmaceutical Compounding – Sterile Preparations.
6	Radiopharmaceuticals Preparation of radiopharmaceuticals.
7	Veterinary Preparation of veterinary pharmaceuticals.

Compounding meets patients' needs that cannot be met with manufactured products. Quite simply, it is not feasible practically or economically for pharmaceutical companies to manufacture all the different dosage forms or dosage strengths required to meet various individual needs. Some examples of individual needs that can be met with compounding are as follows:

- *Noncompliant children.* Children often refuse to take medication. Dosage forms that might appeal to a child include chewing gum, lozenges, lollipops, suckers, puddings, or

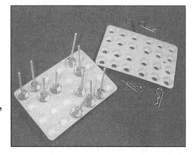

topical ointment. Flavoring and color also can influence a child's compliance.

- *Difficulty in handling or measuring dosages.* Prefilled syringes and prefilled dosage cups are well accepted because the dose is premeasured. Another application is to combine several needed medications into one dosage form (e.g., capsule).

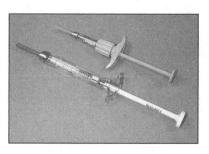

- *Physiological barriers that prevent dosing by one route of administration.* For example, if oral administration is not possible because of a patient's debilitation or inability to swallow, a suppository or topical formulation might be indicated. If the patient cannot swallow a tablet, the tablet can be crushed and placed in a suspension.

- *The need to change dosages frequently, depending on the patient's pharmacokinetic parameters.* With drugs that are therapeutically monitored, dosages are changed based on parameters such as renal function. Adjustments in the dosages can be made quickly and frequently with compounded formulations.

- *Long-term therapy in home-care settings* where the patient does not have access to, or does not require, institutional services.

- *Cases in which a specific commercial drug product is not available in the amount or concentration required for a patient.* A common case would be a pediatric patient needing a medication that currently is available only in an adult formulation.

- *Cases in which drugs have not been formulated into commercial products* (e.g., orphan drugs).

- *A commercial product that has been discontinued.*

- *In the institutional setting, routine use of parenteral dosage formulations such as admixtures, parenteral nutrition solutions, and radiopharmaceuticals prepared on an "as needed" basis.*

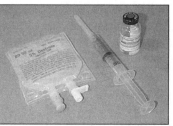

- *In professions other than pharmacy* (e.g., dentistry, veterinary medicine), unique problems that require a compounded intervention.

- *Provide a less invasive formulation such as a topical cream or transdermal gel.* This is an especially good choice for the very young, the mentally or physically challenged, the elderly, and animal patients.

General Compounding Considerations

Compounding considerations are "questions to ask" before, during, and after the compounding process. There must be an initial decision of whether it is necessary to compound the prescription. Then numerous factors have to be considered as the prescription is compounded. Finally, records and checks must be done after the compounding is completed. Below is a summary of some of these considerations.

Decision to compound the formulation:

1. Is the drug on the FDA list of "Drugs That Were Withdrawn or Removed from the U. S. Market for Safety Reasons?" Table 1.2 lists drugs that cannot be used in any compounded formulation.

2. What is the solubility of the active ingredient? Is it soluble in water, oil, or alcohol?
   a. Should the drug be suspended? If so, which suspending agent should be used?
   b. Does a solvent have to be used to wet the drug before suspending?

3. What is the stability of the active ingredient?
   a. Is it unstable in an aqueous solution?
   b. Is it stable in a fixed oil?
   c. What role does pH play in the stability of the final product?
   d. Do certain excipients adversely affect the stability?
   e. How do sweeteners and/or flavors affect the stability or pH?
   f. What are the storage requirements of the final formulation?
   g. Can a beyond use date be determined?

4. Is the active ingredient available for an extemporaneous compounding?
   a. Is the active ingredient available in raw powder form?
   b. Must a commercially available product be the source of the active ingredient?
   c. If the active ingredient is available only as a commercial product, can it be manipulated and still retain its stability?
   d. Which is more cost effective for the patient, the compounded formulation or the manufactured product?
   e. Which of the two preceding options makes a better product with regard to flavor or consistency?

5. What dosage formulations are possible for this specific active ingredient?

Considerations before beginning the compounding process:

- Is the pharmacist qualified to prepare this prescription?
- Are the proper equipment, supplies, facilities, and workspace available?
- Can the drug and ingredient identity, quality, and purity be assured?
- Is literature information available about the formulation to help determine an appropriate beyond use date?
- What basic quality control measures will be used to assure that the prescription is compounded correctly?
- Does the patient have the necessary skills to use and store the prescription?

Considerations as the prescription is being compounded:

- Read and interpret the prescription.
- Determine a preliminary compounding procedure.
- Collect and prepare the required ingredients, drugs, supplies, equipment, and clothing.
- Package the formulation in an appropriate container, and affix appropriate labels.
- Perform quality control procedures.

Considerations after compounding:

- Recheck all work.
- If the compounded formulation is new to the pharmacist, keep a sample or make a second batch to assess its stability or appearance over the expected time of therapy.
- Document the compounding process.
- Deliver the product to the patient with appropriate consultation.
- Return ingredients, supplies, etc. to their proper locations. Perform required maintenance on equipment.

Compounding—Is It for Everyone?

The compounder is responsible for compounding preparations of acceptable strength, quality, and purity with appropriate packaging and labeling in accordance with good compounding practices, official standards, and relevant scientific data and information.[3] Compounders engaging in compounding should have to continually expand their compounding knowledge by participating in seminars, studying appropriate literature, and consulting colleagues.[4]

A pharmacist is legally licensed to compound, but is the pharmacist technically qualified to compound? All

TABLE 1.2: DRUGS THAT WERE WITHDRAWN OR REMOVED FROM THE U.S. MARKET FOR SAFETY REASONS

The list below is a compilation of two lists published by agencies of the federal government. The FDA Compliance Policy Guide 2002 list has 63 items, and the CDER 2003 list has 22 items.

Drug	Products Involved	Drug	Products Involved
Adenosine phosphate	All drug products containing adenosine phosphate	Nitrofurazone	All drug products containing nitrofurazone (except topical drug products formulated for dermatologic application)
Adrenal cortex	All drug products containing adrenal cortex	Nomifensine maleate	All drug products containing nomifensine maleate
Aminopyrine	All drug products containing aminopyrine	Oxyphenisatin	All drug products containing oxyphenisatin
Astemizole	All drug products containing astemizole	Oxyphenisatin acetate	All drug products containing oxyphenisatin acetate
Azaribine	All drug products containing azaribine	Phenacetin	All drug products containing phenacetin
Benoxaprofen	All drug products containing benoxaprofen	Phenformin hydrochloride	All drug products containing phenformin hydrochloride
Bithionol	All drug products containing bithionol	Pipamazine	All drug products containing pipamazine
Bromfenac sodium	All drug products containing bromfenac sodium	Potassium arsenite	All drug products containing potassium arsenite
Butamben	All parenteral drug products containing butamben	Potassium chloride	All solid oral dosage form drug products containing potassium chloride that supply 100 milligrams or more of potassium per dosage unit (except for controlled-release dosage forms and those products formulated for preparation of solution prior to ingestion)
Camphorated oil	All drug products containing camphorated oil		
Carbetapentane citrate	All oral gel drug products containing carbetapentane citrate		
Casein, iodinated	All drug products containing iodinated casein		
Cerivastatin	All drug products containing cerivastatin	Povidone	All intravenous drug products containing povidone
Chlorhexidine gluconate	All tinctures of chlorhexidine gluconate formulated for use as a patient preoperative skin preparation	Phenylpropanolamine	All drug products containing phenylpropanolamine
		Rapacuronium	All drug products containing rapacuronium
Chlormadinone acetate	All drug products containing chlormadinone acetate	Reserpine	All oral dosage form drug products containing more than 1 milligram of reserpine
Chloroform	All drug products containing chloroform		
Cisapride	All drug products containing cisapride	Sparteine sulfate	All drug products containing sparteine sulfate
Cobalt	All drug products containing cobalt salts (except radioactive forms of cobalt and its salts and cobalamin and its derivatives)	Sulfadimethoxine	All drug products containing sulfadimethoxine
		Sulfathiazole	All drug products containing sulfathiazole (except those formulated for vaginal use)
Dexfenfluramine hydrochloride	All drug products containing dexfenfluramine hydrochloride	Suprofen	All drug products containing suprofen (except ophthalmic solutions)
Diamthazole dihydrochloride	All drug products containing diamthazole dihydrochloride	Sweet spirits of nitre	All drug products containing sweet spirits of nitre
Dibromsalan	All drug products containing dibromsalan	Temafloxacin hydrochloride	All drug products containing temafloxacin
Diethylstilbestrol	All oral and parenteral drug products containing 25 milligrams or more of diethylstilbestrol per unit dose	Terfenadine	All drug products containing terfenadine
		3,3',4',5-tetrachlorosalicylanilide	All drug products containing 3,3',4',5-tetrachlorosalicylanilide
Dihydrostreptomycin sulfate	All drug products containing dihydrostreptomycin sulfate	Tetracycline	All liquid oral drug products formulated for pediatric use containing tetracycline in a concentration greater than 25 milligrams/milliliter
Dipyrone	All drug products containing dipyrone		
Encainide hydrochloride	All drug products containing encainide hydrochloride		
Fenfluramine hydrochloride	All drug products containing fenfluramine hydrochloride	Ticrynafen	All drug products containing ticrynafen
Flosequinan	All drug products containing flosequinan	Tribromsalan	All drug products containing tribromsalan
Gelatin	All intravenous drug products containing gelatin	Trichloroethane	All aerosol drug products intended for inhalation containing trichloroethane
Glycerol, iodinated	All drug products containing iodinated glycerol		
Gonadotropin, chorionic	All drug products containing chorionic gonadotropins of animal origin	Troglitazone	All drug products containing troglitazone
		Urethane	All drug products containing urethane
Grepafloxacin	All drug products containing grepafloxacin	Vinyl chloride	All aerosol drug products containing vinyl chloride
Mepazine	All drug products containing mepazine hydrochloride or mepazine acetate	Zirconium	All aerosol drug products containing zirconium
		Zomepirac sodium	All drug products containing zomepirac sodium
Metabromsalan	All drug products containing metabromsalan		
Methamphetamine hydrochloride	All parenteral drug products containing methamphetamine hydrochloride		
Methapyrilene	All drug products containing methapyrilene		
Methopholine	All drug products containing methopholine		
Mibefradil dihydrochloride	All drug products containing mibefradil dihydrochloride		

U. S. Department of Health and Human Services, Food and Drug Administration, Office of Regulatory Affairs, Center for Drug Evaluation and Research. Guidance for FDA Staff and Industry Compliance Policy Guides Manual: Section 460.200 Pharmacy Compounding. Washington, DC: U. S. Department of Health and Human Services Food and Drug Administration; 2002; Issued March 16, 1992; Reissued May 29, 2002. CDER 2003 Report to the Nation: Improving Public Health Through Human Drugs. [U. S. Food and Drug Administration Website] Available at http://www.fda.gov/cder/reports/rtn/2003/rtn2003-3.HTM#Withdraw

pharmacists who make compounding a significant part of their practice must answer that question.[5,6] About one-half of the Schools of Pharmacy in the United States do not offer laboratory instruction in compounding. Programs that do include compounding in the curriculum vary widely in the quantity and quality of instruction. If a pharmacist decides to become a compounding pharmacist, several things require consideration:

- The pharmacist must be willing to be trained and continue their education in this area.
- The pharmacist must be willing to be engaged in a physician/patient/compounder relationship with the intended goal of providing customized medications for patients.
- Financial investment will be required for practice site renovation and purchase of compounding equipment, or an arrangement to have access to the appropriate physical facilities.
- The pharmacist will have to maintain an inventory of raw drug chemicals.
- The pharmacist must have access to or develop compounding formulas.
- The pharmacist must be committed to take the time necessary to compound correctly.

The rewards of the decision to compound can be enormous. Many pharmacists can attest to their renewed enthusiasm and pride when they made compounding a significant part of their practice.[7,8,9,10] But each pharmacist must decide if compounding will be a part of their practice. The decision to compound will carry the pharmacist into a world of seemingly endless possibilities to use their unique knowledge and skills.

Compounding Resources

Numerous agencies, companies, and organizations are available to assist pharmacists in obtaining compounding information, chemicals, supplies, and equipment. Many chemical and supply companies now provide information on compounding incompatibilities and stability. Specialty compounding organizations provide a full line of services, information, and products to the compounding pharmacist. Organizations such as the American

Pharmacists Association (APhA), the American College of Apothecaries (ACA), the National Community Pharmacists Association (NCPA), the National Home Infusion Association (NHIA), and the American Society of Health-System Pharmacists (ASHP), as well as many state organizations, provide continuing education programs in compounding. Table 1.3 provides a list of companies that have an interest in pharmaceutical compounding.

NOTES

1. Gosselin, R. Pharmaceutical Care: Part of TQM? *Drug Topics* 139:10, 1995.
2. Pharmacy Compounding Accreditation Board. Available at http://www.pcab.org/about-pcab.html. Accessed August 9, 2007.
3. <1075> Good Compounding Practices: The United States Pharmacopeia 29/National Formulary 24, The United States Pharmacopeial Convention, Inc., Rockville, MD, 2005, pp. 2903–2906.
4. <795> Pharmaceutical Compounding—Nonsterile Preparations: The United States Pharmacopeia 29/National Formulary 24, The United States Pharmacopeial Convention, Inc., Rockville, MD, 2005, pp. 2731–2735.
5. Allen, L.V., Jr. The Decision to Compound. *International Journal of Pharmaceutical Compounding* 1:72–74, 1997.
6. Newton, G. Should Just Any Pharmacist Compound? *International Journal of Pharmaceutical Compounding* 1:362, 1997.
7. Sundberg, J. A. Extemporaneous Compounding in the Hospital Pharmacy. *International Journal of Pharmaceutical Compounding* 1:314–317, 1997.
8. Climo, D. Compounding Practice Structures. *International Journal of Pharmaceutical Compounding* 3:368–370, 1999.
9. Davis, J. Profile of a Practice. *International Journal of Pharmaceutical Compounding* 3:455–456, 1999.
10. Mathew, B. Profile of a Practice. *International Journal of Pharmaceutical Compounding* 4:448–449, 2000.

ADDITIONAL READING

Allen, L.V., Jr. Preface to the First Edition and Introduction in *The Art, Science, and Technology of Pharmaceutical Compounding*, 2nd edition. American Pharmaceutical Association, Washington, DC, 2002, pp. xv–xxiv.

Douglass, K. Training and Competency Considerations for Pharmacies Providing Compounded Sterile Preparations. *International Journal of Pharmaceutical Compounding* 10:253–261, 2006.

McElhiney, L. F. Education, Training, and Evaluation of Hospital Compounding Personnel. *International Journal of Pharmaceutical Compounding* 10:361–368, 2006.

McElhiney, L. F. Information Resources and Software for the Hospital Pharmacist. *International Journal of Pharmaceutical Compounding* 11:36–41, 2007.

TABLE 1.3: RESOURCES FOR COMPOUNDING

Compounding Chemicals	Telephone Number	Formulas	Telephone Number
Apothecary Products, Inc.	(888) 770-8767	Gallipot, Inc.	(800) 423-6967
B & B Pharmaceuticals	(800) 499-3100	Hawkins Pharmaceutical	(800) 375-0009
Gallipot, Inc.	(800) 423-6967	The Letco Companies	(800) 239-5288
Hawk Biopharma	(714) 879-9172	Paddock Laboratories	(763) 546-4676
Hawkins Pharmaceutical	(800) 375-0009	PCCA	(800) 331-2498
Humco Holding Group, Inc.	(800) 662-3435	RS Software	(877) 290-7774
The Letco Companies	(800) 239-5288	Spectrum Pharmacy Products	(800) 791-3210
LorAnn Oils, Inc.	(800) 862-8620	Transderma Pharmaceuticals, Inc	(604) 472-0744
Mallinckrodt Pharmaceuticals	(800) 325-8888	**QC/QA**	
Medisca	(866) 633-4722	Analytical Research Laboratories	(800) 393-1595
Nutragenica	(818) 883-8708	The Contract Test Service at Associates of Cape Cod	(888) 232-5889
Paddock Laboratories, Inc	(763) 546-4676	DynaLabs	(888) 396-2522
PCCA	(800) 331-2498	Eagle Analytical Services	(800) 745-8916
Pharmaceutical Specialties	(800) 325-8232	Gallipot, Inc.	(800) 423-6967
Spectrum Pharmacy Products	(800) 791-3210	Nova Biologicals, Inc.	(800) 282-5416
Transderma Pharmaceuticals, Inc.	(604) 472-0744	PCCA	(800) 331-2498
X-Gen Pharmaceuticals, Inc.	(866) 390-4411	Pharmaceutical Systems, Inc.	(847) 666-9229
Compounding Machines/Equipment		Q.I. Medical Incorporated	(800) 837-8361
AirClean Systems	(800) 849-0472	Spectrum Pharmacy Products	(800) 791-3210
Air Science USA	(800) 306-0656	**Facility Design and Layout**	
B & B Pharmaceuticals	(800) 499-3100	B & B Pharmaceuticals	(800) 499-3100
Cropharm, Inc.	(203) 877-3859	Flow Sciences, Inc.	(800) 349-8429
Flow Sciences, Inc.	(800) 349-8429	G + M North America	(904) 384-6650
Gallipot, Inc.	(800) 423-6967	Gallipot, Inc.	(800) 423-6967
Health Care Logistics	(740) 477-1686	Gladson Store Design Group	(630) 435-2200
ISO Tech Design, Inc	(800) 476-2010	Integrated Design Resources	(502) 454-0118
The Letco Companies	(800) 239-5288	ISO Tech Design, Inc.	(800) 476-2010
Miele	(800) 991-9380	The Letco Companies	(800) 239-5288
PCCA	(800) 331-2498	PCCA	(800) 331-2498
RS Software	(877) 290-7774	Robert P. Potts & Associates	(214) 821-8747
RxEquip	(866) 951-5847	Spectrum Pharmacy Products	(800) 791-3210
Spectrum Pharmacy Products	(800) 791-3210	Store Planning Associates	(800) 226-4026
Terra Universal	(714) 526-0100	Uniweb	(800) 486-4932

CHAPTER TWO

Regulatory Aspects of Compounding

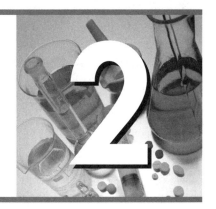

MANY CONSIDERATIONS GO INTO THE DECISION to make compounding a significant part of a pharmacy practice. These issues should be evaluated in light of personal preferences and expectations and also by more global standards or guidelines. Governmental agencies and professional organizations have published several "global" guidelines, addressing topics that range from the definition of compounding to specifications for specialized compounding equipment.

These guidelines are not produced in a vacuum. There is always interplay between federal regulatory authorities, the pharmacy profession, and state boards of pharmacy. Two prominent professional pharmacy organizations are the National Association of Boards of Pharmacy (NABP) and the American Society of Health-System Pharmacists (ASHP). For many years, both of these organizations have developed standards or guidelines pertaining to compounding.[1,2] In more recent years, the US Pharmacopeia (USP) has become the point of origin for many regulations, because it is in the unique position that its guidelines can be legally enforced by the Food and Drug Administration (FDA).

The USP/NF

The USP was established in January 1820 to set uniform standards for the medications prescribed by physicians and to publish compendia of these standards. The National Formulary (NF) was first published in 1888 by the American Pharmaceutical Association, listing standardized formulas including the ingredients and their quantities required for compounding purposes. The USP and NF were both established as official compendia for the United States in the Pure Food and Drug Act of 1906 and the Food, Drug, and Cosmetic Act of 1938, making their standards of strength, purity, packaging, and labeling enforceable under federal law. Today the USP/NF is an independent organization with its scientific work conducted through 60 expert committees by more than 650 volunteers from pharmacy practice, academia, and related support companies.

In 1975 the USP purchased the NF, and in 1980 the first combined USP/NF compendia were published. The combined compendia had been published every 5 years until 2002, when yearly updates were implemented. In the compendia, each general chapter is assigned a number, which appears in brackets along with the chapter name. The general chapters numbered <1> to <999> are considered requirements and official monographs and standards, whereas general chapters numbered from <1000> to <1999> are considered informational, and chapters above <2000> apply to nutritional supplements.

Chapters Related to Compounding

Beginning in the 1980s, pharmaceutical compounding saw a resurgence in the United States, and the USP began to reflect these changes. In 1993 the USP formed two panels—the Expert Advisory Panel and the Review Panel on Pharmacy Compounding Practices. One panel started working on general chapters pertaining to compounding, and the other panel began creating compounding monographs.

With regard to general chapters that pertain to compounding *nonsterile preparations*, the USP published the general information chapter <1161> Pharmacy Compounding Practices, in 1996. Chapter <1161> was changed from the informational chapter to the enforceable chapter, <795> Pharmaceutical Compounding— Nonsterile Preparations with the passage of the 1997 FDA Modernization Act.

With regard to chapters pertaining to compounding *sterile preparations*, the USP issued a draft recommendation entitled <1074> Dispensing Practices for Sterile Drug Products Intended for Home Use, in 1992. In 1995, the final version of <1074> was designated <1206> Sterile Drug Products for Home Use. In 2004, <797> Pharmaceutical Compounding—Sterile Preparations became official.

Because both <795> and <797> are now requirements, pharmacies may be subject to inspection against these standards by state boards of pharmacy, the Food and Drug Administration (FDA), and accreditation organizations such as the Joint Commission on Accreditation of Healthcare Organizations (JCAHO), the Accreditation Commission for Health Care

(ACHC), and the Community Health Accreditation Program (CHAP). Although <795> and <797> have received a great deal of publicity, the USP has implemented many other chapters that either directly or indirectly influence the practice of compounding. Table 2.1 lists many of these relevant chapters.

The USP also has many general chapters that deal with the testing of pharmaceutical products (example chapters shown in Table 2.2). In a compounding pharmacy setting, some of these test chapters are applicable if the analysis is done in-house. If the analytical work is carried out by a contract company, they have to be in compliance with these chapters.

Official Compounded Formulations

Another significant inclusion in the USP consists of monographs of the most commonly compounded preparations used in pharmacy practice. These "official"

TABLE 2.1: USP/NF CHAPTERS APPLICABLE TO PHARMACEUTICAL COMPOUNDING

Chapter Title	Chapter Number
Injections	1
Containers	661
Containers – Permeation	671
Pharmaceutical Compounding – Nonsterile Preparations	795
Pharmaceutical Compounding – Sterile Preparations	797
Radioactivity	821
Radiopharmaceuticals for Positron Emission Tomography – Compounding	823
Biologics	1041
Biotechnology – Derived Articles	1045
Good Compounding Practices	1075
Good Manufacturing Practices for Bulk Pharmaceutical Excipients	1078
Impurities in Official Articles	1086
Labeling of Inactive Ingredients	1091
Medicine Dropper	1101
Microbiological Attributes of Nonsterile Pharmaceutical Products	1111
Nomenclature	1121
Packaging Practice – Repackaging a Single Solid Oral Drug Product into a Unit–Dose Container	1146
Pharmaceutical Stability	1150
Pharmaceutical Dosage Forms	1151
Pharmaceutical Calculations in Prescription Compounding	1160
Prescription Balances and Volumetric Apparatus	1176
Stability Considerations in Dispensing Practice	1191
Teaspoon	1221
Water for Pharmaceutical Purposes	1231

TABLE 2.2: USP/NF CHAPTERS APPLICABLE TO TESTING PHARMACEUTICAL PRODUCTS

Chapter Title	Chapter Number
Thermometers	21
Volumetric Apparatus	31
Weights and Balances	41
Microbial Limit Tests	61
Sterility Tests	71
Bacterial Endotoxins Test	85
Pyrogen Test	151
Thin-Layer Chromatographic Identification Test	201
Elastomeric Closures for Injections	381
Aerosols, Nasal Sprays, Metered Dose Inhalers, and Dry Powder Inhalers	601
Chromatography	621
Completeness of Solutions	641
Deliverable Volume	698
Disintegration	701
Dissolution	711
Loss on Drying	731
Melting Range or Temperature	741
Metal Particles in Ophthalmic Ointments	751
Optical Microscopy	776
Osmolality and Osmolarity	785
Particulate Matter in Injections	788
pH	791
Refractive Index	831
Specific Gravity	841
Uniformity of Dosage Units	905
Viscosity	911
Biological Indicators for Sterilization	1035
Microbiological Evaluation of Clean Rooms and Other Controlled Environments	1116
Monitor Devices – Time, Temperature, and Humidity	1118
Sterile Product Packaging – Integrity Evaluation	1207
Sterility Testing – Validation of Isolator Systems	1208
Sterilization and Sterility Assurance of Compendial Articles	1211
Tablet Friability	1216
Terminally Sterilized Pharmaceutical Products – Parametric Release	1222
Water–Solid Interactions in Pharmaceutical Systems	1241
Weighing on an Analytical Balance	1251

formulations have the advantage of USP testing, quality assurance, and "beyond use date" assignment. Therefore, when a formulation is compounded as described in a monograph, the stability is assumed to be identical to that stated in the monograph, and the beyond use date assignment given in the monograph can be applied to the compounded formulation.

The USP Council of Experts and its expert committees have developed monographs for approximately 150 of the most commonly compounded preparations used in practice today. The number will continue to grow as the USP continues its work. It has been suggested that more than 1,000 other compounded preparations will require a USP monograph.[3]

The inclusion of compounding monographs in the USP is one of several important elements to ensure the quality and benefit of a compounded formulation. It provides uniformity in prescribing and preparing these formulations, as required by law. A prescriber who writes a prescription for a specific compound that appears in the USP has defined the product to be prepared. Pharmacists who adhere to the compendia prepare the product with defined quality standards. When the USP does not contain a monograph for a prescribed compounded preparation or ingredient, pharmacists will have to use their professional judgment in compounding a formulation that conforms to the standards of practice.

Pharmaceutical Compounding— Nonsterile Preparations <795>

Throughout this chapter, a distinction is made between "manufactured products" and "compounded preparations." This differentiates the output of pharmaceutical companies (products) and pharmacies (preparations). The following points highlight many of the major areas within Chapter <795>.

Responsibility of the Compounder

The responsibilities of the compounder (the pharmacist or other licensed health care professional responsible for preparing the compounded preparation) centers on quality assurance of personnel, ingredients, finished preparations, processes, environment, stability, consistency, error prevention and documentation.

Facilities and Equipment

The primary requirements are adequate space with the proper infrastructure for compounding operations, and the availability of appropriate equipment. Equipment must be appropriate in design and size, and suitable for the purpose for which it is used. It should not interact or interfere with the compounded preparation or process. It must be properly maintained, used, calibrated, and cleaned.

Stability of Compounded Preparations

Assigning the beyond use date is the responsibility of the compounder. (Beyond use dates are assigned to compounded preparations; expiration dates are assigned to manufactured products). This section of <795> also requires the compounder to consider the effect of packaging on the stability of the preparation, and addresses sterility concerns.

Compounders can consult appropriate literature and manufacturers and can work with analytical laboratories to determine an appropriate beyond use date. In the event no data are available, the chapter provides guidelines that can be used.[4]

- Solids and nonaqueous liquids prepared from commercially available dosage forms—25% of the remaining expiration date of the commercial product, or 6 months, whichever is earlier.

- Solids and nonaqueous liquids prepared from bulk ingredients—up to 6 months.

- Water containing formulations (prepared from ingredients in solid form)—up to 14 days when stored in a refrigerator.

- All other formulations—up to 30 days or the intended duration of therapy, whichever is earlier.

Sources of Ingredients

USP and NF grade ingredients should be used if they are available. If an ingredient does not have a monograph in the USP or NF, the pharmacist must select a reasonable high-quality grade ingredient from a reliable source. Certificates of analysis can be useful in establishing quality of the ingredients used, both active and excipients.

Acceptable Strength, Quality, and Purity

Five questions are presented to guide a thoughtful consideration of the strength and quality of the compounded preparation. Some are second nature, but others may require further investigation. The questions are:

1. Have the physical and chemical properties and medicinal, dietary, and pharmaceutical uses of the drug substances been reviewed?

2. Are the quantity and quality of each active ingredient identifiable?

3. Will the active ingredients be effectively absorbed, locally or systemically according to the prescribed purpose, from the preparation and route of administration?

4. Are there added substances, confirmed or potentially present from manufactured products, that may be expected to cause an allergic reaction, irritation, toxicity, or undesirable organoleptic response from

the patient? Are there added substances, confirmed or potentially present, that may be unfavorable (e.g., unsuitable pH or inadequate solubility)?

5. Were all calculations and measurements confirmed to ensure that the preparation will be compounded accurately?

Compounded Preparations

The term "compounded preparations" is amplified to include "compounded dosage forms," "compounded drug," and "compounded formulations." But the majority of this section provides quality suggestions, clinical considerations, and technical procedural guidance specific to four groups of compounded preparations:

1. capsules, powders, lozenges, tablets
2. emulsions, solutions, suspensions
3. suppositories
4. creams, topical gels, ointments, pastes

The Compounding Process

Thirteen steps are presented to minimize error and maximize the prescriber's intent. These all should be covered in the standard operating procedures of the pharmacy and are good practice standards to follow.

1. Judge the suitability of the prescription to be compounded in terms of its safety and intended use. Determine what legal limitations, if any, are applicable.
2. Perform necessary calculations to establish the amounts of ingredients needed (see <1160> Pharmaceutical Calculations in Prescription Compounding).
3. Identify equipment needed.
4. Wear the proper attire and wash hands.
5. Clean the compounding area and needed equipment.
6. Compound only one prescription at one time in a specified compounding area.
7. Assemble all necessary materials to compound the prescription.
8. Compound the preparation following the formulation record or prescription, according to the art and science of pharmacy.
9. Assess weight variation, adequacy of mixing, clarity, odor, color, consistency, and pH as appropriate.
10. Annotate the compounding log, and describe the appearance of the formulation.
11. Label the prescription containers to include the following items:
    a. Name of the preparation
    b. Internal identification number
    c. Beyond use date
    d. Initials of the compounder who prepared the label

e. Any storage requirements
f. Any other statements required by law

12. Sign and date the prescription, affirming that all procedures were carried out to ensure uniformity, identity, strength, quantity, and purity.
13. Clean all equipment thoroughly and promptly, and store properly.

Compounding Records and Documents

The purpose of these records is to meet state boards of pharmacy record keeping requirements and to enable another compounder to duplicate the preparation. The *formulation record* generally will be on a computer system, or it may be an individual new prescription or request. The formulation record can be used to prepare the documentation for the compounding record.

The *compounding record* contains the sources and lot numbers of the ingredients, calculations, processes used, results of any testing done, an assigned beyond use date, identification numbers, name of the compounder, quantity of the preparation compounded, and other pertinent information. It contains all relevant information related to the actual compounding of the specific prescription. It is used for checking the final preparation for accuracy. *Material Safety Data Sheets* (MSDSs) may be either hard copy or accessible electronically. They are needed for all drug substances or bulk chemicals located in the compounding pharmacy. If commercial products are used, the package insert can serve this purpose.

Quality Control

All the paperwork from the first step through the final preparation should be reviewed, along with observing the finished preparation. Standard Operating Procedures (SOPs) are documents that describe how to perform routine tasks in the environment of formulation development, purchasing, compounding, testing, maintenance, materials handling, quality assurance, and dispensing. They contain step-by-step instructions to perform tasks reliably and consistently, including how a task will be performed, who will do the task, who is responsible, why it will be performed, and any limits associated with the task.

Verification

Verification involves checking to ensure that all the processes were appropriate and performed accurately.

Patient Counseling

As with any prescription, patient counseling is important. This is especially important with compounded preparations in which the beyond use date may be rather short. Patients should be counseled about use, storage, and evidence of instability (visual changes, odor, etc.).

Pharmaceutical Compounding— Sterile Preparations <797>

The chapter Pharmaceutical Compounding—Sterile Preparations <797> was added to the USP/NF in 2004.[5] The standard grew out of the efforts of the National Association of Boards of Pharmacy (NABP), the USP, and the American Society of Health-Systems Pharmacists (ASHP) over a 20-year period to create a set of guidelines that would be universally accepted by manufacturers and compounders of sterile products.[6] These guidelines were difficult to formulate and slow to be accepted. In a national survey conducted in 2003, only 5.2% of hospitals were in compliance with these guidelines.[7]

The NABP *Model Rules for Sterile Pharmaceuticals* comprised the most general guidelines and did not address some of the key features found in other guidelines. But they enumerated the basic considerations in sterile compounding, as follows.[8]

- Policy and procedure manuals should be established for compounding, dispensing, delivering, storing, administering, using, and disposing of sterile products. These records should be part of a documented, ongoing quality assurance program.
- Pharmacy compounding personnel should be trained and adhere to the basic principles of aseptic techniques.
- Sterile compounding should be done in a designated area with entry restricted to personnel that will be compounding the sterile pharmaceuticals.
- The sterile compounding area should have appropriate environmental control devices capable of maintaining at least ISO Class 5 conditions.
- Records and reports should be maintained on compounded sterile pharmaceuticals, including maintenance schedules, compounding records, and dispensing or distribution records.
- Sufficient reference materials about sterile products should be available.

The ASHP *Technical Assistance Bulletin on Quality Assurance for Pharmacy-Prepared Sterile Products* included language similar to that found in the NABP Model Rules but also designated three levels of patient risk depending upon the complexity of the sterile compounding procedure to be used. Risk Level 1 denotes the least patient risk, and Risk Level 3 the highest. These risk levels were defined, and examples of sterile products were given for each level.[9]

The *Bulletin* included sections on "clean rooms" and "process validation." A clean room was to be a separate room containing laminar air flow hoods and meeting certain standards of airborne particle concentration. Process validation procedures with growth media ("media fills") were included to ensure that the operator, working under the most challenging sterile compounding situation, could consistently produce a sterile product. USP guidelines (found in <1206> Sterile Drug Products for Home Use) contained similar guidelines.[10]

Both the USP standards and the ASHP standards addressed quality assurance activities for compounding sterile products. The major difference was that the ASHP guidelines applied to sterile compounding in various practice settings, whereas USP/NF <1206> pertained to sterile compounding of products that typically were administered in settings other than a professionally staffed health care facility. Comparisons of the two guidelines were published.[11]

Chapter <797> has a final implementation date of January, 2008, to allow time for the various stakeholders to develop and implement a plan to bring their facility into compliance. The standards apply to all health care settings that prepare, store, and dispense sterile preparations and by all disciplines associated with these settings, including physicians, nurses, and pharmacists in office practices, clinics, hospital care units, and main and satellite pharmacies. Enforcement of this chapter by state boards of pharmacy is limited to licensed pharmacies.

Compounded Sterile Preparations (CSPs) are defined as:

- Preparations prepared according to the manufacturer's labeled instructions and other manipulations when manufacturing sterile products that expose the original contents to potential contamination
- Preparations containing nonsterile ingredients or employing nonsterile components and devices that must be sterilized before administration
- Biologics, diagnostics, drugs, nutrients, and radiopharmaceuticals that possess either of the above two characteristics, and include, but are not limited to, baths and soaks for live organs and tissues, implants, inhalations, injections, powders for injection, irrigations, metered sprays, and ophthalmic and otic preparations.

The intent of chapter <797> is

to prevent harm and fatality to patients that could result from microbial contamination (nonsterility), excessive bacterial endotoxins, large content errors in the strength of correct ingredients, and incorrect ingredients in compounded sterile products (CSPs).

The chapter makes the point that sterile compounding differs from nonsterile compounding primarily by requiring a test for sterility. Sterile compounding also requires cleaner facilities, specific training and testing of personnel in principles and practices of aseptic manipulations, air-quality evaluation and maintenance, and sound knowledge of sterilization and stability principles and practices.

The chapter provides the foundation for development and implementation of essential procedures for the safe preparation of CSPs. It does not outline exactly how things are to be constructed or conducted. The chapter provides the foundation (the starting point) for each institution to develop and implement its own procedures that will produce CSPs that provide no harm or fatality.

Responsibilities of Compounding Personnel

Compounding personnel are responsible for the total preparation and dispensing of a CSP. They are to ensure that the CSPs are accurately identified, measured, diluted and mixed, and are correctly purified, sterilized, packaged, sealed, labeled, stored, dispensed, and distributed. The compounder is held accountable for 14 responsibilities that are outlined in this section.

Microbial Contamination Risk Levels

There are three microbial contamination risk levels—low, medium, high. The compounder is responsible for determining the risk level associated with the compounded preparation. The three contamination risk levels are given below including some examples and facility requirements:

Low-Risk Compounding

- Simple admixtures compounded using closed system transfer methods
- Equipment:
  ○ Prepared in International Organization for Standardization (ISO) Class 5 (formerly Class 100) laminar flow hood
  ○ Located in ISO Class 8 (formerly Class 100,000) clean room with anteroom
- Examples:
  ○ Reconstitution of single dose vials of antibiotics or other small volume parenterals (SVP)
  ○ Preparation of hydration solutions
  ○ Using sterile needles and syringe to transfer sterile drugs from the manufacturer's original packaging (vials, ampules)
  ○ Manually measuring and mixing no more than three sterile products to compounded drug admixtures in nutritional solutions

Medium-Risk Compounding

- Admixtures compounded using multiple additives and/or small volumes
- Batch preparations (e.g., syringes)
- Complex manipulations (e.g., TPN)
- Preparations for use over several days
- Equipment:
  ○ Prepared in ISO Class 5 laminar flow hood

  ○ Located in ISO Class 8 clean room with anteroom
- Examples
  ○ Pooled admixtures
  ○ Parenteral nutrition solutions using automated compounders
  ○ Batch compounded preparations that do not contain bacteriostatic components
  ○ TPN fluids compounding using manual or automated devices requiring multiple injections, detachments, and attachments of the nutrients' source products to the device or machine to deliver all the nutritional complements to the final sterile container
  ○ Filling of reservoirs of injection and infusion devices with multiple sterile drug products and evacuation of air from those reservoirs before the filled device is dispensed
  ○ Filling of reservoirs of injection and infusion devices with volumes of sterile drug solutions that will be administered over several days in ambient temperatures between 25° and 40°
  ○ Transfer of volumes from multiple ampules or vials into a single, final sterile container or product

High-Risk Compounding

- Nonsterile (bulk powders) ingredients
- Open system transfers
- Equipment:
  ○ Prepared in ISO Class 5 laminar flow hood
  ○ Located in ISO Class 8 clean room with a separate anteroom
- Examples
  ○ Dissolving nonsterile bulk drugs and nutrient powders to make a solution which will be terminally sterilized
  ○ Sterile ingredients, components, devices and mixtures that are exposed to air quality inferior to ISO Class 5. This includes the storage of opened or partially used packages of manufactured sterile products that lack antimicrobial preservatives in an environment inferior to ISO Class 5
  ○ Measuring and mixing sterile ingredients in nonsterile devices before sterilization is performed

Verification of Compounding Accuracy and Sterilization

The quality (sterility and accuracy) of the CSP depends on the methods used to compound the preparation. CSPs that require some form of terminal sterilization have to be validated to ensure that they are sterile.

Personnel Training and Evaluation in Aseptic Manipulations Skills

Before beginning to prepare products, personnel who prepare compounded sterile products must be provided with appropriate training from expert personnel, audio-video instructional sources, or professional publications.

Personnel shall perform didactic review, written testing, and media fill testing of aseptic manipulative skills initially, and at least annually for low and medium risk levels, and every 6 months for high risk level compounding. Media fill challenge testing will be used to assess the quality of aseptic skills. There are minimum validation challenges for personnel to accomplish and reexamination criteria for personnel to meet depending on the risk levels of the compounding activity.

Validation Minimum Requirements

Low- and Medium-Risk Compounding

- Personnel validation: three consecutive media fills without contamination
- Revalidation: one media fill run annually without contamination
- Failure of revalidation: three consecutive media fills without contamination

High-Risk Compounding

- Personnel validation: three consecutive media fills without contamination
- Revalidation: one media fill run semiannually without contamination
- Failure of revalidation: three consecutive media fills without contamination
- Sterilization process validation: three consecutive media fills without contamination
- Revalidation: one media fill run semiannually without contamination
- Failure of revalidation: three consecutive media fills without contamination

Environmental Quality and Control

The section on environmental quality and control specifies in great detail the physical plant and environmental requirements for each risk level. It discusses the need for laminar air flow work benches, the requirements of an ISO Class 5 environment when a CSP is exposed to air in the physical environment, an ISO Class 8 environment in a clean room, and proper garbing requirements. Some examples of these standards are given below:

Clean rooms
Low- and Medium-Risk Compounding
- Must have an anteroom but need not be separated with a physical wall

- Air classification or quality must meet ISO Class 8 standards
- Physical characteristics of construction:
  ○ Walls, floors, fixtures and ceilings should be smooth, impervious and free of cracks, crevices, and non-shedding.
  ○ Surfaces should be resistant to damage from sanitizing agents.
  ○ Junctures of ceilings to walls should be coved and caulked.
  ○ If ceilings consist of inlaid panels, the panels should be impregnated with a polymer to render them impervious and hydrophobic and they should be caulked around each perimeter to seal them to the support frame.
  ○ Walls may be panels locked together and sealed or they can be made of epoxy coated gypsum board.
  ○ Floors should be overlaid with a wide sheet vinyl flooring with heat sealed seams and coving at the sidewall.
  ○ The anteroom should contain no floor drains.

High-Risk Compounding
- Includes all low- to medium-risk procedures and facilities except that the anteroom must be a separate room.

Gowning
Low- and Medium-Risk Compounding
- Before entering the anteroom, personnel should remove outer lab coats, make-up, and jewelry and thoroughly scrub hands and arms to the elbow.
- After drying hands and arms, they should don clean, non-shedding uniforms consisting of:
  ○ Hair covers
  ○ Shoe covers
  ○ Coveralls or knee-length coats that fit snugly at the wrist and be zipped or snapped in the front
  ○ Appropriate gloves
  ○ Face masks

High-Risk Compounding
- All low- to medium-risk procedures

Processing

Employees must undergo written training and evaluation to ensure that they are knowledgeable and properly trained to prepare CSPs.

Verification of Automated Compounding Devices for Nutrition Compounding

This section gives suggested procedures for ensuring the accuracy and precision of automated compounding devices used in the preparation of parenteral nutrition solutions.

Finished Preparation Release Checks and Tests

All CSPs are required to be checked by a pharmacist prior to being dispensed. Several methods can be used to meet this requirement.

Storage and Beyond Use Dating

Two factors are critical in establishing beyond use dates for CSPs. The first is the chemical stability of the active drug in solution. A number of textbook references are available and should be consulted to determine the chemical stability of medications in solutions. The second factor is the sterility of the CSP. By definition, sterility is the absence of viable microorganisms in the CSP. Because patient injury and death following administration of CSPs have been associated with microbial contamination, sterility testing should be performed with any CSP. If such testing is not conducted, the beyond use date cannot exceed the limits set out in Table 2.3. The beyond use date limit is determined by the storage temperature of the CSP.

TABLE 2.3: BEYOND USE DATES FOR CSPs IN THE ABSENCE OF STERILITY TEST

Risk Level	Room Temp	Refrigeration	Freezer (≤–20°C)
Low	48 hours	14 days	45 days
Medium	30 hours	7 days	45 days
High	24 hours	3 days	45 days

Maintaining Product Quality and Control After the CSP Leaves the Pharmacy

Pharmacists are responsible for ensuring that the quality and integrity of the CSP is maintained during transit and use in its final location. This section gives guidance on the use of appropriate packaging that is capable of maintaining proper temperature and conditions during shipment via common carriers (FedEx, UPS, or USPS).

Patient or Caregiver Training

A formal training program is required to train the patient or caregiver how to store, administer, and dispose of the CSP.

Patient Monitoring and Adverse Events Reporting

This section is directed to clinically monitoring patients who receive CSPs.

Quality Assurance Program

Formalized policies, processes, and procedures must be used when preparing CSPs. A large component of the

program is documentation showing that compounders are really doing what they say they are doing.

Proposed Revisions to Chapter <797>

General Chapter <797> Pharmaceutical Compounding —Sterile Preparations currently is undergoing review for possible revision. The proposed revisions officially appeared in the Pharmacopeial Forum May–June 2006 volume[12] with a call for comments by August 15, 2006. Approximately 2,500 pages of comments from more than 300 participants, including hospitals, professional associations, vendors, stakeholders, and individual practitioners including pharmacists, nurses, physicians, etc., were submitted to the Sterile Compounding Expert Committee.

Because of the number and critical nature of these comments, it is not known when the review of comments to the proposed revisions will be completed and the proposed revisions finalized. USP will post the Expert Committee's responses along with a summary of comments on the USP website. Copies of the proposed revisions can be obtained from the USP website at the following addresses:

- http://www.usp.org/pdf/EN/USPNF/PF797redline.pdf (text with markup of the current version of <797>)
- http://www.usp.org/pdf/EN/USPNF/PF797.pdf (text without markup of the current version of <797>)

Good Compounding Practices <1075>

The USP/NF chapter <1075> Good Compounding Practices is of particular importance because it provides guidance about applying good compounding practices to compounding activities.[13] The chapter has many of the same emphases as <795> and <797> but adds substance to some of the broad overview statements found in those chapters. A summary follows.

Responsibilities of the Compounder

Compounders are responsible for following chapters <795> and <797> as applied to their practices. In addition, compounders are responsible for the entire compounding process, which involves everything from accepting a prescription order to dispensing the final preparation. Compounders also are responsible for ensuring that all equipment is maintained properly, that all personnel are trained adequately, and that all documentation is completed.

Training

This section states that all personnel involved in compounding preparations shall be properly trained but does not provide a list of the training required. As mentioned in the preceding section, the compounder is responsible for ensuring that a training program has been implemented and that training is ongoing.

Procedures and Documentation

All significant compounding procedures will be covered by Standard Operating Procedures (SOPs) and will be documented. All SOPs will ensure accountability, accuracy, quality, safety, and uniformity in the compounding practice.

Drug Compounding Facilities and Drug Compounding Equipment

These two sections state two principles: First, the facilities and equipment must be adequate to carry out the compounding operations and must be in compliance with <797> if dealing with sterile preparations. The second principle states that all the facilities and equipment are to be clean, calibrated, and maintained in good order.

Component Selection Requirements

The compounder is responsible for selecting all components involved in a compounded preparation. This section contains a rank-ordering of the quality of components that should be included in the preparation.

Packaging and Drug Product Containers

All containers and closures for a compounded preparation must meet the requirements of chapter <661> Containers[14] and <671> Containers—Permeation.[15] When compounding sterile preparations, the requirements of <797> apply to the selection of a package or closure.

Compounding Controls

This section gives a multi-step procedure that the compounder must follow to ensure that the finished preparations have the identity, strength, quality, and purity as labeled. Some of the steps state that procedures are to be in place and followed during the compounding process. Other steps give directions about the type of documentation needed for components included in the compounding process.

Labeling

The details to be included on the compounded preparation's label are listed. Also included is the label information that is to be placed on a label for preparations compounded in anticipation of a prescription.

Four other sections of the chapter give brief comments about compounding for a prescriber's office, veterinarian products, and pharmacy generated products. A *pharmacy generated product* is a compounded drug product that can be sold without a prescription.

Enforcement Role of the FDA

In 1997, as part of the Food and Drug Administration Modernization Act (FDAMA), the Food, Drug, and Cosmetic Act of 1938 was amended to clarify the status of pharmacy compounding under federal law. This amendment to the FDCA, however, was legally challenged on the grounds of impermissible regulation of commercial speech. In April 2002, The U. S. Supreme Court ruled that the amendment was invalid in its entirely.

Subsequently, the FDA issued a guidance document describing the factors that the Agency will consider in exercising its enforcement discretion regarding pharmacy compounding (document available on the FDA website[16]). In the Compliance Policy Guidelines, the FDA recognizes that pharmacists traditionally have extemporaneously compounded and manipulated reasonable quantities of drugs upon receipt of a valid prescription from a licensed practitioner for an individual patient. This traditional activity will not be the subject of FDA enforcement. The FDA believes, however, that an increasing number of establishments with retail pharmacy licenses are engaged in manufacturing and distributing unapproved new drugs for human use in a manner that clearly is outside the bounds of traditional pharmacy practice, and that these activities violate the provisions of the FDCA. These establishments and their activities will be the major focus of FDA enforcement.

The Compliance Policy can be summarized as follows. Generally, the FDA will defer to state authorities regarding less significant violations of the FDCA related to pharmacy compounding. But when the scope and nature of a pharmacy's activities raise the kinds of concerns normally associated with a drug manufacturer and result in significant violations of the new drug application, adulteration, or misbranding, the FDA will seriously consider enforcement action. In determining whether to initiate such an action, the FDA will use the following criteria:

1. Compounding of drugs in anticipation of receiving prescriptions, except in limited quantities in relation to the amounts of drugs compounded after receiving valid prescriptions.

2. Compounding drugs that were withdrawn or removed from the market for safety reasons.

3. Compounding finished drugs from bulk active ingredients that are not components of FDA approved drugs without an FDA sanctioned investigational new drug application (IND).

4. Receiving, storing, or using drug substances without first obtaining written assurance from the supplier that each lot of the drug substance has been made in an FDA registered facility.

5. Receiving, storing, or using drug components that and not guaranteed or otherwise determined to meet official compendia requirements.

6. Using commercial scale manufacturing or testing equipment for compounding drug products.

7. Compounding drugs for third parties who resell to individual patients or offering compounded drug products at wholesale to other state licensed persons or commercial entities for resale.

8. Compounding drug products that are commercially available in the marketplace or that are essentially copies of commercially available FDA approved drug products. In certain circumstances, it may be appropriate for a pharmacist to compound a small quantity of a drug that is only slightly different than an FDA approved drug that is commercially available. In these circumstances, FDA will consider whether there is documentation of the medical need for the particular variation of the compound for the particular patient.

9. Failing to operate in conformance with applicable state law regulating the practice of pharmacy.

NOTES

1. National Association of Boards of Pharmacy. Model State Pharmacy Act and Model Rules of the National Association of Boards of Pharmacy. 2007. Accessed August 09, 2007 from http://www.nabp.net/ftpfiles/NABP01/LELReport2007.pdf

2. American Society of Health-System Pharmacists. ASHP Guidelines: Minimum Standard for Pharmacies in Hospitals. *American Journal of Health-System Pharmacy* 52:2711–2717, 1995.

3. Bormel, G., Valentino, J. G., and Williams, R. L. Application of USP-NF Standards to Pharmacy Compounding. *International Journal of Pharmaceutical Compounding* 7:361–363, 2003.

4. <795> Pharmaceutical Compounding—Nonsterile Preparations: The United States Pharmacopeia 29/National Formulary 24, The United States Pharmacopeial Convention, Inc., Rockville, MD, 2005, pp. 2731–2735.

5. <797> Pharmaceutical Compounding—Sterile Preparations: The United States Pharmacopeia 29/National Formulary 24, The United States Pharmacopeial Convention, Inc., Rockville, MD, 2005, pp. 2735–2751.

6. Kastango, E. S. The ASHP Discussion Guide for Compounding Sterile Preparations: Summary and Implementation of USP Chapter <797>. Available at http://www.ashp.org/s_ashp/bin.asp?CID= 483&DID=2216&DOC=FILE.PDF. Accessed August 09, 2007.

7. Morris, A. M, Schneider, P. J., Pedersen, C. A., et al. National Survey of Quality Assurance Activities for Pharmacy-Compounded Sterile Preparations. *American Journal of Health-Systems Pharmacy* 60:2567–2576, 2003.

8. Model Rules for Sterile Pharmaceuticals. National Association of Boards of Pharmacy. Model State Pharmacy Act and Model Rules of the National Association of Boards of Pharmacy. 2007:18–24.

9. American Society of Hospital Pharmacists. ASHP Technical Assistance Bulletin on Quality Assurance for Pharmacy-Prepared Sterile Products. *American Journal of Hospital Pharmacy* 50:2386–2398, 1993.

10. <1206> Sterile Drug Products for Home Use: The United States Pharmacopeia 26/National Formulary 21. The United States Pharmacopeial Convention, Inc., Rockville, MD, 2002, pp. 2417–2429.

11. Lima, H. A. Sterile-Product Compounding: A Comparison of ASHP and USP Guidelines. *International Journal of Pharmaceutical Compounding* 3:270–273, 1999.

12. USP/NF website accessed August 09, 2007, from http://www.usp.org/USPNF/pf/generalChapter797.html

13. <1075> Good Compounding Practices: The United States Pharmacopeia 29/National Formulary 24, The United States Pharmacopeial Convention, Inc., Rockville, MD, 2005, pp. 2903–2906.

14. <661> Containers: The United States Pharmacopeia 29/National Formulary 24, The United States Pharmacopeial Convention, Inc., Rockville, MD, 2005, pp. 2655–2663.

15. <671> Containers—Permeation: The United States Pharmacopeia 29/National Formulary 24, The United States Pharmacopeial Convention, Inc., Rockville, MD, 2005, pp. 2663–2664.

16. Compliance Policy Guide, Compliance Policy Guidance for FDA Staff and Industry, Chapter 4, Sub Chapter 460, Sec 460.200 Pharmacy Compounding, U. S. Department of Health and Human Services, Food and Drug Administration, Office of Regulatory Affairs, Center for Drug Evaluation and Research, May 2002.

ADDITIONAL READING

Allen, L.V., Jr., Okeke, C. Basics of Compounding for the Implementation of United States Pharmacopeia Chapter <797>: Pharmaceutical Compounding—Sterile Preparations, Part 1. *International Journal of Pharmaceutical Compounding* 11:230–236, 2007.

Allen, L. V., Jr., Okeke, C. The Responsibilities of Compounding Personnel in Implementing United States Pharmacopeia Chapter <797>: Pharmaceutical Compounding—Sterile Preparations, Part 2. *International Journal of Pharmaceutical Compounding* 11:314–323, 2007.

Huffman, D. C., Holmes, E. R. Specialty Compounding for Improved Patient Care: A National Survey of Compounding Pharmacists. *International Journal of Pharmaceutical Compounding* 10:462–468, 2006.

Petroff, B. Compounding Issues and Accreditation Agencies. *International Journal of Pharmaceutical Compounding* 5:273–274, 2001.

CHAPTER THREE

An Order to Compound

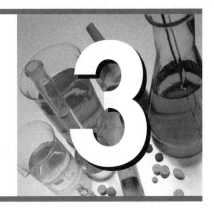

Part of the definition of compounding is the

> …preparation, mixing, assembling, packaging, and labeling of a drug or device in accordance with a licensed practitioner's prescription or medication order under an initiative based on the practitioner/patient/pharmacist/compounder relationship in the course of professional practice.[1]

Prescription and Medication Orders

The prescription drug order generally takes two forms—a written *prescription* or a *medication order*.

Prescriptions and medication orders convey necessary and specific information to the pharmacist, but they typically are used in different patient care settings. Prescriptions generally are used for outpatient care, and medication orders are used in institutional care. A sample prescription is shown in Figure 3.1.

Medication orders are used to order medications for patients in hospitals, nursing homes, and other institutions. Medication orders also contain orders for procedures, laboratory tests, nursing instructions, and discharge instructions. A medication order form may request many different medications, whereas prescription forms usually request only one medication. A sample medication order is shown in Figure 3.2.

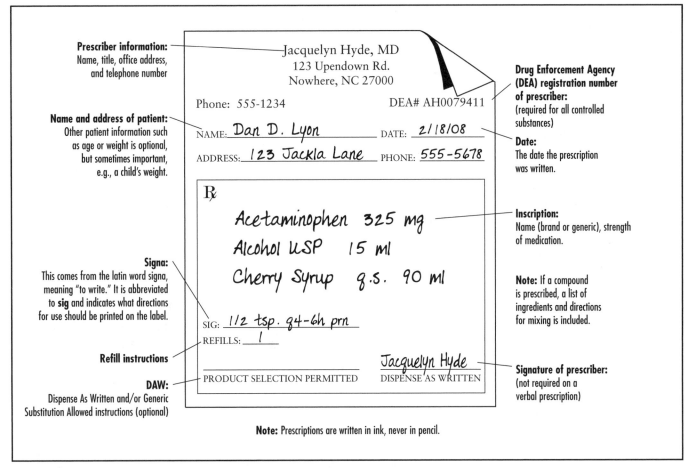

Prescriber information: Name, title, office address, and telephone number

Jacquelyn Hyde, MD
123 Upendown Rd.
Nowhere, NC 27000

Phone: 555-1234   DEA# AH0079411

Drug Enforcement Agency (DEA) registration number of prescriber: (required for all controlled substances)

Name and address of patient: Other patient information such as age or weight is optional, but sometimes important, e.g., a child's weight.

NAME: Dan D. Lyon   DATE: 2/18/08

ADDRESS: 123 Jackla Lane   PHONE: 555-5678

Date: The date the prescription was written.

Rx

Acetaminophen   325 mg
Alcohol USP   15 ml
Cherry Syrup   q.s. 90 ml

Inscription: Name (brand or generic), strength of medication.

Note: If a compound is prescribed, a list of ingredients and directions for mixing is included.

Signa: This comes from the latin word signa, meaning "to write." It is abbreviated to **sig** and indicates what directions for use should be printed on the label.

SIG: 1/2 tsp. q4-6h prn

REFILLS: 1

Refill instructions

Jacquelyn Hyde

DAW: Dispense As Written and/or Generic Substitution Allowed instructions (optional)

PRODUCT SELECTION PERMITTED   DISPENSE AS WRITTEN

Signature of prescriber: (not required on a verbal prescription)

Note: Prescriptions are written in ink, never in pencil.

FIGURE 3.1: SAMPLE PRESCRIPTION

DATE	TIME	DOCTOR'S ORDERS 1	DATE/TIME INITIALS	DATE/TIME INITIALS
1/31/08	2200	Admit patient to 4th floor		
		Pneumonia, Dehydration		
		All: Sulfa-Hives		
		Order CBC, chem-7, blood cultures stat		
		Start LR @ 125 ml/hr IV q8°		
		Dr Johnson x2222		

PATIENT IDENTIFICATION
099999999 675-01
SMITH, JOHN
12/06/1950
DR. P JOHNSON

DOCTOR'S ORDERS

DATE	TIME	DOCTOR'S ORDERS 2	DATE/TIME INITIALS	DATE/TIME INITIALS
2/01/08	300	Tylenol 650mg po q4-6hrs		
		PRN for Temp>38		
		Percocet 5/325 PO q 4 hrs prn		
		break through pain		
		Verbal order Dr Johnson/		
		P. Smith, RN		

DATE	TIME	DOCTOR'S ORDERS 3	DATE/TIME INITIALS	DATE/TIME INITIALS
2/01/08	600	Start ciprofloxacin 500 mg po bid		
		Multivitamin po qd		
		Phenergan 12.5 mg IV q 6 hrs prn nausea		
		Order CXR for this a.m.		
		Dr Johnson x2222		

FIGURE 3.2: SAMPLE MEDICATION ORDER

Although it is not an order form, a *medication administration record* (MAR) also contains important information for pharmacists. It documents when and what medications were administered to a patient. MARs are used extensively in institutional settings where multiple professionals are responsible for a patient's care. Figure 3.3 provides an example.

Review and Interpretation

Once the pharmacist has received an order, the following series of steps must be followed to compound the correct formulation and comply with legal and safety requirements.

1. Review and interpret (translate) the prescription.
2. Accurately weigh and measure all components.
3. Use appropriate compounding techniques to convert individual components into a finished formulation.

COMMUNITY HOSPITAL
Medication Administration Record

Room/Bed: 675-01   From 0730 on 02/01/08 to 0700 on 02/02/08
Patient: SMITH, JOHN
Account #: 099999999   Diagnosis: PNEUMONIA; DEHYDRATION
Sex: M   Height: 5'11"   weight: 75KG
Age: 51Y
Doctor: JOHNSON, P.   Verified by: *Susie Smith, RN*

Allergies: PENICILLIN-->RASH

	0730-1530	1600-2300	2330-0700
LACTATED RINGERS 1 LITER BAG DOSE 125 ML/HR IV Q 8HRS ORDER #2	800 JD	1600 SS	2400
MULTIVITAMIN TABLET DOSE: 1 TABLET PO QD ORDER #4	1000 given @ 9 AM JD		
CIPROFLOXACIN 500 MG TABLET DOSE: 500MG PO BID ORDER #5	1000 JD	2200 SS	
ACETAMINOPHEN 325 MG TABLET DOSE: 650 MG PO Q 4-6 HRS PRN FOR TEMP>38°C ORDER #7	1200 JD		

Init / Signature		Init / Signature
SS / *Susie Smith, RN*		__ / _____
JD / *Jane Doe, RN*		__ / _____
__ / _____		__ / _____

FIGURE 3.3: SAMPLE MEDICATION ADMINISTRATION RECORD (MAR)

4. Properly package and label the formulation.
5. Deliver the formulation to the correct patient with adequate instructions for administration and storage.

Reviewing, interpreting, and labeling the prescription involves a "language" that must be learned and utilized. Part of that language includes abbreviations.

The health care professions use an estimated 10,000 abbreviations. There are no guidelines about which abbreviations can be used in written orders, although many individual institutions have developed some criteria. The pharmacist typically encounters a variety of abbreviations. The types of abbreviations might be grouped into the following categories:

- Latin abbreviations
- Drug name abbreviations
- Medical abbreviations.

Examples of each of these categories are given in Tables 3.1, 3.2, and 3.3.

Many abbreviations are used in only a limited geographical area or institutional setting, so care must be taken when interpreting any abbreviation. For example, the abbreviation T.I.W. can be interpreted as "three times a week" or "twice a week." D/C can be interpreted as "Drug Information Center," "discharge," or "discontinue." HS could mean "at bedtime" or "half-strength."

Some abbreviations are prone to misinterpretation, and their use is not encouraged. Some of the most

TABLE 3.1: LATIN ABBREVIATIONS

Latin Term	Abbreviation	Translation	Latin Term	Abbreviation	Translation
ad	ad	to, up to	dentur tales doses	d.t.d.	give of such doses
	ad lib.	at pleasure	dexter	d.	right
adde	add	add (thou)	diebus alternis	dieb. alt.	every other day
agita	agit	shake, stir	dilutus	dil.	dilute, diluted
alternis horis	alt. h.	every other hour		disp.	dispense
ana	a.a. or aa	of each		div.	divide
ante	a.	before		elix.	elixir
ante cibum	a.c.	before food, before meals	emulsum	emuls.	emulsion
ante meridien	a.m.	morning	et	et	and
	amp.	ampule	ex modo prescripto	e.m.p.	in the manner prescribed; as directed
aqua	aq.	water	fac, fiat, fiant	f.; ft.	let it be made; make
aqua ad	aq. ad	water up to		f.; fl.	fluid
	aq. dest; aqua dist.	distilled water		g.; G.; gm.	gram
auris	aur.; a	ear	granum	gr.	grain
auris dexter	a.d.	right ear	guttae	gtt.	a drop
aurix laevus	a.l.	left ear	hora	h	at the hour of
auris sinister	a.s.	left ear	hora somni	h.s.	at bedtime
auris utro	a.u.	each ear		i.m.; IM	intramuscular
auristillae	aurist	ear drops	injectio	inj.	injection
	a.t.c.	around the clock		i.v.; IV	intravenous
bis	b.	twice		i.v.p.; IVP	intravenous push
bis in die	b.i.d.	twice a day		IVPB	intravenous piggyback
brachium	brach.	the arm	laevus	l.	left
capsula	caps	a capsule	linimentum	lin.	liniment
	c.c.; cc	cubic centimeter	liquor	liq.	a solution
chartulae	charts	powder papers;		lot.	lotion
		divided powders	minimum	min; M$_x$	minum
cibus	cib.; c.	food	misce	m.; M	mix
collunarium	collun	a nose wash		mcg	microgram
collutorium	collut.	a mouth wash		mEq	milliequivalent
collyrium	collyr.	an eye wash		mg	milligram
compositus	comp.	compound		ml	milliliter
congius	cong.; C.	gallon	nocte	n.	at night
cum	c or c̄.	with	naristillae	narist.	nasal drops
cum cibus	c.c.	with food; with meals	nebule	neb.	a spray
dentur	d.	give (thou); let be given	non repetatur	non.rep.	do not repeat

(continued)

TABLE 3.1: LATIN ABBREVIATIONS (CONTINUED)

Latin Term	Abbreviation	Translation	Latin Term	Abbreviation	Translation
octarius	O.	pint	quantum sufficiat ad	q.s. ad	a sufficient quantity to make
oculentum	occulent.	eye ointment	secundum artem	s.a.	according to the art
oculus	o.	eye		S.C.; subc; subq	subcutaneously
oculus dexter	o.d.	right eye	semis	ss	one-half
oculus laevus	o.l.	left eye	signa	Sig.	write, label
oculus sinister	o.s.	left eye	sine	s	without
oculus utro	o.u.	both eyes, each eye	si opus sit	s.o.s.	if necessary
omni mane	o.m.	every morning		sol.	solution
parti affectae applicandus	p.a.a.	to be applied to affected part	statim	stat.	immediately
per os	p.o.	by mouth	suppositorum	supp.	suppository
post cibum	p.c.	after meals	syrupus	syr.	syrup
	p.r.	per rectum	tabella	tab.	tablet
pro re nata	p.r.n.	as needed		tbsp.	tablespoonful
pulvis	pulv.	powder	ter in die	t.i.d.	three times a day
quater in die	q.i.d.	four times a day		tinc.; tr.	tincture
quaque	q.	each, every	trochiscus	troche	lozenge
quaque die	q.d.	every day	tussis	tuss.	a cough
quaque hora	q.h.	every hour	ungentum	ung.	an ointment
quantum sufficiat	q.s.	a sufficient quantity	ut dictum	ut dict.; u.d.	as directed

TABLE 3.2: DRUG NAME ABBREVIATIONS

Abbreviations	Drug Name	Abbreviations	Drug Name	Abbreviations	Drug Name
5-FU	5-fluorouracil	HCL	hydrochloric Acid	NTG	nitroglycerin
6-MP	6-mercaptopurine	HCO_3	bicarbonate	OC	oral contraceptive
6-TG	6-thioguanine	HCTZ	hydrochlorothiazide	PABA	p-amino benzoic acid
$Al(OH)_3$	aluminum hydroxide	I	iodine	PAS	p-aminosalicylic acid
APAP	acetaminophen	INH	isoniazid	PCN	penicillin
Ara-C	cytarabine	ISDN	isosorbide dinitrate	PCP	phencyclidine
ASA	aspirin (acetylsalicylic acid)	K	potassium	PDN	prednisone
AZT	zidovudine	KCl	potassium chloride	PTH	parathyroid hormone
B&O	belladonna and opium	LD	levodopa	PZI	protamine zinc
C	ascorbic acid	LR	Lactated Ringer's solution	RS	Ringer's solution
Ca	calcium	Mg	magnesium	SS	saline solution
Cl	chloride	MgO	magnesium oxide	SSKI	saturated solution of potassium iodide
CO	castor oil	$MgSO_4$	magnesium sulfate	SWI	sterile water for injection
D5W	dextrose 5% in water	MOM	milk of magnesia	T_3	triiodothyroxine, liothyronine
DA	dopamine	MS	morphine sulfate	T_4	levothyroxine
DDAVP	desmopressin acetate	MTX	methotrexate	TCA	trichloroacetic acid
DES	diethylstilbestrol	MVI	multiple vitamin	TCN	tetracycline
DIG	digoxin	Na	sodium	TMP/SMX	trimethoprim/sulfamethoxazole
DW	distilled water	NaCl	sodium chloride	TPN	total perenteral nutrition
ETOH	alcohol	$NaHCO_3$	sodium bicarbonate	U	ultralente insulin
F	fluorine	NO	nitrous oxide	WFI	water for injection
Fe	iron	NPH	Neutral Protamine Hagedorn (insulin)	Zn	zinc sulfate
FeGluc	ferrous gluconate	NS	normal saline solution (0.9% sodium chloride)		
$FeSO_4$	ferrous sulfate	½ NS	one-half normal saline solution (0.45% sodium chloride)		
H_2O_2	hydrogen peroxide				

TABLE 3.3: MEDICAL ABBREVIATIONS

Abbreviation	Term	Abbreviation	Term
AIDS	acquired immunodeficiency syndrome	HCT	hematocrit
AMI	acute myocardial infarction	HDL	high density lipoprotein
ANS	autonomic nervous system	HIV	human immunodeficiency virus
AV	atrial-ventricular	IH	Infectious hepatitis
BM	bowel movement	IO, I/O	fluid intake and output
BP	blood pressure	LDL	low density lipoprotein
BPH	benign prostatic hyperplasia	MDI	metered dose inhaler
BS	blood sugar	MI	myocardial infarction
BSA	body surface area	MRSA	Methicillin-resistant *Staphylococcus aureus* (MRSA) infection
BUN	blood urea nitrogen	N&V	nausea and vomiting
BW	body weight	NK	not known
C	centigrade	NMT	nebulized mist treatment
CA	cancer	NPO	nothing by mouth
CA	cardiac arrest	NVD	nausea, vomiting, and diarrhea
CBC	complete blood count	OD	overdose
CHF	congestive heart failure	OTC	over the counter
CMV	cytomegalovirus	PUD	peptic ulcer disease
CNS	central nervous system	RR	recovery room
COPD	chronic obstructive pulmonary disease	RBC	red blood count or red blood cells
CV	cardiovascular	RSV	respiratory syncytial virus
CVA	cerebrovascular accident	SOB	shortness of breath
DC	discontinue	SVN	small volume nebulization solution
DI	diabetes insipidus	SZ	seizue
DOB	date of birth	T	temperature
DR	delivery room	TB	tuberculosis
DX	diagnosis	TPN	total perenteral nutrition
EC	enteric coated	U	units
EENT	eyes, ears, nose, throat	UA	urinalysis
EKG, ECG	electrocardiogram	URI	upper respiratory infection
ER	emergency room	UTI	urinary tract infection
GERD	gastroesophageal reflux disease	VD	venereal disease
GI	gastrointestinal	VS	vital signs
GYN	gynecology	WBC	white blood count or white blood cells
H	hypodermic	WT	weight
HA	headache	XX	female sex chromosome
HBP	high blood pressure	XY	male sex chromosome

common misinterpreted abbreviations are shown in Table 3.4. The Institute of Safe Medication Practices (http://www.ismp.org) maintains an online resource that provides lists and tools to help prevent medication errors and promote medication safety. A more extensive list of "dangerous abbreviations" is available on the website.

Abbreviations also can be misinterpreted when a designation for a liquid ("fl" or "f") is omitted from a value. For example, if the abbreviation is written as 3 oz., the pharmacist must determine whether a volume or weight measurement is desired. If the abbreviation is written as 3 fl oz., a volume measurement is being prescribed. Some guidelines are helpful in these situations:

- If the ingredient is a liquid in a liquid preparation, the quantity is a volume.
- If the ingredient is a solid, the quantity is a weight.
- In solid preparations, quantities are by weight unless otherwise specified.

Figure 3.4 gives examples of some prescription problems.

TABLE 3.4: ABBREVIATIONS PRONE TO MISINTERPRETATION

Abbreviation	Intended Meaning	Common Error
U	Units	Mistaken as a zero or a four (4), resulting in overdose. Also mistaken for "cc" (cubic centimeters) when poorly written.
µg	Micrograms	Mistaken for "mg" (milligrams) resulting in an overdose.
Q.D.	Latin abbreviation for every day	The period after the "Q" sometimes has been mistaken for an "I," and the drug has been given "QID" (four times daily) rather than daily.
Q.O.D.	Abbreviation for every other day	Misinterpreted as "QD" (daily) or "QID" (four times daily). If the "O" is poorly written, it looks like a period or an "I."
SC or SQ	Subcutaneous	Mistaken as "SL" (sublingual) when poorly written.
T I W	Three times a week	Misinterpreted as "three times a day" or "twice a week."
D/C	Discharged; also Discontinue	Patient's medications have been prematurely discontinued when D/C (intended to mean "discharge") was misinterpreted as "discontinue" because it was followed by a list of drugs.
HS	Half-strength	Misinterpreted as the Latin abbreviation "HS" (hour of sleep).
CC	Cubic centimeters	Mistaken as "U" (units) when poorly written.
AU, AD, AD	Latin abbreviation for both ears; left ear; right ear	Misinterpreted as the Latin abbreviation "OU" (both eyes); "OS" (left eye); "OD" (right eye).
IJ	Injection	Mistaken as "IV" or "Intrajugular."
IU	International Unit	Mistaken as IV (intravenous) or 10 (ten).
MS, MSO4, MgSO4	Confused for one another	Can mean morphine sulfate or magnesium sulfate.

Rx		Rx		Rx		
Zinc Oxide	5.0	Zinc Oxide	5.	Zinc Oxide	5	
Calamine	5.0	Calamine	5.	Calamine	5	
Hydrocortisone	0.5	Hydrocortisone	.5	Hydrocortisone		5
Talc q.s.	50.0	Talc q.s.	50.	Talc q.s.	50	
M.Ft. pulv.		M.Ft. pulv.		M.Ft. pulv.		
Sig: p.a.a. t.i.d.		Sig: p.a.a. t.i.d.		Sig: p.a.a. t.i.d.		

Note: When units are omitted and quantities are expressed in Arabic numbers, it is assumed that the quantities are expressed in the metric system with weight measurements in grams and volume measurements in milliliters. Note that the vertical bar in the last prescription has the same meaning as the decimals in the previous two prescriptions.

Rx			
Potassium iodide			7.2 g
Guaifenesin syrup			
Hydroiodic acid syrup	aa	q.s.	120 ml
M.FT. syrup			
Sig: i tsp q6h			

Rx			
Benadryl elixir			
Nystatin oral suspension	aa.		10 ml
Mylanta suspension		q.s. ad	120 ml
M.Ft. susp			
Sig: 1 Tbl swish and swallow q.i.d, p.c. and h.s.			

Note: The abbreviation aa (or $\overline{aa}$) means "of each." In the first prescription, the prescription is brought to final volume with a mixture of equal parts of the two syrups. In the second, the suspension is prepared by mixing 10 ml each of Benadryl elixir and Nystatin oral suspension, then adding sufficient Mylanta suspension to make a total of 120 ml.

Rx	
Acetaminophen	gr xx
Codeine phosphate	gr v
Lactose q.s.	gr C
M. et ft capsules No. XX	
Sig: i q6h prn pain	

Note: The abbreviation M. et ft. (or M. ft or M. Ft.), meaning "mix and make," tells the pharmacist that a mixture of the ingredients should be prepared in the amounts listed and then divided into the number of dosage forms indicated. In this case, the ingredients would be divided into 20 capsules, each containing 1 gr. of acetaminophen, 1/4 gr. codeine phosphate, and enough lactose to make a total of 5 gr.

Rx	
Acetaminophen	65 mg
Codeine phosphate	10 mg
Lactose q.s.	300 mg
M. Ft. D.T.D. caps #10	
Sig: i q6h prn pain	

Note: Because D.T.D. means "of such doses," this prescription requires that the pharmacist prepare 10 capsules, each containing the listed weights of ingredients. To determine the total weight of each ingredient, the pharmacist multiplies the given weight by the number of dosage forms. Here, the pharmacist would weigh 10 × 65 mg = 650 mg acetaminophen.

FIGURE 3.4: EXAMPLES OF INSCRIPTION, SUBSCRIPTION, AND SIGNA PORTIONS OF THE PRESCRIPTION

Other translation problems come from misreading the actual drug or ingredient name. Many drugs appear similar when they are written, or they sound alike when spoken. A listing of many common "look-alike, sound-alike" drugs is available at the Institute of Safe Medication Practices website (http://www.ismp.org) and at the University of North Carolina School of Pharmacy Pharmaceutical Care Laboratory website (http://pharmacy.unc.edu/carelabs/resources/alike/LookAlike.htm).

Labeling

Proper labeling is one of the most important aspects of dispensing a prescription. The label must comply with state and federal regulations and should convey correctly and clearly all necessary information regarding dosage, mode of administration, and proper storage of the formulation. The quality of labeling is extremely important to the patient's perception of the quality of the product

LOOK-ALIKE AND SOUND-ALIKE DRUGS

Acetohexamide	Acetazolamide	Lasix	Lidex
Alfentanil	Fentanyl, Sufentanil	Lisinopril	Fosinopril
Amitriptyline	Aminophylline	Magnesium Sulfate	Manganese Sulfate
Atenolol	Albuterol	Mellaril	Elavil
Bupropion	Buspirone	Methicillin	Mezlocillin
Cafergot	Carafate	Metolazone	Metaxalone
Capitrol	Captopril	Metoprolol	Metaproterenol
Cefamandole	Cefmetazole	Nifedipine	Nicardipine
Cefotaxime	Ceftizoxime	Oxymorphone	Oxymetholone
Cefoxitin	Cefotaxime	Pancuronium	Pipecuronium
Cephalexin	Cephalothin	Pentobarbital	Phenobarbital
Chlorpropamide	Chlorpromazine	Phenytoin	Mephenytoin
Clomiphene	Clomipramine	Pramoxine	Pralidoxime
Clonazepam	Clofazimine	Prazosin	Prednisone
Clotrimazole	Co-trimoxazole	Prednisone	Prednisolone
Cyclosporine (cyclosporin A)	Cycloserine	Primidone	Prednisone
Dexamethasone	Desoximetasone	Proparacaine	Propoxyphene
Digoxin	Digitoxin	Quazepam	Oxazepam
Diphenhydramine	Dimenhydrinate	Reserpine	Risperidone
Dopamine	Dobutamine	Ribavirin	Riboflavin
Doxazosin	Doxorubicin	Ritodrine	Ranitidine
Encainide	Flecainide	Sucralfate	Salsalate
Enflurane	Isoflurance	Sulfadiazine	Sulfasalazine
Etidronate	Etretinate	Sulfamethizole	Sulfamethoxazole
Flunisolide	Fluocinonide	Testoderm®	Estraderm®
Glyburide	Glipizide	Thyrar®	Thyrolar®
Guanadrel	Gonadoreline	Thyrolar®	Theolair®
Guanfacine	Guaifenesin	Timolol	Atenolol
Halcinonide	Halcion	Torsemide	Furosemide
Hydralazine	Hydroxyzine	Tretinoin	Trientine
Hydrochlorothiazide	Hydroflumethiazide	Triamterene	Trimipramine
Hydrocortisone	Hydrocodone	Vicodin	Hycodan
Kanamycin	Garamycin, Gentamicin	Vincristine	Vinblastine
Neutra-Phos	Neutra-Phos-K	Zantac	Xanax

A comprehensive list can be seen at http://www.pharmacy.unc.edu/carelabs/resources/alike/LookAlike.htm

and may have profound implications on its safe use and compliance with the prescribed regimen.

> The outward appearance of the prescription drug package is often the only tangible basis for the patient's judgment of a pharmacist's care and skill

Required label information includes:

- name, address, and phone number of the pharmacy
- prescription (serial) number
- date of initial dispensing
- patient's name
- directions for use
- name and strength of the active ingredient(s)
- prescriber's name
- name of dispensing pharmacist
- beyond use date.

In addition to the information required by law, the following information is recommended for inclusion on the prescription label:

- number of dosage units or volume of product dispensed
- number of refills allowed.

The actual label format is dictated by many factors, such as the computer software, personal preference,

and institutional guidelines. An example label is given in Figure 3.5.

Directions to the patient about how to use the formulation must be clear and not be subject to mis-interpretation. Some guidelines about wording patient instructions are as follows.

- Indicate the dosage form to be administered:
  "Take one capsule every day" instead of "Take one every day."
- Use words instead of numbers:
  "Take one capsule every day" instead of "Take 1 capsule every day."
- Express quantities to be administered in units that are familiar to the patient, and for which they are likely to have suitable measuring devices:
  "Take two teaspoonfuls every six hours" instead of "Take ten ml every six hours."
- Specify the route of administration if the medication is not intended for oral use:
  "Insert one suppository vaginally every night at bedtime."
- Specify which side is to receive the medication if more than one organ/appendage is present:
  "Instill two drops in left eye daily" instead of "Instill two drops daily."
- Do not use abbreviations:
  "Take two capsules twice a day," not "Take two caps twice a day."

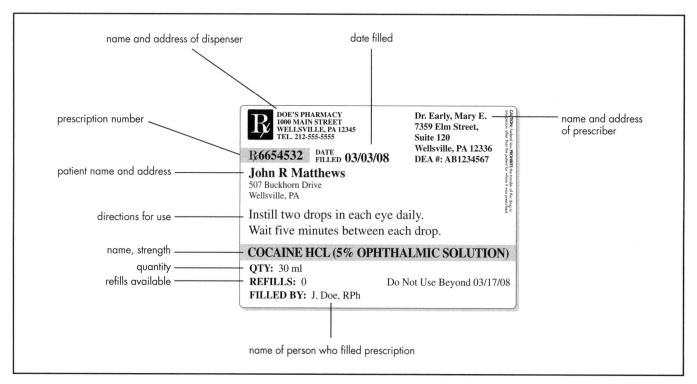

FIGURE 3.5: EXAMPLE OF A PRESCRIPTION LABEL

- Specify all active ingredients in a compounded prescription. Inert bases or vehicles may, but need not, be labeled.

- In general, specify the amount of active ingredient *per dosage unit*:

  Inderal 2 mg/chart, Amoxicillin 250 mg/5ml,
  Phenergan 25 mg/suppository

- When dispensing medications in bulk, such as solutions, suspensions, emulsions, ointments, or creams, express the amounts of active ingredients as a percentage strength:

  Hydrocortisone cream 1% or
  Betadine Solution 2%

Some examples of abbreviations and their translations are given in Table 3.5.

Guidelines for labeling formulations dispensed for inpatients (where the inpatient is not in possession of the formulation) are given in the NABP's Model Rules for Pharmaceutical Care.[2] The label for a single unit package should include:

- the nonproprietary or proprietary name of the drug
- the route of administration, if other than oral
- the strength and volume, where appropriate, expressed in the metric system
- the control number and expiration date
- identification of the repackager by name or by license number
- any special storage conditions.

Labeling parenterals for inpatient use is described in the ASHP's Technical Assistance Bulletin on Quality Assurance for Pharmacy-Prepared Sterile Products.[3] In addition to the labeling requirements listed for inpatient formulations, the following are recommended:

- patient's name, location, identification number
- prescribed administration regimen.

Auxiliary Labels

In addition to the information provided on the typed prescription label or medication order, auxiliary labels sometimes are necessary to provide supplementary information regarding proper and safe administration, use, or storage of the formulation. Example auxiliary labels are shown below.

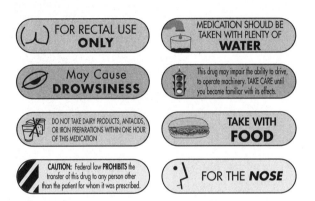

Controlled substances from schedules II, III, and IV must carry an auxiliary label stating, "Caution: Federal law prohibits the transfer of this drug to any person other than the patient for whom it was prescribed."

TABLE 3.5: EXAMPLES OF TRANSLATING ABBREVIATIONS TO LABELING

Abbreviation	Translation
gtts. ii a.u. b.i.d.	Instill two drops in each ear twice a day.
ung. p.a.a. q12h	Apply ointment to affected area (part) every twelve hours.
caps ii stat, then 1 q6h a.t.c.	Take two capsules now (immediately), then one capsule every six hours around the clock.
supp p.r.n. q6h prn N & V	Insert one suppository rectally every six hours as needed for nausea and vomiting.
tabs i q.i.d., 1/2 hr a.c. and h.s.	Take one tablet four times a day, one-half hour before meals and at bedtime.
2 tsp. pulv ex aq p.o. t.i.d., p.c.	Mix two teaspoonfuls of powder in water and take by mouth three times a day, after meals.
tab i ss h.s., p.r.n. sleep. Non rep.	Take one and one-half tablets at bedtime as needed for sleep. Do not repeat.
tab i q.o.d. in am	Take one tablet every other day, in the morning.
gtts i o.d. q.d.	Instill (put) one drop in right eye every day.
4 tbls. in O aq. dist.; gargle 1 fl oz. q4h	Mix four tablespoonfuls in a pint of (distilled) water and use two tablespoonfuls as a gargle every four hours.
M. et. div. caps No. L	Mix and divide into 50 capsules.
M. Ft. elix.; disp O.	Mix and make an elixir; dispense 1 pint.
M. Ft. sol.; disp ss cong.	Mix and make a solution; dispense 1/2 gallon.
M. et. ft. charts No. XL	Mix and make 40 individual powders (papers).
Ft. supp. rect.; disp # xiv	Make 14 rectal suppositories.

NOTES

1. <1075> Good Compounding Practices: The United States Pharmacopeia 29/National Formulary 24, The United States Pharmacopeial Convention, Inc., Rockville, MD, 2005, pp. 2903–2906.

2. Model Rules for the Practice of Pharmacy. National Association of Pharmacy. National Association of Boards of Pharmacy. Model State Pharmacy Act and Model Rules of the National Association of Boards of Pharmacy. 2007:2–4.

3. American Society of Hospital Pharmacists. ASHP Technical Assistance Bulletin on Quality Assurance for Pharmacy-Prepared Sterile Products. *American Journal of Hospital Pharmacy* 50:2386–2398, 1993.

ADDITIONAL READING

Stiles, M. L, Todd, J., Rankin, M., Settle, H., and Hudson, J. The Ten Basic Steps in Filling A Prescription: Then and Now. *International Journal of Pharmaceutical Compounding* 1:14–17, 1997.

Thompson, J. E. Prescription and Medication Orders (chapter 1) in *A Practical Guide to Contemporary Pharmacy Practice,* 2nd edition. Lippincott Williams & Wilkins, Baltimore, MD, 2004, pp. 1.3–1.12.

Thompson, J. E. Labeling Prescriptions and Medications (chapter 2) in *A Practical Guide to Contemporary Pharmacy Practice,* 2nd edition. Lippincott Williams & Wilkins, Baltimore, MD, 2004, pp. 2.1–2.8.

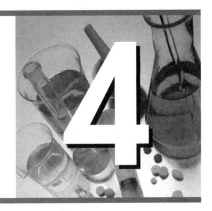

CHAPTER FOUR

Compounding Facilities and Equipment

THE PRACTICE OF EXTEMPORANEOUS COMPOUNDING has changed dramatically over the last decades. This change has been accompanied by an evolution in the "tools of the trade." Pharmacists who decide to make compounding a significant part of their practice will make financial commitments for facilities, equipment, and supplies. The extent of these commitments will depend on the type of compounding the pharmacist will do. Obviously, all pharmacists do not need the most elaborate sterile facilities and compounding equipment available to initiate a compounding practice. Many pharmacists start with a limited inventory of equipment and supplies and then add items or renovations as their practice increases.

Facilities

National Association of Boards of Pharmacy's (NABP) Good Compounding Practices Applicable to State Licensed Pharmacies gives the following guidelines regarding facilities:

> Pharmacies engaging in compounding shall have a specifically designated and adequate area (space) for the orderly placement of equipment and materials to be used to compound medications and to prevent mix-ups or contamination between components, containers, labels, in-process materials, and finished drug products. The drug compounding area for sterile products shall be separate and distinct from the area used for the compounding or dispensing of non-sterile drug products. The area(s) used for the compounding of drugs shall be maintained in a good state of repair and be of suitable construction and location to facilitate cleaning, maintenance, and proper operation. Adequate space and appropriate material flow shall be provided.
>
> Adequate lighting, heating, ventilation, and air conditioning shall be provided in all drug compounding areas to prevent contamination or decomposition of components. Potable water shall be supplied under continuous positive pressure in a plumbing system free of defects that could contribute contamination to any compounded drug product. Adequate washing facilities, easily accessible to the compounding area(s) of the pharmacy, shall be provided. These facilities shall include, but not be limited to, hot and cold water, soap or detergent, and air-dryers or single-use towels.
>
> The area(s) used for the compounding of drugs shall be maintained in a clean and sanitary condition. Sewage,

trash, and other refuse in and from the pharmacy and immediate drug compounding area(s) shall be held and disposed of in a safe, sanitary, and timely manner.[1]

The American Society of Hospital Pharmacists (ASHP) Technical Assistance Bulletin on Compounding Nonsterile Products in Pharmacies gives some refinements such as, "The area should be isolated from potential interruptions, chemical contaminants, and sources of dust and particulate matter."[2] These guidelines also state that "the compounding area should not contain dust-collecting overhangs (e.g., ceiling utility pipes, hanging light fixtures) and ledges (e.g., window sills)."

USP/NF chapter <795> amplifies many of the concepts elaborated in these earlier documents. Overall, the compounding area is to be adequately designed, and isolated so as to avoid unnecessary traffic and air flow disturbances. It is to provide for the proper storage of drugs and supplies under appropriate conditions of temperature, light, moisture, sanitation, ventilation, and security."[3]

Most of these recommended facilities are required by state boards of pharmacy when a pharmacy is built. The one facility component that warrants special consideration is the "specifically designated and adequate area" that will be used exclusively for compounding. If the pharmacy also is to have a sterile compounding area, this will be an additional consideration because the sterile compounding area is to be separated from the compounding area. These two areas—the compounding area and a sterile compounding area—may occupy a significant portion of the available space and may require renovations of the facility.

Ingredients

An ingredient is a chemical or material that is added to a formulation during the formulation process. *Active ingredients* are those chemicals or materials that have therapeutic benefit. USP/NF chapter <795> states that

> Active ingredients usually refers to chemicals, substances, or other components of articles intended for use in the diagnosis, cure, mitigation, treatment, or prevention of diseases in humans or other animals or for use as nutritional supplements.

Inactive ingredients (also called excipients, pharmaceutics ingredients, added substances, and pharmaceutical necessities) are necessary for preparing dosage forms or for enhancing the stability of finished preparations. They do not (or, at least, are not intended to) give a therapeutic response if given alone in the concentration present in the dosage form.

Purity of Ingredients

USP/NF chapter <795> contains the following statements regarding the purity of ingredients used in compounded formulations:

> A USP or a NF grade drug substance is the preferred source of ingredients for compounding all other preparations. If that is not available, or when food, cosmetics, or other substances are or must be used, then the use of another high quality source, such as analytical reagent (AR), certified American Chemical Society (ACS), or Food Chemicals Codex (FCC) grade, is an option for professional judgment.

Therefore, the pharmacist is responsible for choosing appropriate, quality ingredients for compounded drug formulations. Several grades are mentioned by the USP, above. A more complete listing of the chemical grades is given in Table 4.1.

USP/NF chapter <795> prefers that USP or NF grade be the lowest grade of chemical purity used in compounding, and if that grade is not available, that

higher grades of purity can be used if approved by the pharmacist. In selecting chemicals of higher grades of purity, the pharmacist should require a certificate of analysis from the supplier. For any substance used in compounding not purchased from a registered drug manufacturer, the pharmacist should establish purity and safety by reasonable means, which may include lot analysis, manufacturer reputation, or reliability of source.[4]

Sources of Ingredients

Manufactured drug products, such as tablets, capsules, or injections, often are used as sources of active ingredients for compounded preparations. If such a manufactured product is to be used as an active ingredient in compounding, the manufactured drug product must contain a batch control number and the product must be within its stated expiratory date. Additional considerations in using a manufactured drug product as the source of an active ingredient are the following.

- Certain solid dosage forms should not be crushed and used as ingredients for compounding.
  - Controlled release and enteric coated products are specially formulated or coated to give certain desired or required release characteristics. These features may be destroyed by crushing the product.
  - Some drugs are put in capsules, or are formulated into tablets that are sugar or film coated, to mask their unpleasant taste, to protect the mouth or throat from irritation, or to protect the teeth from staining. Crushing the tablets or emptying the contents of the capsules to use these as compounding ingredients destroys this protection.
  - Sublingual or buccal tablets may contain drugs that require this special route of administration for therapeutic activity.
- Special care must be exercised when manipulating chemotherapy drug products as ingredients for compounding. For example, when crushing oral solid dosage forms of cytotoxic drugs, the dosage form should be placed in a sealable plastic bag and crushed with the back of a spoon or with a pestle, taking care not to puncture the bag.
- Care must be exercised when selecting injectable products as ingredients for other routes of administration.
  - Some injectable products use prodrugs to enhance solubility of the active ingredient. These prodrugs may or may not be therapeutically active when used by other routes of administration. For example, if the prodrug is an ester, esterases must be present at the site of administration for the drug to become active.
  - Some drugs that are efficacious when given parenterally may not be therapeutically active orally or topically. This can be caused by factors such as: loss

TABLE 4.1: PURITY GRADES APPLIED TO CHEMICALS

Chemical Grade	Description
USP	Meet or exceed specifications prescribed in current edition of USP
NF	Meet or exceed specifications prescribed in current edition of NF
FCC	Meet or exceed specifications in current edition of Food Chemical Codex
ACS	Meet or exceed specifications in current edition of Reagent Chemicals published by the American Chemical Society
AR	Chemicals of high purity suitable for analytical laboratory work (analytical reagent grade)
Purified	Chemicals of superior quality for which there is no official standard
CP	Chemicals more refined than technical grade, but only partial analytical information available (chemically pure)
HPLC	Very high purity used in high pressure liquid chromatography analytical work
Spectroscopic grade	Very high purity use in spectroscopic analytical work
Primary standard	Highest purity available used in standard solutions for analytical purposes
Technical	Chemicals of commercial or industrial quality (commercial grade)
Food grade	Chemicals that have clearance for use in foods
Cosmetic grade	Chemicals approved for use in cosmetics

Modified from "General Guidelines for the Use of Chemicals for Prescription Compounding," by L. V. Allen, Jr., International Journal of Pharmaceutical Compounding 1:46, 1997.

by first-pass metabolism; degradation in the gastro-intestinal tract or lack of absorption in the gut when the drug product is given orally; or lack of absorption through the skin or mucous membranes when given topically.

- The pharmacist should consider all these factors when deciding to use a manufactured drug product as an ingredient for a compounded drug preparation. The product package insert always should be consulted for helpful information from the product's manufacturer.

Cosmetic grade chemicals are approved for use in cosmetics. The pharmacist should be clear about the differences between a drug product and a cosmetic product because if the pharmacist compounds a cosmetic, the product must comply with standards that are different from those of a drug product.

Equipment and Supplies for Measuring, Mixing, Molding, and Packaging

NABP guidelines state that

> equipment used in the compounding of drug products shall be of appropriate design, adequate size, and suitably located to facilitate operations for its intended use and for its cleaning and maintenance. The types and sizes of equipment will depend on the doage forms and the quantities compounded. Equipment used in the compounding of drug products shall be of suitable composition so that surfaces that contact components, in-process materials, or drug products shall not be reactive, additive, or absorptive so as to alter the safety, identity, strength, quality, or purity of the drug product beyond that desired, which they purport or are represented to possess.

These guidelines in essence say to "use the right equipment" but offer no specific recommendations. ASHP specifies that

> the equipment needed to compound a drug product depends upon the particular dosage form requested. Although Boards of Pharmacy publish lists of required equipment and accessories, these lists are not intended to limit the equipment available to pharmacists for compounding.

This bulletin then lists some specific equipment under the categories of Weighing Equipment, Measuring Equipment, and Compounding Equipment. Under weighing equipment, specifications for torsion and electronic balances and weights are given. Measuring equipment specified includes cylindrical graduates, syringes, micropipets, and conical graduates. Under compounding equipment, the guidelines recommend:

- two types of mortars and pestles, one glass and one Wedgewood or porcelain
- weighing papers, weighing cups, glassine papers

- stainless steel and plastic spatulas
- ointment slab, pill tile, or parchment ointment pad
- suppository molds
- funnels, filter paper
- beakers, glass stirring rods
- a source of heat, a refrigerator, and a freezer.

Another way of determining what compounding equipment is needed is to visualize a compounded formulation as the result of a four-step process:

1. *To measure*: balance, weights, weighing containers, volumetric glassware (cylindrical or conical graduates, calibrated and volumetric pipets, volumetric flasks), syringes, micropipets
2. *To mix*: beakers, Erlenmeyer flasks, spatulas, mortar and pestle, stirring hotplate, homogenizers, blenders, ointment slabs
3. *To mold*: sieves, funnels, suppository molds, capsule shells, ointment slabs, tablet triturate mold
4. *To package*: prescription bottles, capsule vials, ointment jars.

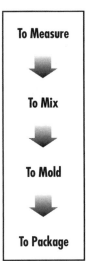

To Measure
↓
To Mix
↓
To Mold
↓
To Package

To Measure

A *balance* is used to determine the weight of a powder, dosage form, liquid, or other substance. The three main types of balances are prescription, triple-beam, and electronic. Most pharmacies have either a Class A prescription balance or an electronic balance. The triple-beam balance is used more often in laboratory work than in pharmacy compounding.

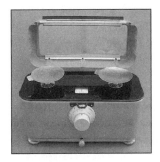

The *Class A prescription balance* has a sensitivity requirement of 6 mg with a minimum weighable quantity of 120 mg. These balances have a maximum weighable quantity of either 60 or 120 grams. They are two pan, torsion type balances that utilize both internal and external weights. The balance has a rider that adds an internal weight to the right pan. The rider always is calibrated in the metric system (grams), but some riders also have calibration marks in the apothecary system (grains).

Class A balances can weigh 120 mg of material with a 5% error; 5% generally is taken as the acceptable error inherent in most pharmaceutical processes. If a formulation calls for an ingredient weighing less than 120 mg, two approaches can be taken.

1. Make a trituration of the ingredient and bulk material such that an aliquot of greater than 120 mg will contain the correct amount of ingredient.

2. Use a balance with a greater sensitivity (i.e., a lower sensitivity requirement).

Electronic balances are available that can weigh quantities as large as 600 g with a sensitivity as little as 1 mg. They come in a variety of

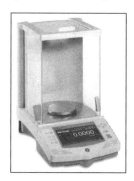

shapes and sizes. Most are top loading. Some electronic balances are enclosed in either glass or Plexiglas. Other balances have removable rings or shields to protect the balance against air drafts and to shield the balance from dust particles.

Weight sets usually consist of brass cylindrical weights ranging from 1 g to 50 g with flat fractional weights ranging from 10 mg to 500 mg. Older sets sometimes contain weights for both the metric system and the apothecary

system, but newer sets contain only the metric system weights. To prevent soiling and erosion of the weights, they should be kept in their designated box and forceps should be used to handle the weights. When used on

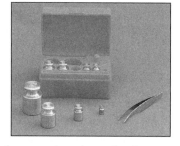

a prescription balance, weights are placed on glassine paper or weighing boats.

Weighing papers or *weighing boats* always should be placed on the balance pans before doing any weighing. These protect the pans from damage and also provide a convenient way to transfer the weighed material from the balance to another vessel. Weighing papers are made of nonabsorbable glassine paper, and weighing boats are made of polystyrene. When using weighing papers, the

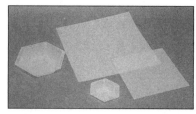

paper should be creased diagonally and then flattened and placed on the pans. This creates a collection trough in the paper. New

weighing papers or weighing boats should be used with each new drug to prevent contamination.

In compounding, liquid drugs, solvents, or additives are measured in volumetric glassware or plasticware. The volume capacity is etched on the side of the vessel, and some devices have graduation marks. Volumetric vessels also are marked as either *TD (to deliver)* or *TC (to contain)*. "To deliver" means that when the vessel is

emptied, it will deliver the total volume measured. "To contain" glassware will hold the total volume measured, but it will deliver more than the total volume if it is completely emptied. An example of a TD vessel is a syringe. Volumetric flasks and cylindrical and conical graduates are TC vessels, although in practice the graduates often are used as TD vessels. Common volumetric vessels include *single volume and calibrated pipets, cylindrical and conical graduates, syringes,* and *volumetric flasks.*

Pipets are thin glass tubes used to deliver volumes less than 25 ml. The two types of pipets are the single volume and the calibrated. The single volume pipet is the most accurate and simplest to use but is limited to measurement of a single fixed volume. These pipets are not capable of partial measuring. Single volume pipets are available in 1, 2, 5, 10, or 25 ml sizes. The calibrated pipet has graduation marks from a point near the tip to the capacity of the pipet. In addition to delivering the entire contents of the pipet, the calibrated pipet can be used to deliver partial volumes with good volumetric precision.

Micropipets generally are used if very small volumes (less than 1 ml) are required. These are available in a variety of sizes. Each micropipet can be adjusted to deliver a volume within a limited range. For example, one micropipet may deliver volumes of 0–20 μl, another 0–100 μl, and yet another 0–1,000 μl. The pharmacist selects the micropipet with the range that would give the

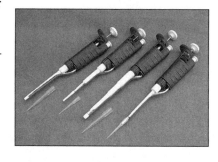

greatest accuracy for the desired volume to be measured. For example, if the pharmacist is going to measure 10 μl, the 0–20 μl micropipet, not the 0–100 μl micropipet, would be used.

A number of adjustable pipeting devices will deliver a fixed volume with each actuation. The Repipet® uses a glass syringe as the measuring device. Each time the plunger is raised, the volume is drawn into the syringe. When the plunger is depressed, the volume is dispensed through the discharge tube. Hand-held pipets operate in a similar manner. These have a large reservoir tip (25–50 ml) that initially is filled with liquid. The dial on the pipet is set to dispense the desired volume. When the pipet is

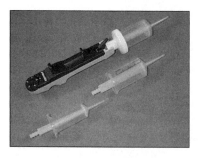

actuated, that volume is dispensed from the reservoir. Hand-held pipets generally are used to dispense 1–5 ml volumes, and the Repipet® is used to dispense larger volumes.

Graduates are used to measure and transfer liquids. They can be made of glass or plastic and are either

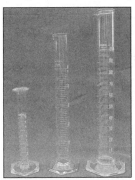

conical or cylindrical in shape. Because cylindrical graduates are more accurate, they are preferred in pharmaceutical compounding. Sizes of the graduates range from 5 ml to 4,000 ml. The pharmacist always should choose the smallest graduate capable of containing the volume to be measured. Measurements of volumes that are below 20% of the capacity of the graduate should be avoided because the accuracy is unacceptable. For example, a 100 ml graduate cannot accurately measure volumes below 20 ml. When measuring small volumes such as 25 ml and less, a syringe or pipet often is preferable.

Syringes range in size from 0.5 ml to 60 ml and are made of either plastic or glass. They are composed of a barrel and a plunger. The barrel has graduation marks for measuring partial volumes. Liquids are drawn into the syringe by pulling back on the plunger while the tip is emerged in the liquid. Syringes are particularly useful when measuring viscous liquids. Most compounding tasks utilize a disposable, nonsterile syringe made of plastic. When preparing sterile products, sterilized plastic syringes are used. As with graduates, the smallest syringe capable of containing the volume to be measured should be used.

Syringes come with four different tips.

1. Insulin syringes have a nonremovable needle molded into the tip syringe.

2. Luer-Lok® hypodermic syringes have a locking mechanism in the tip that secures the needle within a threaded ring.

3. Slip-Tip® hypodermic syringes do not have such a locking mechanism; friction holds the needle in place.

4. Oral syringes have a Slip-Tip® type syringe tip, but the tip is larger than the tip on a hypodermic syringe. These syringes will not hold a needle. They are used to accurately dispense a dose of liquid medication to a patient. They also are used with an Adapt-a-Cap® to

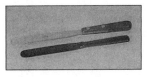

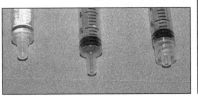
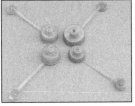

conveniently remove liquids from bottles. Adapt-a-Caps come in a variety of sizes to fit different bottle openings and are designed to accept only oral syringes.

Volumetric flasks have a slender neck and wide bulb-like base. They are single volume glassware and come in sizes ranging from 5 ml to 4,000 ml. Only one calibration

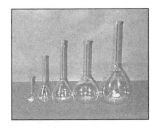

mark is etched on the neck of the flask. When the flask is filled to that mark, the flask contains the volume marked on the flask. Volumetric flasks are difficult to use if dissolving solids in liquid because of the narrowness of the neck. If solids are to be dissolved, the pharmacist should fill the flask partially with liquid, add the solid and complete dissolution, then fill the flask to the calibration mark.

To Mix

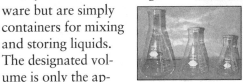

Erlenmeyer flasks, beakers, and *prescription bottles,* regardless of graduation markings on the vessel, are *not* volumetric glassware but are simply containers for mixing and storing liquids. The designated volume is only the approximate capacity of the vessel.

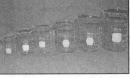

Spatulas are used to transfer solid ingredients. Spatulas are available in a variety of sizes (4, 6, and 8 inch are common) and are made of stainless steel, hard rubber, or plastic. Because stainless steel spatulas can be corroded by certain metals such as iodine, rubber or plastic spatulas should be used to handle these chemicals. The small spatulas are used for handling dry chemicals, for scraping materials from other spatulas, and for scraping materials from the sides of small mortars and pestles.

Because stainless steel spatulas can scratch the sides of a mortar, hard rubber or plastic spatulas should be

used for this purpose. The larger spatulas are used for handling larger quantities of drug chemicals and for mixing or spatulating ointments. Also, various small, double-sided bladed or single-sided cupped microspatulas are useful for withdrawing small amounts of chemicals and drugs from their containers. They are not useful for other purposes.

The *mortar and pestle* are made of three types of materials: glass, Wedgewood, or porcelain. They also come in a variety of common sizes from 2 oz. to 32 oz. Wedgewood and porcelain mortars are earthenware, are relatively course in texture, and are used to grind crystals and large particles into fine powders. Wedgewood generally is reserved for grinding hard powder particles, and porcelain is used for pulverizing soft aggregates or crystals.

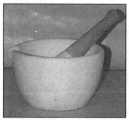 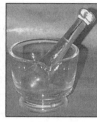

Because these types of mortars are porous, they should not be used with ingredients that stain, are present in small quantities, or are highly potent drugs. Glass mortars and pestles are preferable for mixing liquids and semisolid dosage forms. They are not preferred for making emulsions because it is more difficult to generate adequate shear.

Ointment slabs (sometimes called pill tiles) are made of porcelain or ground glass plates that are square or rectangular in shape. These slabs provide a non-absorbing surface for mixing formulations such as ointments and creams. They also are used to hand punch capsules. Some slabs have an area with a

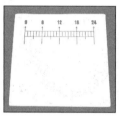 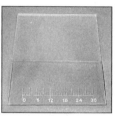

rough surface for reducing powder particle size by comminution. Many slabs have graduated markings on one end for measuring lengths of hand rolled materials used for suppositories or lozenges.

A *stirring hotplate* that uses magnetic stir bars enables the pharmacist to perform other duties while ingredients are dissolving or mixing. If the plate also has a heating element, melting ingredients such as ointments and suppository bases can be blended as they liquefy.

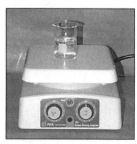

Most solids and semisolids used in compounding formulations will melt by 75°C, so the hotplate has to be a special low temperature (25°C to 120°C) hotplate. Standard laboratory hotplates heat at 125°C to 150°C at their lowest setting. If a low-temperature hotplate is not available, a water bath or a steam bath is a good alternative. Microwave ovens offer a convenient and fast way to heat materials, but these ovens have "hot spots" that produce different temperatures at different places in the oven.

A *vortex mixer* rotates a platform at high speed. When a vessel filled with liquid is placed on the

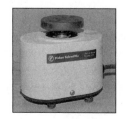

platform, the rotating action produces a mixing vortex in the center of the liquid, resulting in a well-mixed liquid in as little as 15–30 seconds.

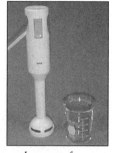

Various *blenders* can be used to mix ingredients. Professional blenders include Braun type blenders and electric homogenizers with interchangeable heads that process different volumes of material. Some blenders are designed to mix and dispense the ingredients in the same container.

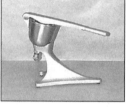

Home type blenders include cabinet top and hand-held mixers. The cabinet type mixer is good for preparing solutions, emulsions, and gels. The hand-held mixer can be used to make lotions, creams, and other semisolid preparations. Kitchen choppers or grinders can be used for reducing particle size and to blend small quantities of powders. Food processors can be used for making ointments and pastes. Laboratory-type blenders can be used in making many formulations. Some are designed to mix the ingredients in a container and then dispense the formulation in the same container.

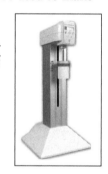

To Mold

Some formulations are fashioned or shaped using a mold. Common molds are those used for suppositories, lozenges, capsules, and tablets.

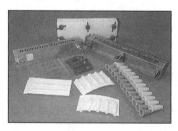

Suppository molds are available to make rectal, vaginal, or urethral suppositories. The molds are metal (aluminum or steel), rubber, or plastic. Metal molds are available in different sizes ranging from 6 to 100 cavities. The mold actually consists of two halves held together with screws when the suppository material is added. After the material has solidified, the screws are removed and the two halves are separated. The suppositories then are removed, wrapped in foil, and placed in a suppository box.

Plastic molds come in long strips and can be torn into any number of shells. Melted suppository formulation is poured into the shells, and when the material has hardened, the open end of the shell is heat sealed. Then the strip is torn into individual shells that are placed in a box. When patients are ready to use the formulation, they peel the shell off the suppository.

Rubber suppository molds come in strips that can be cut if only a few cavities are needed. The suppository material is poured into the mold and allowed to harden. Then the strip is dispensed to the patient, usually in a special box. To administer a suppository, the patient pushes it out of the cavity.

Although capsules can be filled individually by hand, using a capsule filling machine allows the pharmacist to fill up to 300 capsules at one time. The machine comes with a capsule loader that aligns all of the capsules correctly in the machine base. The powder formulation is

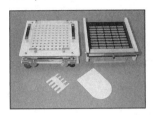

poured onto a base plate, and the pharmacist uses special spreaders and combs to fill the individual capsules. Capsules also can be filled with non-aqueous liquids while they are in the machine. Generally a syringe is used to place the nonaqueous liquid inside the capsule body.

Tablets can be produced by two methods:

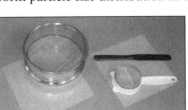

1. A single punch tablet press: A blend of the active drug and excipients are weighed and placed in the die and the handle is lowered, compressing the powder blend into a tablet or pellet.

2. A triturate mold, for making smaller tablets, called tablet triturates: The active drug is incorporated into a blend of sucrose and lactose and wetted with alcohol. The moist powder is pressed into the cavities of the mold, punched out by the posts on the base plate, and allowed to air dry.

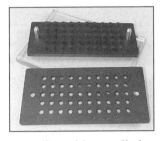

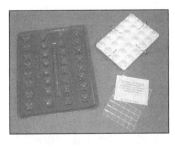

Lozenges and lollipops are made using molds. Both of these dosage forms are intended to dissolve slowly in the mouth. Lollipops are hard candy bases made by heating sugar and other carbohydrates. Lozenges have a softer texture and are made by melting components such as polyethylene glycol (PEG) or gelatin.

Funnels are used when a formulation has to be filtered. They are made of plastic or glass and have either a short stem or a long stem. Funnels come in a variety of sizes from 2 oz. to 32 oz. Some funnels are designed with a

vacuum to aid in filtration. Pre-assembled disposable units contain both the filter and the funnel together. These generally are sterilized and are useful in sterile compounding.

Sieves are used to make a uniform particle size distribution in a

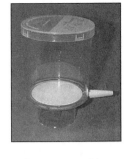

powder or powder mixture by passing the material through a wire mesh screen. Sieves are available in a variety of wire mesh opening sizes from 9.52 mm (size 2) to approximately 0.04 mm (size 400).

To Package

The pharmacist must dispense a compounded formulation in an appropriate package. NABP's Good Compounding Practices Applicable to State Licensed Pharmacies gives the following guidelines for packaging formulations:

> Compounded drug products should be packaged in containers meeting USP standards. The container used depends on the physical and chemical properties of the compounded drug products. Drug product containers and closures shall not be reactive, additive, or absorptive so as to alter the safety, identity, strength, quality, or purity of the compounded drug beyond the desired result for which it purports or is represented to possess.
>
> Components, drug product containers, and closures for use in the compounding of drug products shall be rotated so that the oldest stock is used first. Container closure systems shall provide adequate protection against foreseeable external factors in storage and use that can cause deterioration or contamination of the compounded drug product. Drug product containers and closures shall be clean and, where indicated by the intended use of the drug, sterilized and processed to remove pyrogenic properties to ensure that they are suitable for their intended use.[6]

These guidelines indicate that the container should not react in any manner with the formulation and should protect the formulation against factors that could cause deterioration or destruction of the dosage form. This latter condition suggests that the container must protect the formulation from factors such as humidity (moisture), light, dust and airborne contamination, microorganisms, ingredient loss, and physical damage.

The General Notices of the USP/NF define certain types of containers:[7]

• Light-resistant containers protect the formulation from the effects of light. The light resistant property may be in the container material itself or may be the result of an opaque coating on the container.

Specifications for light-resistant containers are given in the USP/NF chapter <661> Containers.

- Well-closed containers protect the formulation from extraneous solids and from loss of product under normal conditions.

- Tight containers protect the formulation from contamination by extraneous liquids, solids, or vapors, from loss of product, and from efflorescence, deliquescence, or evaporation under normal conditions.

- Hermetic containers are impervious to air or any other gas under normal conditions. Specifications for well-closed, tight, and hermetic containers are in the USP/NF chapter <671> Containers—Permeation.

The materials used for the different types of containers may be paper (plastic or foil coated), metal, glass, or plastic. Different types of glass containers block actinic rays to different extents, as shown in Table 4.2. Amber glass is the preferred glass for compounded formulations.

TABLE 4.2: GLASS TYPES AND ACTINIC RAYS BLOCKED

Glass Type	Actinic Rays Blocked (%)
Amber	98
Blue	41
Green	59
Clear	38

Plastic containers are widely used. The choice of plastic container has to be based on considerations of water and oxygen permeability, potential to leach the active drug out of the formulation, and potential for chemical reactions between the plastic and the formulation. Properties of the various plastics used in containers are summarized in Table 4.3.

After the type of container and/or type of plastic has been selected, the actual package is selected. The package itself may be just a storage container, or it may serve as a device to administer or help administer the formulation. Capsule vials, ointment jars and tubes, and prescription bottles all serve as storage containers. But many other containers are devices for administration. Examples of these devices are:

- atomizers
- dropper bottles
- droptainers
- lip balm tubes
- lozenge molds
- medication sticks
- nebulizers

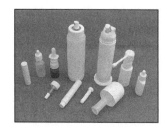

TABLE 4.3: PROPERTIES OF PLASTIC CONTAINERS

Plastic Type	Properties
Polyethylene	Good water barrier
	Poor oxygen barrier
	Not too clear
	Odors, flavors, gases permeate
Polypropylene	Excellent barrier to water, gases
	Not too clear
Polyvinyl Chloride	Clear, rigid
	Good oxygen barrier
	Permeable to water
	Yellows when exposed to heat or UV light
	Used for parenteral solutions
Polystyrene	Rigid
	Crystal clear
	Used for solid dosage forms
Polycarbonate	Clear, transparent
	Rigid
	Possible replacement for glass
	Expensive

- oral syringes
- powder papers
- pressured aerosols
- suppository shells and rubber strip molds.

The storage temperature of the formulation is a part of the packaging process. Storing formulations at increased temperatures generally will increase the rate of chemical reactions or accelerate a decomposition process characteristic of the formulation. Examples are listed in Table 4.4.

TABLE 4.4: EXAMPLES OF ENHANCED REACTIONS WITH INCREASED TEMPERATURES

Formulation	Reaction Properties Enhanced
Solids	Sublimation
Liquids	Solvent loss
Emulsions	Phase separation
Suspensions	Increased sedimentation
Tablets	Increased disintegration times

Storing formulations at decreased temperatures also have adverse effects for formulations, some of which are listed in Table 4.5. Among the adverse effects of freezing formulations are increased risk of container breakage, loss of potency, and alterations in the formulation properties.

The General Notices give several descriptors of storage temperature requirements for pharmacopeial

TABLE 4.5: EXAMPLES OF REACTIONS WITH DECREASED TEMPERATURES

Formulation	Potential Adverse Effects
Solutions	Crystal formation
Emulsions	Phase separation
Suspensions	Increased sedimentation
Tablets	Cracking of sugar coated tablets

articles when stability data have indicated that the storage or distribution at a lower or higher temperature will produce undesirable results (see Table 4.6).

TABLE 4.6: STORAGE TEMPERATURE REQUIREMENTS

Descriptors of Storage Condition	Temperature
Freezer	–25°C to –10°C
Cold	Not exceeding 8°C
Refrigerator	2°C to 8°C
Cool	8°C to 15°C
Room	Prevailing temperature
Controlled room temperature	Thermostatically maintained 20°C to 25°C
Warm	30°C to 40°C
Excessive heat	above 40°C

Equipment Maintenance and Cleaning

Subpart D of the NABP Good Compounding Practices Applicable to State Licensed Pharmacies mentions that equipment used in compounding shall be of "appropriate design, adequate size, and suitably located to facilitate operations for its intended use and for its cleaning and maintenance. The remainder of that section states:

> Equipment and utensils used for compounding shall be cleaned and sanitized immediately prior to use to prevent contamination that would alter the safety, identity, strength, quality, or purity of the drug product beyond that desired. In the case of equipment, utensils, and containers/closures used in the compounding of sterile drug products, cleaning, sterilization, and maintenance procedures as set forth in the NABP Model Rules for Sterile Pharmaceuticals must be followed.
>
> Previously cleaned equipment and utensils used for compounding drugs must be protected from contamination prior to use. Immediately prior to the initiation of compounding operations, they must be inspected by the pharmacist and determined to be suitable for use.
>
> Equipment shall be properly maintained to prevent malfunctions that would alter the drug product's safety, identity, strength, quality, or purity. Equipment shall be subject to maintenance and there shall be cleaning schedules and descriptions of the methods, equipment, and materials used in cleaning and maintenance operations. There shall be methods of reassembling equipment to assure proper cleaning and maintenance.

> Automatic, mechanical, or electronic equipment, or other types of equipment or related systems shall be routinely inspected, calibrated (if necessary), or checked to assure proper performance, as per manufacturer instructions.[8]

Equipment maintenance and cleaning should be a routine part of the compounding operation. Standard operating procedures (SOPs) should be developed for each piece of equipment in the compounding area, with the manufacturer's recommendations as the basis. Keeping a log record that details the history of the equipment's performance is prudent.

Sample SOPs can be found in published references. Examples are:

- glassware washing equipment[9]
- class A prescription balance[10]
- refrigerators[11]
- horizontal laminar air flow[12]
- pH meter.[13]

Sterile Compounding Equipment

Sterile compounding requires that the pharmacist adhere to additional rules and requirements. Those regulations describe additional facilities and specialized equipment needed for this level of compounding.

All sterile compounding areas must have a laminar flow hood capable of providing a "Class 100 environment" (ISO Class 5). A Class 100 environment means an atmospheric environment that contains fewer than 100 particles 0.5 microns in diameter per cubic foot of air. The hoods are to be located in a controlled area that meets "Class 100,000" conditions (ISO Class 8). This means that no more than 100,000 particles 0.5 microns and larger may exist per cubic foot of air.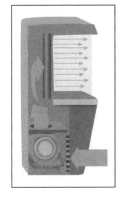

In addition to laminar flow hoods and other specialized equipment, special clothing is required. This garb can consist of aprons, sleeves, gloves, hoods, shoe covers, coveralls, head coverings, lab coats, smocks, shirts/pants, hats/caps, facemasks, and beard covers.

A discussion of all of the aspects involved in sterile compounding is covered in other chapters.

The Bottom Line

As stated at the beginning of this chapter, "pharmacists who decide to make compounding a significant part of their practice will make financial commitments for facilities, equipment, and supplies." This chapter has detailed some of these physical components. Most pharmacists start with a limited inventory of equipment and expand their facilities as the practice increases. This chapter concludes with a partial list of additional equipment and supplies that can be used in a more advanced compounding practice. The list may discourage some pharmacists, but others may see in it almost endless possibilities.

NOTES

1. Good Compounding Practices Applicable to State Licensed Pharmacies. National Association of Boards of Pharmacy. Model State Pharmacy Act and Model Rules of the National Association of Boards of Pharmacy. 2007:24–35.

2. American Society of Hospital Pharmacists. ASHP Technical Assistance Bulletin on Compounding Nonsterile Products in Pharmacies. *American Journal of Hospital Pharmacy* 51:1441–1448, 1994.

3. <795> Pharmaceutical Compounding—Nonsterile Preparations: The United States Pharmacopeia 29/National Formulary 24, The United States Pharmacopeial Convention, Inc., Rockville, MD, 2005, pp. 2731–2735.

4. Allen, L.V., Jr. General Guidelines for the Use of Chemicals for Prescription Compounding. *International Journal of Pharmaceutical Compounding* 1:45, 1997.

5. General Notices and Requirements (Preservation, Packaging, Storage, and Labeling). The United States Pharmacopeia 29/National Formulary 24, The United States Pharmacopeial Convention, Inc., Rockville, MD, 2005, pp. 9–11.

6. Allen, L. V., Jr. Standard Operating Procedure: Washing Glassware and Equipment Used in Compounding Nonsterile Preparations. *International Journal of Pharmaceutical Compounding* 9:470, 2005.

7. Allen, L. V., Jr. Standard Operating Procedure for Performing Class A Prescription Torsion Balance Performance Tests. *International Journal of Pharmaceutical Compounding* 2:166–167, 1998.

8. Allen, L. V., Jr. Standard Operating Procedure: Refrigerator—Installation, Maintenance, Cleaning, and Power Interruptions. *International Journal of Pharmaceutical Compounding* 11:66–67, 2007.

9. Allen, L. V., Jr. Standard Operating Procedure: Labconco Basic 47 Laboratory Hood. *International Journal of Pharmaceutical Compounding* 10:135, 2006.

10. Allen, L. V., Jr. Standard Operating Procedure for the Use, Standardization and Care of a pH Meter. *International Journal of Pharmaceutical Compounding* 1:116–117, 1997.

ADDITIONAL READING

Braverman, B., and Northcon, K. Technology Spotlight: Liquid-Filling Machines. *International Journal of Pharmaceutical Compounding* 6:439–440, 2002.

Kastango, E. S. Using ACDs in the Practice of Pharmacy. *International Journal of Pharmaceutical Compounding* 9:15–21, 2005.

McElhiney, L. F. Equipment, Supplies, and Facilities Required for Hospital Compounding. *International Journal of Pharmaceutical Compounding* 10:436–441, 2006.

SOME ADDITIONAL COMPOUNDING EQUIPMENT AND SUPPLIES

Nonsterile Compounding

Basic

Glass thermometers—not mercury-filled
Hand-held graters (fine, medium, course)
Homogenizer (hand operated)
Low temperature hotplate with magnetic stirrer
pH meters
Refrigerator with freezer
Sieves (assorted sizes)

Advanced

Background light boxes
Capsule filling machine (plates for different capsule sizes)
Carts (plastic or metal)
Digital thermometers with alarms
Dispensing pumps (variable speed and volume)
Drying ovens
Electric mortar and pestle
Enteric coating machine
Hand-held micropipets (small and large volume)
Heat gun, variable heat outputs
Homogenizers (hand-held or electric)
Microwave ovens
Ointment mill
Pipets
Single punch tablet press
Ultrasonic cleaner (sonicator)
Vacuum sealer for bags or suppositories shells
Vial crimper
Water system (high quality)

Sterile Product Compounding

Basic

Apparel
Disposable vacuum filter units
Impulse sealer for plastic overwraps or bags
Laminar flow hood, horizontal or vertical
Pump, pressure and vacuum
Repeating hand-held syringe dispenser with three-way connector and check valve
Sharps disposal containers
Stainless steel pressure filter holders (various capacities)
Sterilizing filters (numerous types/shapes/applications)
Vial crimper
Vial decappers

Advanced

Ampule sealer
Autoclave and supplies
Biohazard disposal equipment and supplies
Particulate testing equipment
Pyrogen test materials
Repeating pump dispenser
Sample transporter coolant (maintains sample at about 5°C–10°C for 30 minutes)
Sterile spatulas and spoons (plastic for weighing and obtaining drugs)
Sterility test equipment
Vial filling machine

CHAPTER FIVE

Quality Assurance

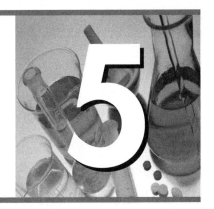

A MAJOR COMPONENT IN OPERATING A COMPOUNDING pharmacy is to establish and maintain a good quality assurance program. Quality assurance (QA) is a series of activities that will ensure that the preparation of a compounded formulation will be a product that meets certain specifications and standards. The specifications and standards most often are defined as an accurately compounded formulation that is safe, stable, and of the proper identity, strength, purity, and quality. Another goal for the pharmacy is to have product uniformity when the formulation is compounded by different pharmacists.[1]

Policies and procedures are developed (and required) to document the operation of the QA program in a compounding pharmacy. This framework gives structure and detail to every important operation in the pharmacy. Each pharmacy or institution develops policies and procedures to meet its specific needs. Several areas, however, are common in any pharmacy:

- pharmacy facilities
- training, monitoring, and evaluating pharmacy personnel performance
- testing, maintaining, and monitoring equipment used in compounding
- acquisition, storage, and handling of supplies
- prescription processing
- compounding nonsterile formulations
- compounding or processing sterile formulations
- monitoring and testing compounded formulations (i.e., quality control)
- prescription labeling
- monitoring and evaluating patient outcomes to ensure efficacy of the compounded formulations
- plan for corrective action if problems are identified by the QA activities
- periodic review of the QA activities for effectiveness.

Documentation in a QA program can be both "active" and "passive." Passive documentation is official information or needed assurances so a judgment can be made about the strength, purity, and quality of a formulation component, that a correct storage container

has been selected, that equipment has been maintained, that the pharmacy personnel have the proper training to complete the compound, etc. Active documentation is completed during the compounding process. It may be a checklist of steps to follow during the compounding process, a record to complete consisting of specific information collected at the time of the compounding (e.g., lot numbers, description of components, beyond use date assigned), equipment calibration results, etc. Both types of documentation have to be assembled and completed for each compounding.

The five types of documentation central to a good QA program are:

1. standard operating procedures (SOPs)
2. formulation records
3. compounding records
4. ingredient records
5. equipment maintenance records.

In addition to these five types of documentation are numerous forms, checklists, analysis results, etc., that each individual pharmacy will include. Thus, each QA program is individualized for each pharmacy and should reflect the overall compounding capability of the pharmacy while giving individual guidance for each compounding.

Standard Operating Procedures (SOPs)

Standard Operating Procedures (SOPs) are step-by-step written instructions about how to conduct specific activities.[2] SOPs cover all important tasks performed in a compounding pharmacy. They also should include log sheets or checklists documenting that the SOPs have been followed.

General examples of SOPs include:

- facility maintenance
- equipment calibration and maintenance
- personnel training and validation
- preparation of compounded formulations
- packaging, labeling, and storage of compounded formulations

• receiving, inventorying, storing, and disposal of supplies.

Figures 5.1 represents the basic information on a SOP record. Commercial vendors have created SOP templates that can be purchased and modified to fit a pharmacy's individual operation. Figure 5.2 shows a SOP that might be supplied by a vendor.

STANDARD OPERATING PROCEDURE

SOP #_____

	Policies and Procedures		
Subject:	Effective Date:	Revision Date:	Revision No.:
	Approved by:	Reviewed by:	
[What the SOP is concerning]			
	[Additional Items]	[Additional Items]	[Additional Items]

Purpose of Procedure:

[The purpose of the procedure should be described.]

Procedure:

[The procedure should be detailed in a step-by-step fashion so it can be easily followed. It should contain sufficient detail and descriptive information to minimize misinterpretation. It also may contain graphs, charts, figures.]

1.

2.

3.

4.

5.

Documentation Forms:

[The results of the SOP may need to be documented on a form or checklist. These should be maintained in a notebook with space available to describe the procedure, and give the date it was done, accountable individual or signature, and the results.]

FIGURE 5.1: SAMPLE STANDARD OPERATING PROCEDURE

STANDARD OPERATING PROCEDURE

SOP #____16____

	Policies and Procedures		
Subject: Prescription Labeling	Effective Date: 12/05/07	Revision Date:	Revision No.:
	Approved by: JT	Reviewed by:	

Purpose of Procedure:

To ensure that all pharmaceutical formulations meet Federal, State, and local pharmacy labeling requirements and provide necessary information for the safe administration, storage, and disposal of the formulations at home.

Procedure:

1.0 Prescription Labeling. A pharmacist shall dispense all prescriptions in a container bearing a label with the following information:

    1.1 Pharmacy Identification.

    1.2 Prescription number.

    1.3 The name of the patient (last and first name).

    1.4 The name of the prescriber.

    1.5 The date of issue.

    1.6 Either the manufacturer's trade name of the drug or the generic name and the name of the manufacturer.

    1.7 The directions for use of the drug.

    1.8 Additives should be recorded as total per bag. The most common metric designation should be used for additives, e.g., "mEq" for electrolyte concentrations, "mMol" for phosphate and "units" for heparin and insulin. Trace elements of combination additives, such as multiple vitamins, may be expressed in volume measurement terms (e.g., "ml"). Concentrations should only be given in total/liter upon MD request.

    1.9 Dextrose, Lipids and Amino Acids: Label should read as the final concentration in percentage or as absolute amounts added.

    1.10 Volume: The prescribed volume per container must be indicated on the label.

    1.11 Prepared by: The initials of the individual compounding the admixture must be placed on the label. If the individual compounding the admixture is not a registered pharmacist, a supervising pharmacist must also initial the label.

    1.12 Beyond use date should follow recommendations for the formulation as set forth in policies and procedures. In those cases where the formulation is not listed, the manufacturer's package insert or other reference may be used to determine the beyond use date.

    1.13 Storage requirements must be specified on the label, e.g., whether the drug should be kept in the refrigerator, freezer, or at room temperature. Any light sensitivity or other unusual storage requirements must also be noted on the label.

    1.14 Disposal Requirements: Any drugs requiring special handling during disposal should be labeled accordingly, e.g., chemotherapeutic agents.

    1.15 Federally controlled substances shall bear the appropriate "transfer" auxiliary label.

2.0 Ancillary Warning Labels shall be attached to the formulation warning the patient of possible harmful effects of taking prescribed drugs in combination with alcohol, or of impairment the drug may cause to a person's ability to drive a motor vehicle or other machinery.

3.0 All legend items must be labeled in accordance with state laws.

4.0 A copy of the prescription label(s) shall be placed in the Patient's chart by affixing it to the Compounding Record.

FIGURE 5.2: A DETAILED SOP

COMMON SOPS

Evaluation of Compounding Personnel for Proper Compounding Process	Job Description—Compounding Pharmacy Technician
Batch Compounding	Determining the Volume of Syringe
Hand Washing and Garb Procedures	Determination of an Emulsion Type
Assigning Beyond Use Dates	Dropper Calibration
Labeling a Compounded Formulation	Geometric Dilution
Final Check of a Compounded Formulation	Filling an Ointment Tube
Quality Assessment of Compounded Formulation	Packing an Ointment Jar
Patient Medication Records System	Sealing a Metal Ointment Tube
Patient Counseling for Compounded Formulations	Wrapping Suppositories
Patient Grievance	Calibration of a Suppository Mold
Incident Report	Calibration of a Lollipop Mold
Reference Library for Compounding	Packing Capsules
Delivery of Compounded Products	Pulverization by Intervention
Ingredient Inventory	Unit Dosing Oral Syringes
Sharps Containers	Preparing an Emulsion
Compounding Area Space	Preparing an Oral Solution
Compounding Area Sanitation	Preparing a Syrup
Compounding Area Temperature and Humidity	Incorporation of Liquids in Ointments
Compounding Area Lighting, Heating, and Ventilation	Preparing Methylcellulose Gel
Compounding Storage Area Monitoring	Preparing Lip Balms
Drug Formulation Refrigerator	Preparing Oil-filled Capsules
Monitoring Drug Formulation Freezer	Preparing Polyethylene Glycol Based Troches
Calibration of a Torsion Balance	Operating a Torsion Balance
Calibration of an Analytical Balance	Operating an Analytical Balance
Calibration of a pH Meter	Operating an Electric Blender
Calibration of a Hot Plate	Using Graduated Cylinders
Handling of Hazardous Drug Materials	Using a pH Meter
Disposing of Hazardous Drug Waste	Using a Capsule Machine
Hazardous Drug Spills	Using a Sieve
Delivery and Storage of Hazardous Drug Materials	Using an Electronic Mortar and Pestle
Hazardous Drug Training for Personnel	Using an Ointment Mill
Personnel Training Verification	Meeting HIPPA Requirements in a Compounding Pharmacy
Medication Records System	OSHA Regulations Pertinent to a Compounding Pharmacy
Job Description—Compounding Pharmacist	State Board Rules and Regulations

Formulation Records

Formulation Records are specific step-by-step instructions on how to prepare a compound.[3] The formulation record ensures that pharmacy personnel will prepare the compound in a consistent manner. It should include the following information:

- *Name, strength, and dosage form of the preparation.* The name, strength, and dosage form actually serve as the title of the product or recipe. The title should express the essence of the product as clearly and succinctly as possible, avoiding common or local institution names.

- *All ingredients and their quantities.* Individual ingredients and their quantities should be listed. Presenting this data in tabular form is helpful.

- *Equipment required to compound the preparation.* Using different equipment yields different results. Therefore, it is necessary to list the exact equipment to be used so that the compounded formulation will be uniform in appearance and activity.

- *Pertinent calculations.* Sample calculations required in the compounding procedure can be included for illustration purposes.

- *Step-by-step mixing instructions.* Precise mixing instructions are required to produce acceptable and uniform formulations. Mixing instructions include the order of mixing and any environmental or other conditions that should be monitored, such as the temperature, duration of mixing, and so forth. If the mixing order is important, this order should be listed and explained in detail. Any pharmaceutical necessities (e.g., levigating agents, solubilizing agents) also should be cited and described.

- *Quality control procedures.* Quality control procedures should be described, and a data sheet provided to document results obtained when performing the quality control procedures.

- *Reference citation or source of the recipe.* The source of the recipe should be included. If the recipe or formula came from the literature, a copy of the article should be appended to the formulation record.

- *Beyond use date.* The beyond use date is assigned based upon the best available knowledge. If a literature citation is the source of information, a copy of the citation should be appended to the formulation record.

- *Container or device used to dispense the formulation.* The container to be used should be listed on the formulation record to ensure uniformity of packaging and stability. Because much of the stability information is predicated upon a certain type or composition of container, any change in the storage container may change the beyond use date.

- *Storage requirements.* Storage requirements for the finished product should also be listed.

Figure 5.3 gives a sample Formulation Record.

Compounding Records

The Compounding Record contains the information about what actually happened when the formulation was made.[4] It should contain a list of the ingredients actually used, their lot numbers, and the quantity that was measured or weighed. It also includes the signature of the person who made the formulation, the date of preparation, the assigned beyond use date, and the results of any quality control procedures that were carried out.

In some pharmacies the Formulation Record is modified to become the Compounding Record worksheet. The Formulation Record is prepared so it can be photocopied, and space is left on it for the information required for the Compounding Record. This practice speeds up the record keeping process.

FORMULATION RECORD

Name of Formulation: _____

Strength: _____

Dosage Form: _____

Route of Administration: _____

Date of Last Review or Revision: _____

Person Completing Last Review or Revision: _____

Formula:

Ingredient	Quantity	Physical Description	Solubility	Therapeutic Activity

[The formula and all of the information about the individual ingredients are described.]

Example Calculations:

[Examples of calculations that must be made each time the formula is compounded are shown.]

Equipment Required:

Method of Preparation:

1. [The method is a step-by-step sequence in the correct order of mixing.]

2. [The description should be clear and detailed so all personnel can complete the steps in exactly the same manner.]

3. [The description also can consist of graphs, tables, charts, etc.]

Description of Finished Product:

Quality Control Procedures:

[Details of all quality control tests to be performed on final formulation.]

Packaging Container:

Storage Requirements:

Beyond Use Date Assignment:

[The criteria that is used to assign a beyond use date, and the date assigned.]

Label Information:

[To include auxiliary labels]

Source of Recipe:

Literature Information:

[Copies of relevant references or primary literature.]

FIGURE 5.3: SAMPLE FORMULATION RECORD

COMPOUNDING RECORD

Name of Formulation: _____

Strength: _____

Dosage Form: _____

Route of Administration: _____

Quantity Prepared: _____

Date of Preparation: _____

Person Preparing Formulation: _____

Person Checking Formulation: _____

Formula:

Ingredient	Manufacturer and Lot Number	Purity Grade	Description	Quantity Required	Actual Quantity Used

[This information is completed at the time of compounding.]

Calculations:

[Calculations performed at the time of compounding.]

Equipment Operation:

[Equipment performance notes or alternate equipment used.]

Method of Preparation:

[Description of any deviation from the Formulation Record method of preparation.]

Description of Finished Product:

Quality Control Procedures:

[Details of quality assurance test results and data.]

Beyond Use Date Assignment:

[The beyond use date assigned, and reasons for difference from Formulation Record, if applicable.]

FIGURE 5.4: SAMPLE COMPOUNDING RECORD

Compounding Records should contain the following information:

- Name, strength, and dosage form of the formulation
- Quantity of formulation prepared (i.e., weight, volume, or number of units prepared)
- Signature of pharmacist or support person preparing the product
- Signature or initials of the pharmacist responsible for supervising the preparation and conducting in-process and final checks of the compounded formulation

- Date of preparation
- Individual ingredients, the manufacturer's name, lot number, and expiration date, and the actual quantity measured or weighed
- Assigned internal identification number, if applicable
- Assigned beyond use date
- Results of the quality control procedures.

Figure 5.4 is an example of a Compounding Record.

Ingredient Records

The pharmacy should maintain records of ingredients purchased, certificates of analysis for purity of chemicals, and Material Safety Data Sheets (MSDSs). MSDSs also should be maintained for any drug substance or bulk chemical used in the pharmacy. The information in MSDSs consists mainly of physicochemical properties, toxicity, and handling requirements. Precautions, information about other potential hazards, and shipping instructions are included. This information should be reviewed for the protection of the pharmacist and pharmacy personnel, as well as the patient.

MSDSs can be obtained without charge from suppliers and can be easily filed in three-ring binders. They are commonly shipped with chemicals, often packed in the same carton. They also can be obtained from the Internet or through fax from the suppliers.

Certificates of Analysis are supplied when raw ingredients are shipped from manufacturers. These documents indicate the results of the assay or analytical information about the ingredient. A complete Certificate of Analysis gives the contact information of the laboratory performing the assay and the complete contact information of the client or the person who submitted the sample to be tested, including their address, fax, or any appropriate contact information. This record also should include the type of test performed—sterility, endotoxin, HPLC assay, etc. Sample information included on the Certificate of Analysis includes product name, labeled amount, assayed amount, and percent difference.

NOTES

1. Kupiec, T. C. Ensuring Compounding Excellence: Quality Control or Quality Assurance? *International Journal of Pharmaceutical Compounding* 6:160, 2002.

2. Ashworth, L. D. Quality-Control: Standard Operating Procedures—An Essential Tool for Developing Quality Preparations. *International Journal of Pharmaceutical Compounding* 11:226–229, 2007.

3. Allen, L. V., Jr. Standard Operating Procedure: Basic Compounding Documentation—The Master Formula Form. *International Journal of Pharmaceutical Compounding* 11:240–241, 2007.

4. McElhiney, L. F. Records and Record-Keeping for the Hospital Compounding Pharmacist. *International Journal of Pharmaceutical Compounding* 11:136–141, 2007.

ADDITIONAL READING

Kupiec, T. C., Okeke, C., Allen, L.V., Jr., and Denison, C. Quality Control Analytical Methods: Glossary of Quality Control/Quality Assurance Terms in Pharmaceutical Compounding. *International Journal of Pharmaceutical Compounding* 9:300–302, 2005.

CHAPTER SIX

Drug Product Stability

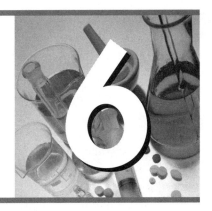

THE TERM *DRUG PRODUCT STABILITY* HAS MANY CON-notations. One connotation is that the active drug must remain stable, i.e., be present in the intended form and concentration as indicated on the product labeling. This implies that the active drug has not decreased in quantity, has not undergone any chemical change or formed any toxic products, and will have the same bioavailability as when it was originally manufactured. Stated another way, a stable drug product will have the same identity, strength, quality, and purity at the time of use.

Another connotation is that the entire drug product remains stable. In this case, the expectation is that the product will retain all of the properties of the original product. For example, if the original product was a clear solution, the solution remains clear, i.e., does not develop a color or turn cloudy. If the original product was a suspension, the suspension retains its suspending properties. If the product was originally sterile, sterility is maintained.

A third connotation is that the drug product remains stable when used. For example, if the product is mixed with another product and some instability occurs, the original drug product might be referred to as, "unstable in the other product." This last connotation often is referred to as an "incompatibility" rather than "instability." The overall effect of an incompatibility, however, can be the same as product instability.

Stability is defined as "the extent to which a dosage form retains, within specified limits, and throughout its period of storage and use (i.e., its shelf life), the same properties and characteristics that it possessed at the time of its manufacture."[1]

Types of Stability

The instability of each formulation can have many sources.

> Each ingredient, whether therapeutically active or pharmaceutically necessary, can affect the stability of drug substances and dosage forms. The primary environmental factors that can reduce stability include exposure to adverse temperatures, light, humidity, oxygen, and carbon dioxide. The major dosage form factors that influence drug stability include particle size (especially in emulsions

and suspensions), pH, solvent system composition (i.e., percentage of "free" water and overall polarity), compatibility of anions and cations, solution ionic strength, primary container, specific chemical additives, and molecular binding and diffusion of drugs and excipients.[2]

The lack of product stability can result in a wide range of changes from *visible* signs such as precipitation, cloudiness or haziness, color change, viscosity change, effervescence (evolution of a gas), or formation of immiscible layers, to *invisible* changes such as drug degradation, microbial growth, or formation of toxic substances that generally are detected only through analytical techniques. The rate of these changes can vary widely for different products that undergo the same type of instability. It is important to recognize that many degradation mechanisms also are occurring at room temperature or below, so degradation pathways may take weeks or months to become significant. The USP/NF chapter <1191> section for Criteria for Acceptable Levels of Stability gives the five causes of instability as

1. physical (i.e., retains its original physical properties)
2. chemical (i.e., retains its chemical integrity and labeled potency)
3. microbiological (i.e., retains its sterility or resistance to microbial growth)
4. therapeutic (i.e., retains the therapeutic effect)
5. toxicological (i.e., has no significant increase in toxicity).

The most common causes of instability are the failure to maintain physical, chemical, and microbiological stability. If these three stabilities are maintained, therapeutic and toxicological stabilities almost always will be ensured.

Physical Instabilities

Examples of physical instabilities are

- a drug precipitating out of solution
- a drug adsorbing to a container wall
- two solid drugs forming a eutectic mixture when triturated together
- drugs that absorb or release waters of hydration (efflorescent, hygroscopic, or deliquescent drugs)

- a drug or adjuvant that vaporizes from a solution by volatilizing through the container
- a complexation reaction between an ion and the drug in solution.

Chemical Instabilities

Chemical instabilities include hydrolysis, oxidation, and photolysis. The USP/NF Chapter <1191> adds epimerization, decarboxylation, and dehydration to the list of chemical instability mechanisms and comments on the influence of pH, inter-ionic compatibility, and temperature on product stability.

Hydrolysis, Oxidation, Photolysis

Hydrolysis is a process in which chemicals interact with water molecules and yield reaction products. Hydrolysis is a subset of solvolysis because solvents other than water (e.g., ethanol, polyethylene glycol) can react with chemicals. The most common hydrolysis reactions involve chemicals with labile carbonyl groups such as esters, lactones, lactams, and substituted amides.[3] For example, aspirin combines with water molecules and hydrolyzes to one molecule of salicylic acid and one molecule of acetic acid.

Hydrolysis can be prevented by several methods. An obvious way is to reduce or eliminate water from the formulation. In liquid preparations, water frequently is reduced or replaced by using glycerin, propylene glycol, or ethanol. In injectables, anhydrous vegetable oils may be substituted for water.

Other methods to prevent hydrolysis are to suspend the drug in a non-aqueous vehicle or supply the drug in a dry powder form to be reconstituted before administration. If powders in solid dosage forms have to be protected from humidity, a waterproof coating can be applied. Storing formulations under refrigeration will slow the rate of hydrolysis.

Controlling the pH through the use of buffers can prolong the stability of a formulation. Most hydrolytic reactions have a pH where the rate is slowest. If the formulation is created at that pH, the product stability can be increased. For many drugs, this pH is between pH 5 and 6.

The *oxidative process* affects many different chemical classes of drugs including aldehydes, alcohols, phenols, sugars, alkaloids, and unsaturated fats and oils. Oxidation involves the loss of electrons from one chemical atom or molecule and the receipt of electrons by another chemical atom or molecule. With inorganic chemicals, oxidation increases the positive valence of an element; for example, ferrous ($+2$) oxidizes to ferric ($+3$). With organic chemicals, oxidation generally results in the loss of a hydrogen atom from the molecule.

Further, the oxidative process frequently involves free radicals, molecules or atoms containing one or more unpaired electrons as molecular oxygen ($\cdot$O-O$\cdot$) or free hydroxyl ($\cdot$OH). These free radicals take electrons from the formulation components, thereby oxidizing them. Oxidation is more likely to occur when molecules are not in a dry state and when they are exposed to oxygen or light. Many oxidation reactions are characterized by a change in color, precipitation, or odor.

Many pharmaceutical products undergo *auto-oxidation*. These spontaneous reactions can be initiated by the presence of molecular oxygen or trace amounts of metal ion impurities introduced into the formulation by the drug, solvent, or container. The reaction proceeds slowly at first, but as the chemical and the initiating substance combine, additional free radicals are created, propagating the reaction, which proceeds more rapidly as the process continues.

Oxidation is prevented by adding antioxidants to the formulation. These chemicals have electrons or available hydrogen atoms that are preferentially oxidized by the free radicals, so the chain reaction is diverted from the other formulation components. The antioxidants used most frequently in aqueous formulations are sodium sulfite, sodium bisulfite, hypophosphorous acid, and ascorbic acid. Alpha-tocopherol, butylhydroxyanisole, and ascorbyl palmitate are used in non-aqueous formulations.

If the oxidation reaction results from the presence of trace metal ions, chelating agents such as calcium disodium edetate or ethylenediamine tetraacetic acid (EDTA) can be added to the formulation to complex the metal and remove it as a potential initiator. If molecular oxygen is the initiator, the product might be packaged in a sealed container where the oxygen has been replaced by an inert gas such as nitrogen.

Photolytic reactions (catalyzed by normal sunlight or room light) often cause oxidation-type reactions but are not limited to that type of decomposition. The energy from light radiation can be absorbed by a number of chemical classes such as aromatic hydrocarbons and their heterocyclic analogues, aldehydes, and ketones. Chemicals that absorb light at wavelengths below 280 nm generally undergo decomposition in sunlight, and those absorbing light above 400 nm can be degraded by either sunlight or room light.

The manufacturer usually packages light-sensitive drugs in appropriate light-resistant or opaque containers. The instability is seen most often when the drug is removed from the packaging and placed in a new environment that does not have appropriate light protection.

Polymerization, Racemization, Decarboxylation, Deamination, and Dehydration

Chemical instabilities and incompatibilities can be caused by other processes, such as polymerization, racemization, decarboxylation, deamination, dehydration, and pH changes. These processes occur less frequently than hydrolysis, oxidation, and photolysis and generally are limited to a small group of chemical substances.

Drug *polymerization* is a reaction between two or more identical molecules that results in a new, and generally larger, molecule. Formaldehyde is capable of polymerization in solution and forms paraformaldehyde $(CH_2O)_n$, which is a white crystalline substance that causes the solution to become cloudy.

Many drugs are present in a pharmaceutical product as a *racemic mixture*, in which one racemate has significantly different absorption, distribution, metabolism, excretion, and therapeutic characteristics than the other. Re-proportioning of the racemate mixture can adversely affect the product's therapeutic efficacy. Examples of drugs that have the potential of such a racemization reaction include epinephrine, pilocarpine, ergotamine, and tetracycline.

Polymorphic compounds can be viewed as having the same type of interaction potential as racemic compounds. Polymorphs are different crystalline structures of the same molecule; each form exhibits differences in solubility, dissolution rate, etc. A conversion of the metastable form to the stable form in the product formulation could cause a significant change in the physical characteristics and therapeutic efficacy of the product.

Decarboxylation and *deamination* are examples of degradation reactions that remove a functional group from a molecule. Decarboxylation removes a carbonyl group from an organic acid, and carbon dioxide gas is formed as a byproduct of this reaction. Deamination reactions remove nitrogen-containing groups from an organic amine.

Dehydration reactions occur when drug molecules eliminate waters of hydration from their chemical structure. In many of these dehydration processes, the anhydrous molecule has different properties than the hydrated form.

pH Changes

Another source of instability is a change in the *acid-base environment* in solution. The acid–base environment can be changed when diluting a solution, adding another chemical (e.g., an antioxidant), or changing the type of packaging container. Temperature also has an effect on pH. The pH of a solvent (or solution) is an important determinant in a chemical's solubility in that solvent. Therefore, changes in the pH can cause a chemical to precipitate from the solvent, or it might cause a chemical to dissolve into the solvent, which could be undesirable if the chemical was to remain as a solid particle in the solution.

Changes in solubility brought about by alterations in solvent pH can be predicted by the pHp equation. The pHp is the pH below which an acid or above which a base will begin to precipitate.

$$pHp = pKa + \log \frac{S - S_o}{S_o} \qquad \text{(for a weak acid)}$$

$$pHp = pKw - pKb + \log \frac{S_o}{S - S_o} \qquad \text{(for a weak base)}$$

where

S_o = the molar solubility of the undissociated acid or base

S = the molar concentration of the salt form of the drug initially added

pKa = dissociation constant of the acid

pKw = dissociation constant of water

pKb = dissociation constant of the base ($pKa + pKb = pKw$)

In addition to changing the solubility, pH has a significant influence on the rate of chemical degradation. In a specific acid-catalyzed reaction or specific base-catalyzed reaction, the presence of hydrogen ions or hydroxyl ions accelerates the decomposition of a chemical. There is a specific pH at which the rate of degradation is minimized. Therefore, creating a formulation that establishes and maintains that pH is important in formulation development.

To investigate a specific acid-catalyzed reaction, the degradation rate of a chemical is studied at several different pHs in the acidic pH range. The pHs are established by using buffer systems. The observed degradation rate of the chemical (k_{obs}) will be proportional to the hydrogen ion concentration at the different pHs:

$$k_{obs} = k_{acid}[H^+]$$

Taking the logarithm of the equation gives

$$\log k_{obs} = \log k_{acid} + \log [H^+]$$

Recognizing that pH is defined as $-\log [H^+]$

$$\log k_{obs} = \log k_{acid} - pH$$

This equation suggests that a plot of $\log k_{obs}$ versus pH will be linear with a slope of -1 and a y-intercept of $\log k_{acid}$.

Using the same derivation for a specific base-catalyzed reaction,

$$\log k_{obs} = \log k_{base} + \log [OH^-]$$

Relating the hydroxyl ion concentration to the hydrogen ion concentration with the ionization constant of water (Kw):

$$\log k_{obs} = \log k_{base} + \log Kw + pH$$

Therefore, a plot of log k_{obs} versus pH in the alkaline region would yield a straight line with a slope of $+1$ and a y-intercept of log $k_{obs} + $ log Kw.

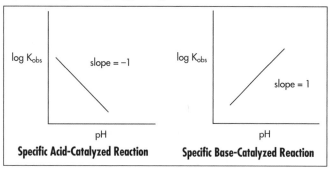

Specific Acid-Catalyzed Reaction   **Specific Base-Catalyzed Reaction**

A complete log k_{obs} versus pH profile for a drug should appear similar to the illustration below. At relatively low pH values, the acid-catalyzed reaction predominates, and at relatively high pHs, the base-catalyzed hydrolysis predominates. The pH at which the minimum rate of degradation occurs is a function of the relative magnitudes of the specific rate constants k_{acid} and k_{base}. If $k_{base} > k_{acid}$, the minimum pH will be in the acidic region. If $k_{base} = k_{acid}$, the expected minimum rate would be expected to occur at pH 7.

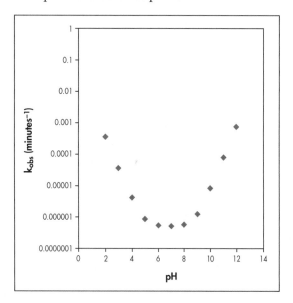

Variations in this basic pH-rate profile will occur if additional catalytic components are in the system. One component might be the solvent itself (e.g., water). Components of buffer systems also can serve as catalysts, and these decompositions are termed *general acid-catalysis* or *general base-catalysis* depending on whether the components are acidic or basic. Metal ions, undissociated acids and bases, and some anions also catalyze chemical decompositions. When these additional catalytic components operate in a pharmaceutical system, the profile of k_{obs} versus pH generally deviates from the profiles seen when specific acid- or specific base-catalysis is the only responsible mechanism.[4]

Microbiological Instabilities

An example of a microbiological instability is the presence of microorganisms in a sterile product. In nonsterile products, microbial growth is to be expected and typically is controlled by the addition of a preservative. Instability in such a nonsterile product would be uncontrolled growth or growth outside of acceptable limits.

Determination of a Manufactured Product Expiration Date

As mentioned above, drug products are subjected to numerous stability tests during their development and manufacturing processes. One of the most important outcomes of these tests is assigning an *expiration date*—the date when the amount or concentration of the active drug no longer equals the labeled value. Sometimes the expiration date is referred to as the "shelf life" of the product. Expiration dates are written as the month and year the product will "expire" or cease to equal the labeled value and typically are written on the immediate container of the product and the outer retail package.

One method of estimating the expiration date of a product is to take repeated samples over the normal time the product is expected to remain in stock and in use. This could be several years, so this method clearly is both time-consuming and uneconomical.

Another method is to accelerate the instability of the product to shorten the testing period and then use those study results to predict the normal time that would be required to produce the same instability. These "accelerated" studies commonly are done by subjecting the product to elevated temperatures, humidity, and/or light. For example, an initial stress study might be conducted for 6 months at 40°C and 75% relative humidity. If significant decomposition is seen under these conditions, a second study might be done using milder conditions (e.g., 30°C and 60% relative humidity).

Temperature is a variable in these accelerated studies, not because the products are expected to be maintained at temperatures greater than room temperature (though this might happen) but because the rate of many chemical reactions increases when temperature is elevated. A generally held rule is that the rate will increase two to three times with each 10°C rise in temperature. In 1889, Arrhenius derived a largely empirical relationship called the *Arrhenius equation*, that summarizes the influence of temperature on chemical reactions as:

$$k = Ae^{\frac{-E_a}{RT}}$$

where

    k   =   the specific reaction rate

    A   =   a constant (Arrhenius factor or frequency factor)

E_a = the Arrhenius activation energy
R = the gas constant (1.987 calories/deg mole)
T = the absolute temperature (°K)

According to collision theory, E_a is the difference between the average energy of reactive molecules and the minimum energy required for reactants to form products. When molecules collide and form reactants, there must be enough energy (i.e., the activation energy) to overcome the repulsion between the molecules and allow the molecules to get close enough to allow bonds to rupture and new bonds for the products to form. As the activation energy increases, the reaction rate will decrease because there is a smaller fraction of collisions that will attain the required activation energy. $e^{\frac{-E_a}{RT}}$ is the probability that a collision will have energy equal to or greater than E_a to result in the formation of products.

The Arrhenius equation, in its logarithmic form, suggests how accelerated studies can be conducted at elevated temperatures:

$$\ln k = \ln A - \frac{E_a}{R}\frac{1}{T}$$

Obtain the Reaction Rate Constant

In several studies the product is subjected to different temperatures and the reaction rate (k) is determined for each temperature. Generally, the study is conducted at four different temperatures that show significant differences in the product reaction profiles. But the range of temperatures allowed is restricted by limitations of the Arrhenius equation. One restriction is that the reaction mechanism cannot change over the range of temperatures. Another assumption is that the reaction is a thermally activated mechanism with activation energies of about 10 – 30 kcal/mole. If the reaction mechanism is based on diffusion, photochemical, freezing, microbial contamination, or excessive agitation, etc., the Arrhenius equation has no predictive power. In general, elevated temperature studies also cannot be used with products containing suspending agents that coagulate on heating, proteins that may denature, and ointments and suppositories that may melt.

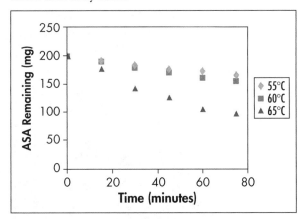

These reaction rates (k's) are plotted against the reciprocal of the absolute temperature ($\frac{1}{T}$) in the Arrhenius plot.

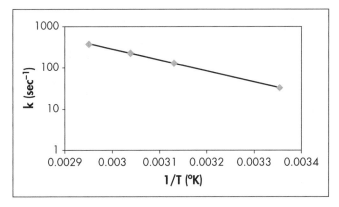

The slope of the curve equals ($-\frac{E_a}{R}$) and is used to determine E_a. The intercept on the vertical axis equals ln A and is used to determine A. Once E_a and A are known, the reaction rate at room temperature can be calculated by substituting these parameters back into the Arrhenius equation and using the absolute temperature that corresponds to room temperature.

A derivation of the Arrhenius equation allows E_a to be calculated for the situation when the reaction rate constants at two different temperatures is known:[5]

$$\ln \frac{k_2}{k_1} = \frac{E_a}{R}\frac{T_2 - T_1}{T_2 T_1}$$

where

k_1 and k_2 = the observed rate constants at T_1 and T_2, respectively

T_1 and T_2 = the absolute temperatures at which the reaction studies were conducted

This rearrangement provides another method of determining the reaction rate constant at room temperature. Two stability studies are conducted at elevated temperatures (T_1 and T_2) and the reaction rate constants are determined (k_1 and k_2). The activation energy (E_a) then is calculated using the given equation. That calculated E_a then is used in a back calculation where one of the temperatures and its corresponding reaction rate constant are taken to be at room temperature. The other temperature and its reaction-rate constant will be data from one of the initial stability studies.

Calculate the Expiration Date

Products are required to be stable—they must maintain the active drug above or at the labeled value for a length of time. Products generally are regarded as stable when the active drug is greater than 90% of the labeled value (but there are exceptions). Expiration dating then is defined as the time period the product will remain stable when stored under recommended conditions. Most manufactured products require an expiration date of at least 2 years to ensure adequate stability at the time of consumption by the patient.

Using the reaction rate constant predicted for room temperature determined from the Arrhenius plot, the *expiration date* can be determined. If the loss of drug is independent of the concentration of the reactants and constant with respect to time, the reaction rate is called "zero order" and usually is expressed as:

$$k_o = \frac{-dC}{dt}$$

where

k_o = the zero order reaction rate constant

$\frac{dC}{dt}$ = the rate of change in the concentration as a function of time

The integrated form of the expression is more useful:

$$C = -k_o t + C_o$$

where

C_o = the initial concentration at time = 0

The k_o is taken from the Arrhenius plot (i.e., the reaction rate at room temperature), and the equation is rearranged to:

$$t = \frac{C - C_o}{-k_o}$$

The C_o in the product is known because it is the labeled concentration on the product. The concentration C is taken as $0.9C_o$ because that will be the concentration when the product has reached 90% of its labeled value. The calculated t value will be the time for C_o to fall to 90% of that value—the expiration date.

EXAMPLE: A drug product is subjected to an accelerated stability study. Using the Arrhenius plot, the reaction rate constant (k_o) at room temperature is determined to be 0.02 mg/ml/day for the zero-order reaction. Determine the expiration date if the initial concentration is 500 mg/ml in a 20 ml package.

$$t_{90} = \frac{0.9C_o - C_o}{-k_o} = \frac{-0.1C_o}{-k_o} = \frac{-0.1(500 \text{ mg/ml})}{-0.02 \text{ mg/ml/day}}$$

$$= 2{,}500 \text{ days}$$

In this example, the product would be stable (i.e., within 90% of the labeled value) for a period of about 7 years. Clearly, this formulation shows a good stability profile.

A similar derivation can be developed for reaction rates that are other than zero order. The equivalent expression to calculate the t value when the reaction rate is first order can be shown to be:

$$t = \frac{\ln C - \ln C_o}{k}$$

where

k = the first order reaction rate constant

When the Reaction Rate is Not Known

There is a method to determine the expiration date that does not require a knowledge of the reaction rate order. The Q_{10} *method* estimates the shelf life at a new temperature when the shelf life at an original temperature is known.[6] The estimation assumes an E_a at room temperature. The general expression is:

$$Q_{10} = e^{\left[\frac{E_a}{R}\left(\left(\frac{1}{T}+10\right)-\frac{1}{T}\right)\right]}$$

Q_{10} values of 2, 3, and 4 are commonly used and are related to different E_a's that occur at room temperature. For example, a Q_{10} of 2 corresponds to an E_a of 12.2 (kcal/mol), 3 corresponds to an E_a of 19.4 (kcal/mol), and a Q_{10} value of 4 corresponds to an E_a of 24.5 (kcal/mol).

The shelf life estimate at a new temperature is calculated as:

$$t_{90}(T_2) = \frac{t_{90}(T_1)}{Q_{10}^{\left(\frac{\Delta T}{10}\right)}}$$

where

$t_{90}(T_1)$ = the shelf life at the original temperature

$t_{90}(T_2)$ = the estimated shelf life at the new temperature

ΔT = $T_2 - T_1$

T_1 = the original temperature

T_2 = the new temperature

EXAMPLE: A solution has a shelf life of 6 hours at room temperature (25°C). Calculate the estimated shelf life if the solution is stored in a refrigerator (5°C). Use 3 as the estimate of Q_{10}.

$$t_{90}(T_2) = \frac{t_{90}(T_1)}{Q_{10}^{\left(\frac{\Delta T}{10}\right)}} = \frac{6 \text{ hours}}{3^{\left(\frac{5-25}{10}\right)}} = \frac{6 \text{ hours}}{3^{(-2)}} = 54 \text{ hours}$$

Therefore, it is estimated that this solution would have a shelf life of 54 hours if refrigerated.

In addition to the accelerated stability studies, drug products are subjected to *long term-stability studies* under the usual conditions of transport and storage expected during product distribution. In conducting these studies, the different climatic zones and expected variances in temperature and humidity are included in the study design. Geographic regions of the world are defined by climatic zones:

zone III = "temperate"
zone III = "subtropical"
zone III = "hot and dry"
zone IV = "hot and humid"

A drug product may encounter more than one climatic zone during its production and shelf life.

Further, the drug product may be warehoused, transported, placed on retail shelves, and subsequently in the patient's residences for varying time periods and over a wide range of temperature and humidity conditions. These long-term (12 months minimum) studies, however, generally are conducted at 25°C ± 2°C and at a relative humidity of 60% ± 5%. Products may be kept under these conditions for periods of 5 years or longer. These studies, in concert with the accelerated stability studies, provide a more precise determination of drug products' stability and actual shelf life.

Stability of Compounded Formulations

With manufactured products, stability studies initially are conducted in the preformulation phase and are continued throughout the manufacturing process. As might be expected, different studies are conducted at different phases during the development process. The sum total of these studies, however, identifies the various types of instabilities, helps develop the manufacturing process, assists in establishing proper packaging and storage conditions, serves as the basis for the expiration date assigned to the product, and helps to develop administration recommendations.

These studies are conducted with the entire pharmaceutical product—i.e., the active drug in its complete formulation, in its specific container or closure system, and under the environmental conditions expected in shipment, storage, and handling. Expiration dates are required on commercially manufactured products and are determined by extensive study of the product's stability. Most expiration dates are in the order of years.

The stability of an extemporaneously prepared formulation should be determined in the same manner as the stability of commercially manufactured products. But the truth is that this is not done on any routine basis. Therefore, stability dating must be assigned by some other method. Stability of compounded preparations is assigned as a *beyond use date*.[7] A beyond use date is the date after which a compounded preparation should not be used. The beyond use date is different from an expiration date. beyond use dates generally are in the order of days or months.

Assigning a Beyond Use Date

The major problem for the pharmacist is that the stability of a compounded preparation is generally not known. Many instabilities can occur in a preparation and cannot be detected without the use of analytical equipment. Most pharmacies do not have the equipment or the knowledge or resources to conduct stability studies on their compounded preparations. A manufacturer's expiration date cannot be used to extrapolate or estimate a beyond use date for a compounded preparation. The compounded preparation probably will not be identical to the manufactured product; it may have a different drug concentration, use different diluents, be a different fill volume, and be packaged in a different type of container.

- When possible, beyond use dates should be in accordance with the manufacturer's approved labeling. This means that the preparation was formulated according to the manufacturer's directions, or that the formulation contains the same concentration of drug, in the same diluent, in the same packaging, for the same intended period of use, and so on. If the formulation is an official USP/NF compounded preparation, the beyond use date and packaging requirements are given in the monograph.

- When the above is not possible, use drug-specific and general stability documentation and literature from reference books or the primary literature. When assigning a beyond use date, consider the nature of the drug and its degradation mechanism, the container in which it is packaged, the expected storage conditions, and the intended duration of therapy. A growing number of references sources contain stability information, and the pharmacist should have ready access to this material. Some of the more common resources are:
  - Trissel's Stability of Compounded Formulations
  - Trissel's Handbook of Injectable Drugs
  - AHFS Drug Information
  - United States Pharmacopeia
  - Remington: The Science and Practice of Pharmacy
  - USP Dispensing Information
  - Journal of Pharmaceutical Sciences
  - American Journal of Health-System Pharmacy
  - International Journal of Pharmaceutical Compounding
  - Chemical Companies
  - Monographs of AHFS Drug Information
  - Lippincott's Hospital Pharmacy

- Many times the published references do not evaluate exactly the same formulation, or the study did not examine the stability for a long enough period of time. In this case, the USP/NF Chapter <795> gives the following maximum recommended beyond use dates for nonsterile compounded drug preparations packaged in tight, light-resistant containers when stored at controlled room temperature, unless otherwise noted:

Non-aqueous liquids and solid formulations:

- If the source of the ingredient(s) is a manufactured drug product, the beyond use date is not later than 25% of the time remaining until the original product's expiration date, or 6 months, whichever is earlier.

- If the source of the ingredient(s) is a USP or NF substance, the beyond use date is not later than 6 months.

Water containing formulations:

- When prepared from ingredients in solid form, the beyond use date should be not later than 14 days when stored at cold temperature.

For all other formulations:

- The beyond use date is not later than the intended duration of therapy or 30 days, whichever is earlier.

Observable Signs of Instability

The USP/NF chapter <1191> Stability Considerations in Dispensing Practice details visual signs of instability that can be monitored by a pharmacist. The premise is that a pharmacist ordinarily cannot detect chemical degradation because it requires analytical equipment, but that excessive chemical degradation sometimes is accompanied by observable physical changes. Some of these changes might be changes in color and odor, formation of a precipitate, or clouding of a solution. Excessive microbial growth and/or contamination also may appear as a physical change.

As an example of physical changes that might be observed in "Hard and Soft Gelatin Capsules":

> Since the capsule formulation is encased in a gelatin shell, a change in gross physical appearance or consistency, including hardening or softening of the shell, is the primary evidence of instability. Evidence of release of gas, such as a distended paper seal, is another sign of instability.

An example for physical changes in "Emulsions":

> The breaking of an emulsion (i.e., separation of an oil phase that is not easily dispersed) is a characteristic sign of instability; this is not to be confused with creaming, an easily redispersible separation of the oil phase that is a common occurrence with stable emulsions.

For creams (semisolids), the following information is given:

> Unlike ointments, creams usually are emulsions containing water and oil. Indications of instability in creams are

emulsion breakage, crystal growth, shrinking due to evaporation of water, and gross microbial contamination.

Some of the signs of instability that might be observed for several types of dosage forms are summarized in Table 6.1.

The USP/NF chapter <795> recommends that written policies and procedures be established for determining and documenting the beyond use dates assigned to its compounded products. As part of these policies and procedures, the following additional information should be included:

- Copies of product-specific stability studies based on a stability indicating analytical procedure

- Copies of letters from manufacturers certifying the beyond use dating

- Predictive materials such as publications, charts, and tables

- In-house quality control data collected for compounded formulations.

Incompatibilities

Incompatibility refers to physicochemical phenomena such as concentration-dependent precipitation and acid-base reactions that result in a visually evident change in the product. These changes might include precipitation, cloudiness or haziness, color change, viscosity change,

TABLE 6.1: SIGNS OF INSTABILITY IN COMPOUNDED FORMULATIONS

Dosage Form	Signs of Instability
Solutions	Precipitation, discoloration, haziness, gas formation resulting from microbial growth
Suspensions	Caking, difficulty in resuspending; crystal growth
Gels	Shrinkage, separation of liquid from the gel, discoloration, microbial contamination
Emulsions	Breaking, creaming
Creams	Emulsion breakage, crystal growth, shrinkage caused by evaporation of water; gross microbial contamination
Ointments	Change in consistency and separation of liquid, if contained, and formation of granules or grittiness; drying
Capsules	A change in the physical appearance or consistency of the capsule or its contents, including hardening or softening of the shell; also, any discoloration, expansion, or distortion of the gelatin capsule
Powders	Caking or discoloration instead of free flowing; release of pressure upon opening, indicative of bacterial or other degradation
Suppositories	Excessive softening, drying, hardening, shriveling; evidence of oil stains on packaging
Troches	Softening or hardening, crystallization, microbial contamination, discoloration
Sterile Products	Discoloration, haziness, precipitation

Adapted from "Stability of Compounded Products," by L. V. Allen, Jr., (chapter 4) in The Art, Science, and Technology of Pharmaceutical Compounding, 2nd edition (Washington, DC: American Pharmaceutical Association, 2002), pp. 43–52.

BEYOND USE DATE FLOW CHART

Title of Formulation _____   Assigned Beyond Use Date _____
(Name, Strength, Dosage Form)

TYPE OF DOSAGE FORM   **BEYOND USE DATE**

Solid ▬▬▬ Yes ▬▬▬ Active ingredient ▬▬▬ Yes ▬▬▶ 25% of time remaining
                  from a manufactured product   until product's expiration date
                                                     or 6 months, whichever is earlier

No   No

                    6 months (if from a *USP/NF* substance)

Liquid ▬ Yes ▬ Nonaqueous ▬ Yes ▬ Active ingredient ▬▬ Yes ▬▶ 25% of time remaining until
                                  from a manufactured product   product's expiration date
                                                                   or 6 months, whichever is earlier

No   No

                                  6 months (if from a *USP/NF* substance)

              No ▬▬▬▬▬ Prepared from ingredients ▬▬ Yes ▬▶ 14 days at 5°C
                        in solid form

                                       No

                              30 days or intended duration of therapy, whichever is less*

All other dosage forms ▬▬▬▬▬▬▬▬▶ 30 days or intended duration of therapy, whichever is less

*Note: These beyond use date limits may be exceeded when there is supporting valid scientific stability information that is directly applicable to the specific preparation (i.e., same drug concentration range, pH, excipients, vehicle, water content, etc.). This includes preparations that have been commercially available.

Documentation/References

1. _____

2. _____

3. _____

4. _____

From "Assessment of a Beyond Use Date for Compounded Preparations," by L. V. Allen, Jr., International Journal of Pharmaceutical Compounding 4:474–475, 2000.

effervescence (evolution of a gas), or the formation of immiscible layers.[8]

The factors that cause incompatibilities are pH, solubility, concentration, complexation, and light.[9] Most often the incompatibility occurs when a drug has been dissolved or dispersed in an aqueous solution. The factor most responsible for incompatibilities is a change in the acid–base environment of the drug. The pH factor is a critical parameter in a drug's solubility and its stability.

The pH solubility profiles and pH degradation rate profiles are determined early in a drug's development. Although this information is crucial for the preclinical and clinical studies that will be conducted with the drug, they are not necessarily related directly. For example, increasing the pH might increase the solubility of a drug but also cause it to degrade faster. Of course, the three other possible variables also could be true, depending on the drug. The acid–base environment of a drug can be altered when diluting, admixing, adding another drug, or adding ingredients such as antioxidants. Temperature also has an effect on pH.

The incompatibilities expected when a drug is put into an aqueous solution can be different than if the drug is dissolved in a non-aqueous solvent. Non-aqueous solvents may have very different viscosities compared to water. Some drugs must be formulated in co-solvent mixtures for dissolution, and the effect of the environment and other drugs or ingredients may be difficult to predict. Some of these non-aqueous solvents include alcohol, propylene glycol, glycerin, polyethylene glycols, and oils such as corn, cottonseed, and peanut.

Some drug products are compatible at selected concentrations but not at other concentrations. Generally, the more concentrated a drug solution, the greater is the likelihood that an incompatibility will occur. But this rule has the following exceptions:

- The complexation of tetracycline in the presence of calcium ions is a classic example of a complexation incompatibility.
- Light-sensitive drugs generally are packaged by the manufacturer in appropriate light-resistant containers. The incompatibility comes when the drug is removed from that container and placed in a new environment that does not afford the necessary light protection.

NOTES

1. <795> Pharmaceutical Compounding—Nonsterile Preparations: The United States Pharmacopeia 29/National Formulary 24, The United States Pharmacopeial Convention, Inc., Rockville, MD, 2005, pp. 2731–2735.

2. <1191> Stability Considerations in Dispensing Practice: The United States Pharmacopeia 29/National Formulary 24, The United States Pharmacopeial Convention, Inc., Rockville, MD, 2005, pp. 3029–3031.

3. Guillory, J. K., and Poust, R. I. Chemical Kinetics and Drug Stability (chapter 6) in G. S. Banker and C. T. Rhodes, editors, *Modern Pharmaceutics*, 4th edition. Marcel Dekker, New York, NY, 2002, pp. 139–166.

4. Martin, A. Kinetics (chapter 12) in *Physical Pharmacy*, 4th edition. Lea & Febiger, Philadelphia, PA, 1993, pp. 284–323.

5. Allen, L. V., Jr., Popovich, N. G., and Ansel, H. C. Dosage Form Design: Pharmaceutical and Formulation Considerations (chapter 4) in *Ansel's Pharmaceutical Dosage Forms and Drug Delivery Systems*, 8th edition. Lippincott Williams & Wilkins, Baltimore, MD, 2005, pp. 92–141.

6. Allen et al., Note 5.

7. Lima, H. A. Drug Stability and Compatibility: Special Considerations for Home Health Care. *International Journal of Pharmaceutical Compounding* 1:301–305, 1997.

8. Allen, L. V., Jr. Parenteral Admixture Incompatibilities: An Introduction. *International Journal of Pharmaceutical Compounding* 1:165–167 (1997).

9. Thompson, J. E. Compatibility and Stability of Drug Products and Preparations Dispensed by the Pharmacist (chapter 34) in *A Practical Guide to Contemporary Pharmacy Practice*, 2nd edition. Lippincott Williams & Wilkins, Baltimore, MD, 2004, pp. 34.3–34.31.

ADDITIONAL READING

Chan, D. S. Stability Issues for Compounding Extemporaneously Prepared Oral Formulations for Pediatric Patients. *International Journal of Pharmaceutical Compounding* 5:9–12, 2001.

Newton, D. W. Three Drug Stability Lives. *International Journal of Pharmaceutical Compounding* 4:190–193, 2000.

Thompson, J. E. Expiration and Beyond Use Dating (chapter 4) in *A Practical Guide to Contemporary Pharmacy Practice*, 2nd edition. Lippincott Williams & Wilkins, Baltimore, MD, 2004, pp. 4.1–4.8.

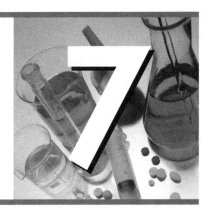

CHAPTER SEVEN

Weighing and Measuring

Introduction to Measurement Systems

THE ACCURATE MEASUREMENT OF INGREDIENTS IN A formulation is a critical part of compounding. Formulation ingredients mostly are solids or liquids, but their amounts or volumes can be expressed in more than one system of measurement. The three most common systems used in compounding are the metric system, the apothecary system, and the avoirdupois system.

The Metric System

The metric system is the preferred system of measurement in all of the health care sciences. This system is based on multiples or fractions of 10. The three basic units of measure are the gram (weight), liter (volume), and meter (length). The nomenclature to indicate multiples of 10 is deca-, hecto-, and kilo-, and fractions of 10 are expressed as deci-, centi-, milli-, and micro-. Table 7.1 shows these relationships.

The Apothecary System

In the past, pharmacists and physicians commonly used the apothecary system for prescribing and dispensing medications. Although it has been largely replaced by the metric system, pharmacists still encounter these symbols in practice. The apothecary system of fluid measure is still commonly used in commercial products as fluid ounce, pint, quart, and gallon.

Quantities of ingredients in the apothecary system are commonly written in Roman rather than in Arabic numerals:

ss or s̄s̄	= 1/2
i	= 1
V or v	= 5
X or x	= 10
L or l	= 50
C or c	= 100

D or d	= 500
M or m	= 1000

Table 7.2 shows the units of measure and conversion relationships.

TABLE 7.1: METRIC UNITS OF MEASURE AND ABBREVIATIONS

Unit	Commonly Used Abbreviation	Equivalent to Basic Unit
Microgram	μg (mcg)	1/1,000,000 gram
Milligram	mg	1/1,000 gram
Centigram		1/100 gram
Decigram		1/10 gram
Gram	g	1 gram
Dekagram		10 grams
Hectogram		100 grams
Kilogram	kg	1,000 grams
Liquid		
Microliter	μl	1/1,000,000 liter
Milliliter	ml	1/1,000 liter
Centiliter		1/100 liter
Deciliter	dl	1/10 liter
Liter	l	1 liter
Dekaliter		10 liters
Hectoliter		100 liters
Kiloliter		1,000 liters
Length		
Micrometer	μm (micron)	1/1,000,000 meter
Millimeter	mm	1/1,000 meter
Centimeter	cm	1/100 meter
Decimeter		1/10 meter
Meter	m	1 meter
Dekameter		10 meters
Hectometer		100 meters
Kilometer	km	1,000 meters

TABLE 7.2: UNITS OF MEASURE IN THE APOTHECARY SYSTEM

Unit	Symbol	Conversions
Gallon	gal	1 gal = 4 qt
Quart	qt	1 qt = 2 pt
Pint	pt	1 pt = 16 fl oz
Ounce	fl oz	1 fl oz = 8 fl dr
Fluid dram	fl dr	1 fl dr = 60 min
Minim	min or M_x	

The Avoirdupois System

The avoirdupois system is a system of weight measurement only. Its basic unit of measure, the *grain*, is the same as in the apothecary system. The avoirdupois ounce and pound differ in weight and symbols from those in the apothecary system. The avoirdupois pound is the pound to which we are accustomed in our daily lives. It also is the weight measure in which bulk chemicals and over-the-counter pharmaceuticals are bought and sold. Table 7.3 shows the units of measure in the avoirdupois system.

TABLE 7.3: UNITS OF MEASURE IN THE AVOIRDUPOIS SYSTEM

Unit	Symbol	Conversions
Pound	lb	1 lb = 16 oz
Ounce	oz	1 oz = 437.5 gr
Grain	gr	1 gr = 64.8 mg

THE GRAIN

The grain is the same weight in several different measurement systems: Apothecary, Avoirdupois, and Troy. It is said to have been established as a unit of weight in 1266 by King Henry III of England when he required the English penny to weigh the equivalent of 32 dried grains of wheat. On the metric scale, one grain equals 64.8 milligrams. However, this is often rounded to 65 milligrams.

Table 7.4 shows several of the important conversions between the three systems of measurement. These conversions are used daily in compounding practice and should be committed to memory.

TABLE 7.4: COMMON CONVERSIONS BETWEEN SYSTEMS OF MEASUREMENT

Common Conversions					
1 L	=	33.8 fl oz	1 lb	=	453.59 g
1 pt	=	473.17 ml	1 oz	=	28.35 g
1 fl oz	=	29.57 ml	1 g	=	15.43 gr
1 kg	=	2.2 lb	1 gr	=	64.8 mg

Introduction to Weighing

To determine the accurate weight of an ingredient, a balance will be required. Various balances are available. Each type has a procedure for the proper operation, testing, and/or calibration of the equipment.

Accuracy in Weighing

Many pharmacies use a Class A prescription balance for their compounding work. The USP/NF chapter <1176> states:

> In order to avoid errors of 5% or more that might be due to the limit of sensitivity of the Class A prescription balance, do not weigh less than 120 mg of any material.[1]

This *least weighable quantity (L.W.Q.)* can be determined for a Class A (or any other) balance from the following equation:

$$L.W.Q. = \frac{\text{sensitivity requirement}}{\% \text{ error tolerated}} \times 100\%$$

EXAMPLE: What is the least weighable quantity that will result in an error of 5% or less on a Class A prescription balance?

The sensitivity requirement of a Class A balance is 6 mg.

$$L.W.Q. = \frac{6 \text{ mg}}{5\%} \times 100\% = 120 \text{ mg}$$

If the sensitivity requirement of a balance is known, the percentage of possible error can be calculated when any amount of the substance is weighed by rearranging the equation to:

$$\% \text{ error} = \frac{\text{sensitivity requirement}}{\text{quantity weighted}} \times 100\%$$

EXAMPLE: The Class A prescription balance has a sensitivity requirement of 6 mg. What % error would result in weighing 50 mg of a drug on the balance?

$$\% \text{ error} = \frac{6 \text{ mg}}{50 \text{ mg}} \times 100\% = 12\%$$

So if a Class A balance is used to weigh 50 mg of material, the possible error would be 12%, which is greater than the required 5%. Therefore, a Class A balance should not be used to weigh that small a quantity of material.

Balances

Two types of balances commonly used are the Class A prescription balance and the electronic balance.

Class A Balances

A *Class A prescription balance* is a two-pan torsion type balance that must have the following:

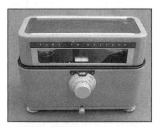

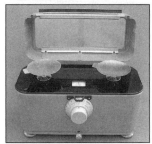

- A metal identification plate indicating the serial number, model number, sensitivity requirement, and maximum capacity of the balance

- Removable weighing pans of equal weight and free of dirt and corrosion

- A device, usually leveling screws, that may be used for leveling the balance

- A lid to protect the balance from dust and permit draft-free weighing

- A mechanical beam (oscillation) arrest to allow the operator to add or remove weight without damaging the balance

- A graduated beam, equipped with a rider, or calibrated dial capable of measuring 1 g in 0.01 g increments. The beam or dial must have a "Stop" at the zero point

- An appropriate index and pointer to determine rest points.

The Class A balance has a *sensitivity requirement* of 6 mg, meaning that as much as 6 mg can be added to or removed from the pan before the pointer on the balance marker plate will move 1 division. The smallest readable amount on the balance's calibrated dial or rider beam— referred to as *readability*—is 0.01 g, or 10 mg. The calibrated dial or rider will give up to 1 g of weight to the right pan. The maximum capacity of the balance— referred to as *capacity range*—may be 60 g or 120 g. That information is supplied with the individual balance. When no information is given, the capacity is assumed to be at least 15 g. Weighing more than 15 g–30 g on a torsion balance is not practical because the volume of that much ingredient is difficult to contain on glassine papers or weighing boats.

To obtain an accurate weight of components on the prescription balance, appropriate techniques must be used. The following procedure details how to level the balance and correctly weigh materials on the prescription balance.

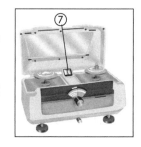

1. Set the internal weights to zero by turning the calibrated dial to zero.

2. Lock the balance by turning the arrest knob. Level the balance front to back by turning the leveling screw feet all the way into the balance and then moving them the same direction until the four sides of the base of the balance are equidistant from the bench top. For balances with leveling bubbles, move the leveling screw feet until the bubble is in the middle of the tube.

3. Unlock the balance and level it left to right by adjusting the leveling screw feet. To shift the pointer left, grasp both the screw feet between the thumbs and

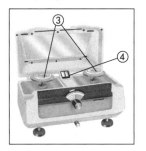

forefingers and rotate so the thumbs move inward. To shift the pointer to the right, rotate both screw feet so the forefingers move toward the back of the balance. Continue adjusting the screw feet slowly until the pointer rests at the center of the marker plate.

4. Lock the balance. Fold glassine weighing papers diagonally, then gently flatten and place one on each weighing pan. Or use weighing boats instead.

5. Unlock the balance by releasing the arrest knob. If the pointer does not rest at the center of the marker plate, the balance will have to be leveled from left to

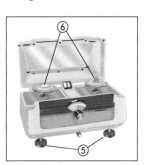

right again to correct for any difference in the weighing papers or boats.

6. Lock the balance and place the required weights on the weighing paper on the right pan, or use the calibrated dial, which also adds the weight to the right pan. Place the material to be weighed on the weighing paper on the left pan.

7. Unlock the balance and note the shift of the pointer on the marker plate. If the pointer shifts left, too much of the drug is on the pan and a portion should be removed. If it shifts right, too little drug is on the pan and more should be added. Each time you add or remove drug from the pan, lock the balance to protect the mechanism inside the balance.

8. Once you are satisfied that you have made an accurate measurement, double-check to be sure you have weighed the correct substance (check the label) and that you have used the correct weights (both in the pan and on the calibrated dial).

Testing the Prescription Balance

Prescription balances must be tested to ensure that they are operating properly. They should be tested in the location where they are used. Testing should be conducted monthly, or more often if the balance is used extensively. Chapter <1176> specifies four tests to be performed on Class A balances. A balance is acceptable if it passes all four tests. If the balance fails any test, it is not to be used until it has been repaired and meets the test conditions. The four tests are:

1. sensitivity requirement
2. arm ratio test
3. shift test
4. rider and graduated beam tests

Sensitivity Requirement The sensitivity requirement is to determine the minimum amount of weight required to move the pointer on the marker plate one division. The balance should have a maximum sensitivity of 6 mg with no load and with a load of 10 g on each pan. Many weight sets do not have a 6 mg weight, so the test can be modified and conducted using 10 mg weights.

6 mg procedure:

1. Level the balance.
2. With the pans empty, adjust the balance until the pointer is in the middle of the marker plate.
3. Place a 6 mg weight on one of the empty pans. The pointer should shift no less than one division.
4. Place a 10 g weight in the center of each empty pan. Adjust the balance until the pointer is in the middle of the marker plate.
5. Place a 6 mg weight on one of the pans. The pointer should shift no less than one division.

10 mg procedure:

1. Level the balance.
2. With the pans empty, adjust the balance until the pointer is in the middle of the marker plate.
3. Place a 10 mg weight on one of the empty pans.
4. When the balance comes to rest, record the number of divisions the 10 mg weight shifted the pointer from zero.
5. Place a 20 mg weight on the same empty pans.
6. When the balance comes to rest, record the number of divisions the 20 mg weight shifted the pointer from zero.
7. Place a 30 mg weight on the same empty pans.
8. When the balance comes to rest, record the number of divisions the 30 mg weight shifted the pointer from zero.

9. Make a plot of the "number of divisions" versus "weight" for the three determinations. A sample plot is shown below. By using a linear regression fitting program found on many hand-held calculators or spreadsheets, the best fit line equation can be calculated. The sensitivity requirement can be determined by solving the equation of the line for x by assigning y = 1 (one division). The solution will tell how much weight is needed to move the pointer one division. This sensitivity requirement must be less than 6 mg.

10. Place a 10 g weight in the center of each empty pan. Adjust the balance until the pointer is in the middle of the marker plate.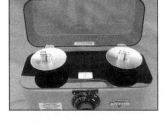

11. Repeat the procedure with the 10 mg, 20 mg, and 30 mg weights.

12. Plot the "number of divisions" versus "weight" for the three determinations and determine the sensitivity requirement from the slope of the line.

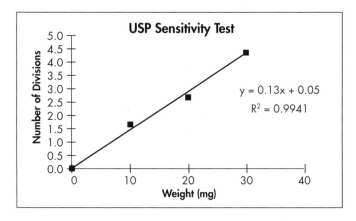

USP Sensitivity Test

$y = 0.13x + 0.05$
$R^2 = 0.9941$

The balance passes the sensitivity requirement if the sensitivity requirement is 6 mg or less with and without the 10 g load.

Arm Ratio Test The arm ratio test will determine if the length of both arms of the balance is equal.

1. Level the balance.
2. With the pans empty, adjust the balance until the pointer is in the middle of the marker plate.
3. Place 30 g of weights in the center of each pan.
4. When the balance comes to rest, record the rest point.

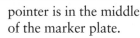

5. If the rest point has changed from the middle of the marker plate, place a 20 mg weight on the lighter side.

6. When the balance comes to rest, this new rest point should either return to or go farther than the middle of the marker plate.

Shift Test The shift test checks the mechanics of the arm and lever components of the balance.

1. Level the balance.

2. With the pans empty, adjust the balance until the pointer is in the middle of the marker plate.

3. Place a 10 g weight in the center of the left pan and place another 10 g weight successively toward the right, left, front, and back side of the right pan, noting the rest point in each case.

4. In any case where the rest point has changed from the center of the marker plate, add a 10 mg weight to the lighter side.

5. When the balance comes to rest, this new rest point either should return to or go farther than the middle of the marker plate.

6. Level the balance and adjust the balance until the pointer is in the middle of the marker plate.

7. Repeat the procedure with the 10 g weight in the center of the right pan, and vary the position of the 10 g weight on the left pan.

8. Level the balance and adjust the balance until the pointer is in the middle of the marker plate. Make several observations in which both 10 g weights are shifted simultaneously to off-center positions on their pans (i.e., both toward the inside, both toward the outside, one front and the other back, etc.). If in any case where the rest point is shifted from the middle of the marker plate, the addition of a 10 mg

weight on the lighter side should equalize or overcome the shift.

Rider and Graduated Beam Test The rider and graduated beam test checks the accuracy of the calibrated dial or rider on the balance.

1. Level the balance.

2. With the pans empty, adjust the balance until the pointer is in the middle of the marker plate.

3. Place a 500 mg weight on the left pan and move the dial or rider to the 500 mg point.

4. When the balance comes to rest, record the rest point.

5. If the rest point has changed from the middle of the marker plate, place a 6 mg weight on the lighter side.

6. When the balance comes to rest, this new rest point should either return to or go farther than the middle of the marker plate.

7. Follow the same procedure using a 1 g weight on the left pan and the dial or rider on the 1 g point. If the new rest point is shifted from the middle of the marker plate, a 6 mg weight to the lighter side should equalize or overcome the shift.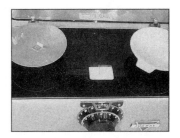

Electronic Balances

Electronic balances have digital displays, and many have internal calibration capabilities. These may be either top-loading or encased in a housing to protect the balance from drafts and dust. Electronic balances generally have a larger capacity range than Class A balances. Most electronic balances have the same readability as the Class A balances, but some increase the readability by a factor of 10 (i.e., to 1 mg). The term *sensitivity requirement* is used with torsion balances. For electronic balances, the analogous term is *precision, absolute error*, or *linear accuracy*. The *absolute error* is the constant weight error inherent in the balance for every weighing. One term unique to electronic balances is *repeatability*. This is the standard deviation of a standard weight or amount of material weighed several times on the balance.[2]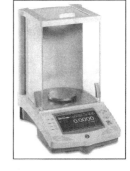

General Guidelines for Using Balances

• Always use the balance on a level surface and in a draft-free area.

• Always cover pans with weighing papers, or use weighing boats. These protect the pans from abrasions,

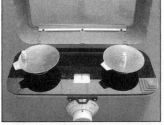 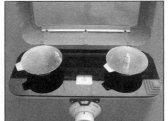
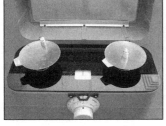 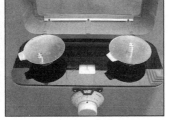

eliminates the need for repeated washing, and reduces loss of drug to porous surfaces. Weighing papers should be folded diagonally to help keep ingredients on them. Weighing papers and boats should be placed on each pan so they do not interfere with free movement of the pans and do not "hit" the balance lid when it is closed.

- Use a clean paper or boat for each new ingredient to prevent contamination of components.

- Always readjust the balance when using new weighing papers or weighing boats. Weighing papers taken from the same box can vary in weight by as much as 65 mg. Large weighing boats can vary as much as 200 mg.

- Always arrest the torsion balance before adding or removing weight or ingredients from either pan to protect the working mechanism of the balance and maintain its accuracy.

- Place external weights on the right-hand pan of torsion balances. The calibrated dial or rider adds weight to this side.

- Use a spatula to add or remove ingredients from the balance. Do not "pour" ingredients out of the bottle.

- Always close the lid or close the sliding glass doors for each weighing. This is absolutely essential to the final weight determination.

- Always clean the balance and close the lid or close the sliding glass doors between uses. Some balances have a plastic protective cover for this purpose.

- Calibrate balances at least monthly, and keep a log.

- Each year, have the balance serviced by a service technician for protective maintenance.

It is always prudent to have SOPs for the use and maintenance of balances. Two sample SOPs have been published and can serve as a starting point to develop individual or institutional SOPs.[3,4]

Weights

Weights come as a set and are stored in a rigid, compartmentalized box. All weights are to have cylindrical construction. Although most weight sets contain only metric weights, some older weight sets also include apothecary weights. All weight sets include a pair of forceps in the box to handle the weights. To prevent soiling and erosion of the weights, the fingers should not be used.

Of the several classes of weights, USP/NF chapter <1176> recommends analytical weights (Class P or better) for prescription compounding. The designation "P" refers to design specifications of weights such as density of materials, surface finish, corrosion resistance, precision, and so on. Class P weights are described as moderate precision weights.[5] Class P weights should be used when weighing quantities of more than 100 mg.

Introduction to Liquid Measurements

The pharmacist is concerned with accurate liquid measurements from two perspectives. The first is to measure liquid components while compounding a formulation, and the second is to have the patient measure liquid dosages after the compound is complete. The techniques used to measure liquids are probably the simplest of the operations related to prescription compounding. At the same time, they are the most susceptible to errant selection and unprofessional execution leading to inaccuracies.

Guidelines for Selecting Liquid Measurement Devices

The first step is to select the appropriate liquid measuring device.

- Always select the smallest device that will accommodate the desired volume of liquid, to minimize the potential for errors of measurement associated with misreading the scale.

- Use a graduated pipet, syringe, or calibrated dropper to measure volumes less than 1 ml.

- Consider using a disposable syringe or measuring by weight rather than volume for oily and viscous liquids, as they are difficult to remove from graduated cylinders and pipets, and at best require a long drainage time.

- Never use prescription bottles, nonvolumetric flasks, beakers, or household teaspoons as measurement devices unless they are calibrated prior to their use.

- When small (less than 5 ml) or very accurate doses are required, provide the patient with a calibrated dropper, oral syringe, or similar device to ensure proper dosing.

- When liquids are poured into containers, they have a *meniscus*—a concave or crescent shaped surface that bulges downward. If the container is very narrow, the meniscus can be quite noticeable. When reading a volume of a liquid against a graduation mark, read the bottom of the meniscus. If the true bottom of the meniscus is difficult to see, hold the container against a broad black band on a white background.

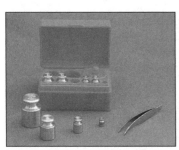 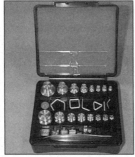

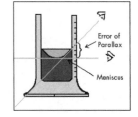

Volumetric Glassware
"To Deliver" or "To Contain"

Volumetric glassware is used to measure and deliver exact volumes of liquids. The capacity of the vessel (1 ml, 50 ml, 1,000 ml, etc.) is etched on the glassware wall, and some glassware has calibration marks for measuring partial or multiple volumes. Some glassware is not volumetric glassware but is simply a container for storing and mixing liquids. Erlenmeyer flasks, beakers, and prescription bottles are not volumetric glassware. The volume inscribed on these types of glassware is an approximation of the vessel capacity.

Volumetric glassware is marked as either "TD" or "TC," indicating "to deliver" or "to contain." "To deliver" glassware means that when the vessel is emptied, it will deliver the total volume measured. Single-volume pipets, burets, syringes, and droppers are TD glassware. Volumetric flasks and cylindrical or conical graduates are TC glassware. "To contain" glassware means that the vessel will hold the total volume measured but it will deliver more than the total volume when emptied. Even though graduated cylinders are TC, they often are used in practice as TD vessels for volumes of 20 ml or more.

The pharmacist must *pay close attention to the glassware itself and not necessarily the inscription.* Some glassware indicates that it is TC when clearly it is TD, and vice versa. TC glassware can be easily recognized, as it has calibration marks on the vessel to account for

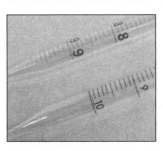

all of the volume of the glassware. For example, a 10 ml calibrated pipet (TC) will have marks for 1 ml, 2ml, and 10 ml inscribed on the glassware. A 10 ml TD calibrated pipet will have marks for 1 ml, 2 ml, …, and 9 ml. There will be no calibration mark for the 10 ml volume; the last 1 ml is contained between the 9 ml mark and the tip of the pipet.

Table 7.5 lists common glassware used in compounding, according to its type.

Volumetric Glassware and Other
Devices Intended "To Deliver"

The devices "to deliver" discussed below are pipets, syringes, and medicine droppers.

TABLE 7.5: TYPES OF GLASSWARE USED IN COMPOUNDING

To Deliver	To Contain	Nonvolumetric
Single volume pipet	Graduated cylinder	Erlenmeyer flask
Syringe	Volumetric flask	Beaker
Calibrated pipet	Calibrated pipet	Prescription bottle

Pipets Pipets are recommended for the delivery of all volumes. Of the several types of pipets, the *single volume* is the most accurate and simplest to use but it obviously is limited to measuring a fixed single volume. They are available in 1, 2, 5, 10, and 25 ml sizes, and deliver their volume when completely emptied.

Single volume pipets have only one graduation mark, and that is the nominal volume of the pipet. The steps in using a single volume pipet are as follows.

1. Draw the liquid into the pipet until it is above the desired graduation mark.

2. Slowly empty the pipet until the liquid attains the desired mark.

3. Be sure to account for any *meniscus* in the pipet lumen.

4. Remove the pipet from the stock solution.

5. Wipe the end of the pipet with a tissue or Kimwipe®.

6. While holding the pipet in a vertical position, release the pressure on the bulb and allow the liquid to flow out of the pipet into the vessel. Remove droplets that remain suspended from the tip by touching the tip of the pipet to the inside of the vessel.

7. Allow the pipet to drain for 30 seconds while touching the tip of the pipet to the inside of the vessel (for viscous liquids, see discussion on page 60).

The *calibrated pipet* has several graduation marks inscribed on the glassware. Thus, it can deliver multiple volumes of liquid with good volumetric precision. For example, if a 10 ml calibrated pipet is filled to the 10 ml graduation, it can be used to deliver ten 1 ml volumes, or two 5 ml volumes.

The calibrated pipet is used in the same manner as the single volume pipet except that fractional volumes may be transferred by noting the meniscus level before and after delivery. For example, 1.50 ml can be delivered if the initial volume is at the 8.50 ml graduation mark and liquid is allowed to flow out of the pipet until the meniscus reaches the 7.00 ml mark. A second delivery could be made by allowing the meniscus to reach 5.50 ml.

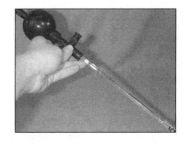

Liquids are drawn up in single volume and calibrated pipets using a respirator (rubber bulb) for suction. There are many types of rubber bulbs. Some are simple bulbs that do not allow any control of suction or emptying beyond the user's hand pressure. Some have sections on the device that are pressed to allow for expelling air from the bulb (A), filling the pipet by suction (S), and emptying the pipet (E).

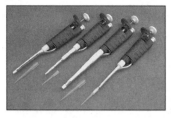

The *micropipet* (hand-held pipet) comes in two parts—a handle (or hand piece) section and a disposable tip attached to the handle section. The handle section usually has a turn-screw that is adjusted to set the volume of liquid that will be drawn into the pipet tip.

Micropipets offer the pharmacist a variety of options, but the devices are much more expensive than single volume and calibrated pipets. Some micropipets are designed to hold 25 ml or 50 ml of liquid and dispense the volume in smaller volumes, such as 1 ml, 5 ml, 10 ml. Some micropipets are intended for delivering volumes that are fractions of a milliliter. Because micropipets can be adjusted to an almost infinite number of volumes, their use in laboratory settings is essential. Pharmacists, too, are finding the utility of these devices in their compounding practice.

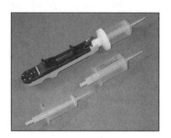

Dispensers have a reservoir and an adjustable hand piece or volume container that can be repeatedly filled with liquid. Like micropipets, dispensers offer a variety of options, but the purchase cost is a consideration. Some are not automated and consist of a glass or plastic container with the dispenser piece attached as a cap. This dispenser piece must be hand actuated each time a volume of liquid is needed. Other dispensers are automated and deliver a preset volume of liquid each time a foot pedal is used or the actuation button is pressed.

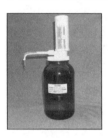

Syringes The pharmacist typically has available a combination of pipeting devices to cover various compounding needs. Many times, however, a syringe is used instead of a pipet for convenience. *Hypodermic syringes* come in a variety of sizes ranging from 0.5 ml (calibrated in 0.01 increments) to 60 ml (calibrated in 2 ml increments) and are made of plastic. Glass syringes are still available but generally are not used in compounding. Syringes may be used to deliver liquid volumes with a high degree of accuracy. Syringes also are useful for measuring and delivering viscous liquids. Table 7.6 indicates that measurements made with syringes are more accurate than those made with cylindrical graduates.

Tips on the syringe provide a point of attachment for a needle. Two common types of tips found on hypodermic syringes are:

1. Slip-Tip® syringe, which has a tip that holds a needle by friction; it is conical shaped with no locking hub.

TABLE 7.6: VOLUME OF WATER DELIVERED BY GRADUATED CYLINDER AND PLASTIC SYRINGE

Nominal Volume	Actual Volume Delivered	
(ml)	10 ml Graduated Cylinder	10 ml Plastic Syringe
1.0	0.94 ± 0.03[a]	1.01 ± 0.02
5.0	4.94 ± 0.04	4.98 ± 0.03
10.0	9.75 ± 0.03	9.95 ± 0.02
10.0		9.98 ± 0.02

[a]Standard deviations were obtained from five trials, except the last entry, for which five different syringes were used with one trial each.

2. Luer-Lok® syringe, which has a conical shaped tip with a locking hub; a needle is rotated as it is placed on the syringe, and the threads of the hub lock the needle securely on the syringe.

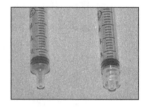

Syringes can be used in compounding, either alone or with a needle (cannula) attached. In most nonsterile compounding, needles are not necessary because most operations involve using the syringe only as the measuring and delivery device. In sterile compounding, needles are necessary to puncture septas on vials, bags, and so forth. Needles come in a variety of sizes, in both length and diameter.

Pulling back on the plunger pulls fluids into the syringe. The tip of the syringe (or needle, if used) must be fully submerged in the fluid to avoid drawing air into the syringe. An excess of solution is drawn into the syringe so any air bubbles may be expelled by holding the syringe tip end up, tapping the air bubbles up into the hub, and depressing the plunger to expel the air. This also ensures that the hub and needle will be completely filled with solution and the volume of delivery will be accurate. Serious errors in dosage can result from failing to consider the volume of solution contained in the hub and needle of the syringe.

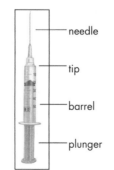

- needle
- tip
- barrel
- plunger

The tip of the plunger inside the syringe barrel usually is covered by black latex. The point at which the latex presses against the wall of the syringe barrel forms a line or guide that is lined up with the graduation marks on the side of the barrel to determine

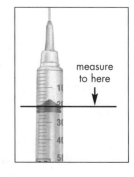

measure to here

the volume that will be delivered when the plunger is depressed.

Oral syringes are available for accurately dispensing a dose of liquid medication to the patient. These are especially useful when administering non-standard doses. Oral syringes have a tip that is larger than Slip-Tip® tips on hypodermic syringes, so needles cannot be placed on these syringes. After the dose is drawn into the syringe,

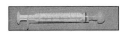

a syringe cap is placed on the tip to prevent leakage and prevent contamination. The patient must be counseled to remove the tip cap before dispensing the contents of the syringe.

Oral syringes also can be used with a device called an "Adapt-a-Cap®." The Adapt-a-Cap device will not work with hypodermic syringe tips. The Adapt-a-Cap screws onto a bottle or reservoir, and the oral syringe is inserted into the cap's opening. When the bottle is inverted, liquid can be withdrawn by pulling back on the plunger of the syringe. When the required volume has been withdrawn, the bottle is

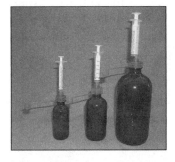

righted, the syringe is removed from the Adapt-a-Cap, and the liquid then can be dispensed. These devices are especially useful when measuring and dispensing viscous liquids.

Medicine Droppers Medicine droppers are described in chapter <1101> of the USP/NF[6]. Droppers are to be constructed so they deliver between 45 mg and 55 mg of water in each drop. Obviously, different volumes would be delivered for liquids other than water. Personal factors can contribute to the inaccuracy of droppers. Two individuals dispensing the same liquid from identical droppers may produce drops of different sizes because of variations in hand pressure, speed of dropping, and angle at which the dropper is held.

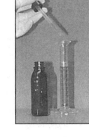

If a medicine dropper is to be used to administer a formulation, it must be calibrated. The calibration should be done with the formulation at the time of delivery to maximize the accuracy of dosing. To calibrate a medicine dropper, slowly drop the formulation into a small graduated cylinder (10 ml) and count the number of drops needed to add several milliliters (ml) to the graduated cylinder. Calculate the average number of drops per ml. This information must be communicated to the patient clearly on the prescription label.

Volumetric Glassware Intended "To Contain"

Volumetric glassware "to contain" includes flasks and graduates of various types.

Flasks *Volumetric flasks* have slender necks and wide bulb-like bases. Volumetric flasks are single volume glassware and come in sizes ranging from 5 ml to 4,000 ml. One calibration mark is etched on the neck of the flask, When the flask is filled to that mark, the flask contains the volume indicated on the flask. Volumetric flasks are hard to use if dissolving solids in liquid because the neck is so narrow. If solids are to be dissolved, the flask is partially filled with liquid to effect dissolution, then filled with more liquid to the calibration mark.

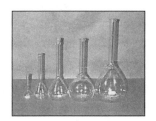

Graduates *Conical and cylindrical graduates* are "to contain" glassware but are used in compounding "to deliver" desired volumes of liquids. Cylindrical graduates (also called graduated cylinders) are more accurate than conical graduates because of the constant diameter of the cylinder. Both types of graduates come in a variety of sizes to accommodate different volumes. Commonly

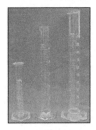

used sizes are 10, 50, 100, and 500 ml, but cylindrical graduates are available from 5 ml to 4,000 ml.

Graduated cylinders may be used to measure and deliver volumes more than 20 ml of most liquids with an acceptable level of accuracy. When the measurement of smaller volumes is required, smaller graduated cylinders could be used, but syringes or pipets are more accurate.

Measuring volumes is less accurate when the lower portions of a graduate are used. A general rule is not to measure volumes that are less than 20% of the capacity of the graduated cylinder. Table 7.7 gives the minimum volumes that can be measured for a given percentage error. For example, using a 50 ml cylinder, a 2.5% error would occur if 15.8 ml were measured, but a 5.0% error would occur if 7.9 ml were measured. Therefore, approximately 15 ml is the lowest volume that should be measured in a 50 ml cylinder to maintain an acceptable error.

When using graduates, the following steps should be followed to maximize measuring accuracy:

1. Hold the graduated cylinder by the base and elevate it so the desired mark is at eye level.

2. Hold the stock bottle with the label face up, and pour the liquid to be measured into the center of

TABLE 7.7: MINIMUM VOLUME TO MEASURE IN GRADUATED CYLINDERS

Capacity of Graduated Cylinder (mL)	Minimum Volume to Measure (mL) with Percent Error	
	2.5%	5.0%
5	3.0	1.5
10	4.4	2.2
25	11.8	5.9
50	15.8	7.9
100	20.9	10.5
250	36.3	18.2
500	66.5	33.2
1,000		200.2

the graduated cylinder to avoid the measuring error resulting from the material adhering to the wall (especially with viscous liquids).

3. As the surface of the liquid approaches the desired mark, decrease the flow rate or use a dropper or pipet to bring to final volume. Determine the final volume by aligning the bottom of the meniscus with the desired graduation mark. Either failing to account for the meniscus or to perceive its true bottom is a common source of error. If the bottom of the meniscus is difficult to see against a light background, use a broad black band on a white background.

4. When transferring the liquid from the graduated

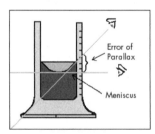

cylinder, allow about 15 seconds for aqueous and hydroalcoholic fluids to drain. Allow approximately 60 seconds (or more) for more viscous liquids, such as syrups, glycerin, propylene glycol, and mineral oil, to drain.

Some special precautions when using graduated cylinders are as follows:

1. Although graduates are volumetric devices, they are *not* mixing devices. Do not use them as the container to dissolve solids in liquids. Instead, prepare a solution in a beaker or flask and then return into the graduate for final adjustments in volume.

2. *Do not* assume that the final volume of a prescription will be the sum of the individual volumes of

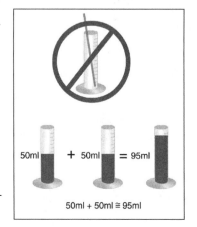

ingredients. This is particularly important with the admixture of aqueous and non-aqueous solutions such as alcohol and water. When these solutions are mixed, the volume actually shrinks and the total volume is less than the numeric sum of the two volumes.

Nonvolumetric Glassware and Devices

Erlenmeyer flasks, beakers, and *prescription bottles* are not volumetric devices and should not be used to measure liquids. The graduation marks inscribed on these containers are only approximations of their capacity. These devices should be used only to mix or store liquid preparations unless they are calibrated to a known volume.

To calibrate a vessel, measure the desired volume of liquid with a graduated cylinder and add the liquid to the vessel. Make a mark on the outside of the vessel with a special marking pen. Empty out the liquid, add the other formulation ingredients to the vessel, and then add sufficient liquid to bring the final product to the calibration mark.

Transfer pipets are useful when transferring liquids from one container to another if an accurate transfer volume is not required. These pipets (sometimes called

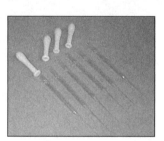

Pasteur pipets) are hollow glass tubes tapered at one end. A rubber bulb is attached to the other end and is used to draw liquid into and expel liquid out of the pipet.

The *teaspoon* and the problem concerning the actual volume of liquid contained in a "teaspoonful" has existed for many years. The USP/NF chapter <1221> provides the following statement:[7]

> For household purposes, an American Standard Teaspoon has been established by the American National Standards Institute as containing 4.93 ± 0.24 ml. In view of the almost universal practice of employing teaspoons ordinarily available in the household for the administration of medicine, the teaspoon may be regarded as representing 5 ml.

Household teaspoons are far from standard. Teaspoons can be found with capacities ranging from 3 ml to 7 ml, and the volume of liquid that a given teaspoon can hold varies with the viscosity and surface tension of the liquid. Therefore, accurate dosages cannot be assured with a teaspoon. Calibrated medicine droppers, oral syringes, or other calibrated measuring device should be used instead.

NOTES

1. <1176> Prescription Balances and Volumetric Apparatus: The United States Pharmacopeia 29/National Formulary 24, The United States Pharmacopeial Convention, Inc., Rockville, MD, 2005, pp. 3020–3021.

2. Newton, D. W. Balances and Weighing Accuracy. *International Journal of Pharmaceutical Compounding* 2:376–377, 1998.

3. Allen, L.V., Jr. Standard Operating Procedure for Performing Class A Prescription Torsion Balance Performance Tests. *International Journal of Pharmaceutical Compounding* 2:166–167, 1998.

4. Allen, L.V., Jr. General Standard Operating Procedure for Electronic Balance Maintenance/Calibration. *International Journal of Pharmaceutical Compounding* 1:44–45, 1997.

5. <41> Weights and Balances: The United States Pharmacopeia 29/National Formulary 24, The United States Pharmacopeial Convention, Inc., Rockville, MD, 2005, p. 2499.

6. <1101> Medicine Dropper: The United States Pharmacopeia 29/National Formulary 24, The United States Pharmacopeial Convention, Inc., Rockville, MD, 2005, p. 2969.

7. <1221> Teaspoon: The United States Pharmacopeia 29/National Formulary 24, The United States Pharmacopeial Convention, Inc., Rockville, MD, 2005, p. 3047.

CHAPTER EIGHT

Overview of Solutions

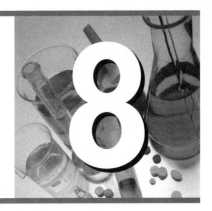

SOLUTIONS ARE USED AS THERAPEUTIC AGENTS, OR AS vehicles for therapeutic agents in almost every route of administration. Depending on what is contained in the solution, they also can be used as flavorings, buffers, preservatives, or suspending agents. Concentrated stock solutions often serve as drug sources for compounded formulations. Test solutions play an important role in the analysis of pharmaceutical products. Each chemical dissolved in the solution, however, will provide a unique contribution to the total solution. Examples of chemical substances that can be dissolved in a solution are

active drugs	colorants
buffers	emulsifying agents
preservatives	suspending agents
isotonicity adjustment agents	antioxidants
co-solvents	chelating agents
flavors	viscosity enhancing
sweeteners	agents

One definition of a solution is a homogenous liquid system with one or more chemical substances, called *solute(s)*, dissolved in a suitable *solvent* or mixture of solvents. Solutions are homogenous systems in which the solute is dispersed throughout the solvent in molecule-sized particles. Water is the most common solvent for oral solutions. Alcohol, glycerin, and propylene glycol also are used. For topical solutions, other solvents may be added, such as acetone, isopropanol, polyethylene glycols, collodion, and various oils and polymers.

Solvents

Solvents are considered to be polar, nonpolar, or semipolar. *Polar solvents* dissolve ionic and other polar solutes. *Nonpolar solvents* dissolve nonpolar solutes. "Likes dissolve likes" is a rule that describes these observations. *Semipolar solvents* may induce a certain degree of polarity in nonpolar molecules and, thus, may improve their miscibility in polar solvents.

Polar Solvents

The solubility of drugs and other polar compounds in polar solvents is related to three factors:

1. polarity of the solvent
2. ability to form hydrogen bonds
3. structural or chemical composition.

Polar solvents will dissolve ionic and polar solutes. For example, water will mix freely with low molecular-weight alcohols, sugars, polyhydroxy compounds, and many salts. The ability of solutes to form hydrogen bonds with polar solvents is the mechanism of water dissolving alcohols, ketones, aldehydes, acids, and amines. Hydrogen bonding occurs in a molecule between a hydrogen atom and an oxygen atom. The weak inter-molecular forces play a significant role in the solubility in many molecules in polar solvents.

The structural and chemical composition of the solution components also influences the interactions between solvents and solutes. For example, straight chain alcohols, aldehydes, and acids with more than five carbons are only slightly soluble in water. This is because the long chain structures prevent the formation of hydrogen bonding between the component and the water molecules.

Nonpolar Solvents

Ionic and polar solutes are not soluble or only slightly soluble in nonpolar solvents. Nonpolar solvents cannot decrease the attraction between ions of strong and weak electrolytes, or break covalent bonds. Nonpolar compounds can be dissolved in nonpolar solvents by inducing dipole interactions and establishing weak *vander Waals forces*. Through this mechanism, oils, fatty acids, and alkaloids will dissolve in nonpolar solvents such as chloroform, dichloromethane, benzene, and mineral oils.

Semipolar Solvents

Semipolar solvents (ketones, ethers, alcohols, glycols) can induce some polarity in nonpolar molecules so the latter will become soluble (or miscible) in polar solvents. Acetone, for example, will increase the solubility of ether in water. Propylene glycol, a semipolar solvent, increases the miscibility of water in peppermint oil.

Available Solvents

Several solvents are available for use in compounded formulations. Table 8.1 lists solvents that have monographs in the USP/NF. Table 8.2 lists oleagenous solvents. Both tables give properties of the solvents.

Solutes

When a solute is dissolved in a solvent, the properties of the solution will change. Solutes can be classified as either *nonelectrolytes* or *electrolytes*, according to whether the solutes dissociate or remain unchanged when dissolved

in the solvent. Nonelectrolytes in solvents will not dissociate (ionize) and, therefore, the solutions will not conduct electricity. Examples of nonelectrolytes are dextrose, sucrose, glycerin, glycol, ethanol, chloroform, and urea.

Electrolytes are compounds that will dissociate or ionize when dissolved in a solvent, and these solutions will conduct electricity. Some electrolytes are sodium hydroxide, sodium chloride, potassium chloride, nitric acid, and sulfuric acid. *Strong electrolytes* are solutes that almost completely dissociate in a solvent. *Weak electrolytes* dissociate to a lesser extent. Examples of strong electrolytes are hydrochloric acid, sulfuric acid, potassium hydroxide, and sodium chloride. Some weak electrolytes are acetic acid, ammonia, phosphoric acid, and the majority of drugs.

Weak electrolytes can be further subdivided into *weak acids* and *weak bases*, depending on their chemical structure. One way to determine if a compound is a weak

TABLE 8.1: PHYSICOCHEMICAL CHARACTERISTICS OF OFFICIAL SOLVENTS

Solvent	Miscibility			General Use		Specific Gravity
	Water	Alcohol	Oil	External	Internal	
Acetone	M	M		Yes	—	0.789
Alcohol	M	M		Yes	Yes	—
Alcohol, diluted	M	M		Yes	Yes	0.936
Amylene hydrate	M	M	—	—	—	0.805
Benzyl benzoate	I	M	—	Yes	Yes	1.118
Butyl alcohol	M	M		Yes	Yes	—
Corn oil	I	SS	M	Yes	Yes	0.918
Cottonseed oil	I	SS	M	Yes	Yes	0.918
Diethylene glycol monoethyl ether	M	M	Par	Yes	—	0.991
Ethyl acetate	M	M	M	Yes	—	0.896
Glycerin	M	M	I	Yes	Yes	1.249
Hexylene glycol	M	M	—	—	—	0.919
Isopropyl alcohol	M	M	—	Yes	—	0.785
Methyl alcohol	M	M	—	Yes	—	—
Methylene chloride	—	M	M	Yes	—	1.320
Methyl isobutyl ketone	SS	M	—	Yes	—	—
Mineral oil	I	I	M	Yes	Yes	0.870
Peanut Oil	I	VSS	M	Yes	Yes	0.916
PEG 300	M	M	—	Yes	Yes	1.12
PEG 400	M	M	—	Yes	Yes	1.12
PEG 600	M	M	—	Yes	Yes	1.12
Propylene glycol	M	M	I	Yes	Yes	1.036
Sesame oil	—	SS	—	Yes	Yes	0.918
Water	M	M	I	Yes	Yes	1.00

M = miscible   I = immiscible   Par = partially miscible   SS = slightly soluble   VSS = very slightly soluble

Adapted from "Featured Excipient: Official Solvents," by L. V. Allen, Jr., International Journal of Pharmaceutical Compounding 4:139–142, 2000.

TABLE 8.2: PHYSICOCHEMICAL CHARACTERISTICS OF OLEAGINOUS SOLVENTS

Substance	Specific Gravity	Refractive Index	Acid Value*	Iodine Value†	Saponification Value‡
Alkyl (C$_{12}$–C$_{15}$) benzoate	0.915–0.935	1.483–1.48	70.5		169–182
Almond oil	0.910–0.915		95–105		190–200
Corn oil	0.914–0.921		102–130		187–193
Cottonseed oil	0.915–0.921		109–120		
Ethyl oleate	0.866–0.874	1.443–1.450	≤ 0.5	75–85	177–188
Isopropyl myristate	0.846–0.854	1.432–1.436	≤ 1		202–212
Isopropyl palmitate	0.850–0.855	1.435–1.438	≤ 1		183–193
Mineral oil	0.845–0.905	—	—	—	—
Mineral oil, light	0.818–0.880	—	—	—	—
Octyldodecane	—	—	≤ 5	≤ 8	≤ 5
Olive oil	0.910–0.915	—	—	79–88	190–195
Peanut oil	0.912–0.920	1.462–1.464	—	84–100	185–195
Safflower oil	—	—	—	135–150	—
Sesame oil	0.916–0.921	—	—	103–116	188–195
Soybean oil	0.916–0.922	1.465–1.475	—	120–141	180–200
Squalane	0.807–0.810	1.451–1.452	≤ 0.2	≤ 4	≤ 2

* Acid value is the number of milligrams of potassium hydroxide required to neutralize the free acids in 1 g of the substance. It is a measure of acidity of the oil.

† Iodine value is the number of grams of iodine absorbed, under the prescribed conditions, by 100 g of the substance; it is a measure of the unsaturation of the oil.

‡ Saponification value is the number of milligrams of potassium hydroxide required to neutralize the free acids and saponify the esters contained in 1 g of the substance.

Adapted from "Featured Excipient: Oleaginous Vehicles," by L. V. Allen. Jr., International Journal of Pharmaceutical Compounding 4: 470–472, 2000.

acid or base is to examine the different salts the chemical has. If the salt form is a sodium, potassium, or calcium ion, the chemical is an acid. For example, sodium phenytoin, sodium carbonate, and sodium phenobarbital indicate that phenytoin, carbonic acid, and phenobarbital are weak acids. If the salt form is a sulfate, hydrochloride, or tartrate, the chemical is a base. For example, morphine sulfate, tetracaine hydrochloride, and metoprolol tartrate indicate that morphine, tetracaine, and metoprolol are weak bases.

Solubility

The solubility of a solute indicates the maximum concentration a solute will have when dissolved in a solvent. When a solvent has dissolved the maximum amount of solute, it is a *saturated solution*. Solutions also may be *unsaturated* or *supersaturated*. An unsaturated solution contains the dissolved solute in a concentration less than the saturate concentration. A supersaturated solution contains more dissolved solute than a saturated solution. Supersaturated solutions may be formed by dissolving the solute at elevated temperature and slowly cooling the solution while maintaining the solute in solution. Supersaturated solutions can be made to precipitate the excess solute and return to a saturated solution by adding

a crystal to the solution, by vigorous shaking, or by scratching the walls of the solution container.

Solubilities of many chemicals are given in standard references such as USP/NF, Remington's The Science and Practice of Pharmacy, Merck Index, Martindales: The Extra Pharmacopeia, USPDI Volume III, The Pharmacist's Pharmacopeia, Material Safety Data Sheets, and from various websites on the Internet. The solubility may be described in a variety of ways. References generally express solubility in terms of the volume of solvent required to dissolve one gram of the solute at a specified temperature. A small distinction, but an important one, has to be made about these solubility values: The solubilities are given as grams of solute per milliliter of solvent, not per milliliter of final solution. If the concentration is going to be close to the solubility, this distinction may be relevant. Solubilities also may be expressed in more subjective terms, as found in the USP/NF and shown in Table 8.3.

Factors Affecting Solubility

Many factors influence the solubility of a solute in a solvent. These factors have to be understood and used correctly when compounding solution formulations.

Temperature

Solubility is a function of temperature. Many compounds have greater solubility at elevated temperatures,

TABLE 8.3: SOLUBILITIES EXPRESSED IN SUBJECTIVE TERMS

Descriptive Terms	Parts of Solvent Needed for One Part Solute
Very soluble	< 1
Freely soluble	1–10
Soluble	10–30
Sparingly soluble	30–100
Slightly soluble	100–1,000
Very slightly soluble	1,000–10,000
Practically insoluble or insoluble	> 10,000

but some have greater solubilities at lower temperatures. This aspect of solubility is useful in the preparation and storage of a solution. Selecting the correct temperature will cause the solution to hold the required amount of drug in solution and also will increase the speed at which a drug dissolves. Knowing the influence of temperature on solubility, too, will help the pharmacist know the correct formulation storage conditions.

Looking at this relationship in another way suggests two situations that the pharmacist should consider.

1. When heating drugs to increase the speed of dissolution, do not use concentrations higher than the solubility at room temperature. When the solution cools, the drug will precipitate if a higher concentration was used.

2. If the solution is to be stored or used at a temperature other than room temperature, consider the solubility of the drug at that temperature.

Presence of Multiple Solutes

The aqueous solubility of nonelectrolytes is nearly always affected in some way by the addition of an electrolyte. Three terms are relevant here:

1. *Salting-out* is the precipitation of organic solutes from an aqueous solution by the addition of an electrolyte or a salt. This is attributed to a competition between solute molecules for the solvent and is dependent upon the size and valence of the electrolyte.

2. *Salting-in* is the increase in solubility of an organic solute upon addition of an electrolyte. The mechanism of this phenomenon is poorly understood and rarely encountered. As an example, globulins are more soluble in dilute salt solutions than in water.

3. *Complexation formation* occurs when an insoluble solute reacts with a soluble substance to form a soluble complex. An example is the complexation of the soluble potassium iodide (KI) to the insoluble iodine molecule (I_2) to form a soluble triiodide complex (KI_3).

Solute pKa and Solvent pH

According to the Henderson-Hasselbach equation, the relationship between pH, pKa, and relative concentrations of an acid and its salt is:

$$pH = pKa + \log \frac{[A^-]}{[HA]}$$

where

$[A^-]$ = the molar concentration of the salt (dissociated species)

$[HA]$ = the concentration of the undissociated acid

pKa = the dissociation constant of the drug

When the concentrations of salt and acid are equal, the pH of the system equals the pKa of the acid. As the pH decreases, the concentration of the undissociated acid increases and the concentration of the salt decreases. This has some interesting implications regarding the aqueous solubility of the acid because the undissociated form usually is much less soluble than its salt. The undissociated acid, however, is what more readily penetrates biological membranes and creates the therapeutic effect. Thus, some balance must be found between the more soluble salt form and the biologically active undissociated acid form.

Changes in solubility brought about by alterations in solvent pH can be predicted by the pHp equation. The pHp is the pH below which an acid or above which a base will begin to precipitate.

$$pHp = pKa + \log \frac{S - S_o}{S_o} \qquad \text{(for a weak acid)}$$

$$pHp = pKw - pKb + \log \frac{S_o}{S - S_o} \qquad \text{(for a weak base)}$$

where

S_o = the molar solubility of the undissociated acid or base

S = the molar concentration of the salt form of the drug initially added

pKa = dissociation constant of the acid

pKw = dissociation constant of water

pKb = dissociation constant of the base ($pKa + pKb = pKw$)

EXAMPLE: Calculate the pHp of a 1% sodium phenobarbital solution.

From Merck Index:

phenobarbital mol. wt. = 232.32

solubility of phenobarbital = 1 g/L

phenobarbital Ka = 3.9×10^{-8}; pKa = 7.4

phenobarbital sodium mol. wt. = 254.22

S_o = molar solubility of phenobarbital = 1 g/L $\times$ 1 mole/232.32 g = 0.0043 moles/L or 0.0043 M

S = 1 g/100 ml $\times$ 1000 ml/L $\times$ 1 mole/254.22 g = 0.0393 moles/L or 0.0393 M

$$pHp = 7.4 + \log \frac{0.0393\ M - 0.0043\ M}{0.0043\ M} = 8.3$$

Therefore, 1% phenobarbital will precipitate at or below a pH of 8.3.

Tables 8.4 and 8.5 list common acids and bases and their corresponding pKa, along with other properties. Tables 8.6 and Table 8.7 list acidifying agents and alkalizing agents, respectively. These agents are used in compounded formulations to establish a pH for the solution. Compatibility with other ingredients in the formulation must be considered.

Co-Solvent Systems

The solubility of a drug in a given solvent is largely a function of the polarity of the solvent. This relationship between polarity and solubility may be used to alter the solubility of a drug in a solution.

One approach is to alter the polarity of the solute by shifting it between its undissociated and ionic (dissociated) states. A shift toward the ionic form improves the solubility of the solute in water and other polar solvents. A shift toward the molecular species improves solubility in nonpolar solvents. These shifts may be produced by altering the pH of the solution or using the salt form of the compound.

Another approach is to mix solvents of different polarities to form a solvent system of optimum polarity to dissolve the solute. This method is referred to as *solvent blending*, or *co-solvency*. The solvents obviously must be miscible. Diazepam Injection, Digoxin Injection, and Phenytoin Sodium Injection all use a co-solvent mixture that contains 40% propylene glycol, 10% ethanol, and 50% Water for Injection. Paclitaxel Injection uses a Cremphor® EL (polyoxyethylated castor oil) and dehydrated alcohol co-solvent.

One method used to extemporaneously determine a co-solvent system is to use dielectric constants as a guide

TABLE 8.4: IONIZATION CONSTANTS OF WEAK ACIDS AT 25°C

Weak Acid	Mol. Wt.	Ka	pKa	Weak Acid	Mol. Wt.	Ka	pKa
Acetaminophen	151.16	1.20×10^{-10}	9.92	Phenobarbital	232.23	3.9×10^{-8}	7.41
Acetic acid	60.05	1.75×10^{-5}	4.76	Phenol	95.12	1×10^{-10}	10.0
Acetylsalicylic acid	180.15	3.27×10^{-4}	3.49	Phenytoin	252.26	7.9×10^{-9}	8.1
p-Aminobenzoic acid	137.13	$K_1\ 2.24 \times 10^{-5}$	4.65	Phosphoric acid	98.00	$K_1\ 7.5 \times 10^{-3}$	2.12
		$K_2\ 1.58 \times 10^{-5}$	4.80			$K_2\ 6.2 \times 10^{-8}$	7.21
Amobarbital	226.27	1.15×10^{-8}	7.94			$K_3\ 2.1 \times 10^{-13}$	12.67
Ascorbic acid	176.12	$K_1\ 5.0 \times 10^{-5}$	4.3	Picric acid	229.11	4.2×10^{-1}	0.38
		$K_2\ 1.6 \times 10^{-12}$	11.8	Propylparaben	180.20	4.0×10^{-9}	8.4
Barbital	184.19	1.23×10^{-8}	7.91	Salicylic acid	138.12	1.06×10^{-3}	2.97
Barbituric acid	128.09	1.05×10^{-4}	3.98	Succinic acid	118.09	$K_1\ 6.4 \times 10^{-5}$	4.19
Benzoic acid	122.12	6.30×10^{-5}	4.20			$K_2\ 2.3 \times 10^{-6}$	5.63
Benzyl penicillin	334.38	1.74×10^{-3}	2.76	Sucrose	342.30	2.4×10^{-13} (19°C)	12.62
Boric acid	61.84	$K_1\ 5.8 \times 10^{-10}$	9.24	Sulfacetaminde	214.24	1.35×10^{-6}	5.87
Caffeine	194.19	1.0×10^{-14}	14.0	Sulfadiazine	250.28	3.3×10^{-7}	6.48
Citric acid monohydrate	210.14	$K_1\ 7.0 \times 10^{-4}$	3.15	Sulfamerazine	264.30	8.7×10^{-8}	7.06
		$K_2\ 1.66 \times 10^{-5}$	4.78	Sulfapyridine	249.29	3.6×10^{-9}	8.44
		$K_3\ 4.0 \times 10^{-7}$	6.40	Sulfathiazole	255.32	7.6×10^{-8}	7.12
α-D-Glucose	180.16	8.6×10^{-13}	12.1	Sulfaisomidine	278.34	3.4×10^{-8}	7.47
Glycine (protonated cation)	75.07	$K_1\ 4.5 \times 10^{-3}$	2.35	Sulfisoxazole	267.30	1.0×10^{-5}	5.0
		$K_2\ 1.7 \times 10^{-10}$	9.78	Tartaric acid	150.09	$K_1\ 9.6 \times 10^{-4}$	3.02
Methylparaben	152.14	4.0×10^{-9}	8.4			$K_2\ 4.4 \times 10^{-5}$	4.36
Monochloroacetic acid	94.50	1.40×10^{-3}	2.86	Tetracycline	444.43	$K_1\ 5.01 \times 10^{-4}$	3.30
Penicillin V	350.38	1.86×10^{-3}	2.73			$K_2\ 2.09 \times 10^{-8}$	7.68
Pentobarbital	226.28	1.0×10^{-8}	8.0			$K_3\ 2.04 \times 10^{-10}$	9.69

TABLE 8.5: Ionization Constants of Weak Bases at 25°C

Weak Base	Mol. Wt.	Kb	pKb	pKa (conjugate acid)	Weak Base	Mol. Wt.	Kb	pKb	pKa (conjugate acid)
Acetanilide	135.16	4.1×10^{-14} (40°C)	13.39	0.61	Papaverine	339.39	8×10^{-9}	8.1	5.9
Ammonia	35.05	1.74×10^{-5}	4.76	9.24	Physostigmine	275.34	$K_1\ 7.6 \times 10^{-7}$	6.12	7.88
Acetanilide	135.16	4.1×10^{-14} (40°C)	13.39	0.61			$K_2\ 5.7 \times 10^{-13}$	12.24	1.76
Ammonia	35.05	1.74×10^{-5}	4.76	9.24	Pilocarpine	208.25	$K_1\ 7 \times 10^{-8}$	7.2	6.8
Apomorphine	267.31	1.0×10^{-7}	7.00	7.00			$K_2\ 2 \times 10^{-13}$	12.7	1.3
Atropine	289.4	4.5×10^{-5}	4.35	9.65	Procaine	236.30	7×10^{-6}	5.2	8.8
Benzocaine	165.19	6.0×10^{-12}	11.22	2.78	Quinacrine dihydrochloride	472.88	1×10^{-6}	6.0	8.0
Caffeine	194.19	$K_1\ 3.98 \times 10^{-11}$	10.4	3.6	Quinine	324.41	$K_1\ 1.0 \times 10^{-6}$	6.00	8.00
		$K_2\ 4.07 \times 10^{-14}$	13.4	0.6			$K_2\ 1.3 \times 10^{-10}$	9.89	4.11
Cocaine	303.35	2.6×10^{-6}	5.59	8.41	Reserpine	608	4×10^{-8}	7.4	6.6
Codeine	299.36	1.6×10^{-6}	5.8	8.2	Scopolamine	303.35	1.6×10^{-6}	5.8	8.2
Ephedrine	165.23	2.3×10^{-5}	4.64	9.36	Strychnine	334.40	$K_1\ 1 \times 10^{-6}$	6.0	8.0
Epinephrine	183.20	$K_1\ 7.9 \times 10^{-5}$	4.1	9.9			$K_2\ 2 \times 10^{-12}$	11.7	2.3
		$K_2\ 3.2 \times 10^{-6}$	5.5	8.5	Theobromine	180.17	$K_1\ 7.76 \times 10^{-7}$	6.11	7.89
Erythromycin	733.92	6.3×10^{-6}	5.2	8.8			$K_2\ 4.8 \times 10^{-14}$	13.3	0.7
Ethylenediamine	60.10	7.1×10^{-8}	7.15	6.85	Theophylline	180.17	$K_1\ 1.58 \times 10^{-9}$	8.80	5.20
Glycine	75.07	2.3×10^{-12}	11.65	2.35			$K_2\ 5.0 \times 10^{-14}$	13.3	0.7
Morphine	285.33	7.4×10^{-7}	6.13	7.87	Tolbutamide	270.34	2.0×10^{-9}	8.7	5.3
Nalorphine	311.37	6.3×10^{-7}	6.2	7.8	Urea	60.06	1.5×10^{-14}	13.82	0.18

Adapted from "Appendix," by E. L. Parrott and W. Saski. Experimental Pharmaceutics, 4th edition (Minneapolis, MN: Burgess Publishing Co., 1977), pp. 315–319.

TABLE 8.6: Physicochemical Characteristics of Acidifying Agents

Acidifying Agents	% Strength	Solubility		Specific Gravity	Solution pH (% aqueous solution)
		Water	Alcohol		
Acetic acid NF	36.5	M	M	1.04	
Acetic acid, glacial USP	100	M	M	1.05	
Citric acid USP	100	VS	FS	—	2.2 (1%)
Fumaric acid NF	100	SS	S	—	2.45 (sat)
Hydrochloric acid NF	37.5	M	M	1.18	0.1 (10%)
Hydrochloric acid, diluted NF	10	M	M	1.06	0.1
Lactic acid	88	M	M	1.21	
Malic acid NF	100	VS	FS	—	2.35 (1%)
Nitric acid NF	70	M	M	1.41	
Phosphoric acid NF	87	M	M	1.71	
Phosphoric acid, diluted NF	10	M	M	1.06	
Propionic acid NF	100	M	M	0.99	
Sodium phosphate monobasic USP	100	FS	PI	—	4.3 (5%)
Sulfuric acid NF	98	M	M	1.84	
Tartaric acid NF	100	VS	FS	—	2.2 (1.5%)

M = miscible   VS = very soluble   FS = freely soluble   S = soluble   SS = slightly soluble   PI = practically insoluble

Adapted from "Featured Excipient: Acidifying Agents," by L. V. Allen, Jr., International Journal of Pharmaceutical Compounding 3:309–310, 1999.

TABLE 8.7: PHYSICOCHEMICAL CHARACTERISTICS OF ALKALYZING AGENTS

| Alkalyzing Agents | % Strength | Solubility | | Specific Gravity | Solution pH (aqueous concentration) |
		Water	Alcohol		
Ammonia solution, strong NF	29	M	M	0.90	
Ammonium carbonate NF	100	FS	—	—	
Diethanolamine NF	100	M	M	1.088	11 (0.1N)
Monoethanolamine	100	M	M	1.012	12.1 (0.1N)
Potassium hydroxide NF	100	FS	FS	—	FS
Sodium bicarbonate USP	100	S	I	—	8.3 (0.1M)
Sodium borate NF	100	S	I	—	
Sodium carbonate NF	100	FS	—	—	
Sodium hydroxide NF	100	FS	FS	—	
Sodium phosphate, dibasic, USP	100	FS	SS	—	9.1 (1%)
Trolamine NF	100	M	M	1.12	10.5 (0.1N)

M = miscible   FS = freely soluble   S = soluble   I = insoluble   SS = slightly insoluble

Adapted from "Featured Excipient: Alkalizing Agents," by L. V. Allen, Jr., International Journal of Pharmaceutical Compounding 3:404–405, 1999.

to developing the system. The dielectric constant (δ) of a solvent is an index of its polarity. Solvents of increasing polarity will show a similar increase in dielectric constant, as indicated in Table 8.8.

Solvents can be classified according to their dielectric constants as polar ($\delta > 50$), semipolar ($\delta = 20 - 50$), or nonpolar ($\delta = 1 - 20$). The value of the dielectric constant for a solution is obtained by multiplying the volume fraction of each solvent times its dielectric constant and summing. So the combined dielectric constant of solvents A and B is:

$$\delta_{(A+B)} = f_A\delta_A + f_B\delta_B$$

where

$\delta_{(A+B)}$ = dielectric constant of the co-solvent mixture

f_A = volume fraction of solvent A

f_B = volume fraction of solvent B

δ_A = dielectric constant of solvent A

δ_B = dielectric constant of solvent B

A co-solvent system for a drug can be determined experimentally. Solutions are prepared containing varying concentrations of absolute alcohol (for example) in water ranging from 0 to 100%. The concentration of drug that will be in the final formulation is added to each solution, the solutions are refrigerated overnight, and the solutions then are viewed for precipitation.

TABLE 8.8: DIELECTRIC CONSTANTS OF VARIOUS SOLVENTS

Solvent	Dielectric Constant (δ) at 20°C	Solvent	Dielectric Constant (δ) at 20°C
N-methylformamide	190	Polyethylene glycol 400	12.4
Water	80	Chloroform	5.0
Sorbitol solution (70% w/w)	62	Castor oil	4.6
Syrup	56	Ethyl ether	4.3
Glycerol (glycerin)	46	Sucrose	3.3
Methanol	33	Olive oil	3.1
Propylene glycol	32	Sesame oil	3.1
Absolute alcohol	25	Benzene	2.2
n-Propyl alcohol	22	Carbon tetrachloride	2.2
Acetone	21	Octane	1.9

SAMPLE RESULTS:

Absolute Alcohol v/v%	0	10	20	30	40	50	60	70	80	90	100
Precipitation Present	+	+	+	+	+	+	—	—	—	—	—

In this example, at least 60% v/v absolute alcohol was required to solubilize the drug. Because the dielectric constant of this solvent system can be determined, the solution can be reformulated so the drug will still dissolve and the solution will be more pleasing from a flavoring standpoint.

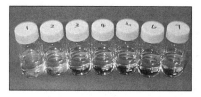

EXAMPLE: Using the sample results above, reformulate the solvent system to contain water, glycerin, and absolute alcohol.

The calculated dielectric constant of the 60% v/v solvent system is:

$$
\begin{aligned}
f_{(Water)}\, \delta_{(Water)} &= 80 \times 0.40 = 32 \\
f_{(Absolute\ Alcohol)}\, \delta_{(Absolute\ Alcohol)} &= 25 \times 0.60 = \underline{15} \\
\delta &= \overline{47}
\end{aligned}
$$

Glycerin often is used for both its solubility properties and its sweetening properties. To use glycerin as part of the new co-solvent system, the appropriate concentration of alcohol first must be determined. If 20% is taken as the new alcohol concentration in the formulation (for preservation), the needed percentages of water and glycerin can be calculated from the dielectric constants of the three solvents, as follows: $\delta_{(Absolute\ Alcohol)} = 25$, $\delta_{(Water)} = 80$, $\delta_{(Glycerin)} = 46$):

$$(0.2)(25) + (X)(80) + (0.8-X)(46) = 47$$
$$5 + 80X + 36.8 - 46X = 47$$
$$34X = 5.2$$
$$X = 0.15$$
$$0.8 - x = 0.65$$

Thus, the vehicle is 20% v/v Absolute Alcohol, 15% v/v water, and 65% v/v glycerin.

If using a co-solvent system consisting only of water and one other solvent, the following equation might be used to determine the solubility of the drug in the new system:[1]

$$\log S_T = f_{water} \log S_{water} + f_{sol} \log S_{sol}$$

where

S_T = total concentration of drug in the solution

S_{water} = solubility of the drug in water

S_{sol} = solubility of the drug in the chosen co-solvent

f_{water} = volume fraction of water

f_{sol} = volume fraction of co-solvent

Speed of Dissolution (Rate of Solution)

The solubility of a solute (drug) in the solvent is a property of that system. The solubility, however, does not give any indication of how fast the drug will dissolve or

go into solution in the solvent. Though the general rule, "the more soluble the drug, the faster the solution into the solvent" holds for many drugs, others require intervention to increase the speed of solution. Some solids may have to be triturated to reduce the particle size; others may require that the solvent be heated. Sometimes vigorous shaking, stirring, or *sonication* is required to increase the speed of solution.

The mechanism of dissolution has been explained by assuming that solid solute particles undergo dissolution in a two-step process:

1. The solid solute particle dissolves at the interface of a static thin layer of solvent (called the aqueous diffusion layer) that forms around the particle. (x = 0)
2. The dissolved molecules diffuse through the aqueous diffusion layer to the bulk of the solvent. (x = h)

In this mechanism of dissolution, the first step is fast and the second step is slower and becomes the rate limiting step.

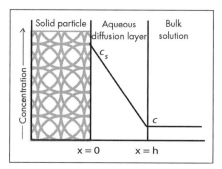

The rate of dissolution (or the rate of solution) is given by the following expression:

$$\frac{dc}{dt} = \text{rate of dissolution} = KS(C_s - C)$$

where

K = the dissolution rate constant of the drug in the solvent

S = surface area of the drug mass

C_s = solubility of the drug in the solvent

C = concentration of drug in the solvent at time t

Standard references show the derivation of the following relationships:

$$K = \frac{D}{hV}$$

where

D = diffusion coefficient of the drug in the solvent

$$D = \frac{kT}{6\pi\eta r}$$

k = Boltzmann constant (gas constant R divided by Avogadro's number)

T = absolute temperature

η = viscosity of the solvent

r = radius of the drug particle

h = thickness of unstirred layer around the drug particle

V = volume of solvent into which the drug is dissolving

These relationships indicate what parameters the pharmacist might control to increase the rate of solution. It is important to recognize that every rule has exceptions.

1. *Temperature.* As temperature increases, D increases, so the rate of dissolution increases. Therefore, most solutes will dissolve faster at elevated temperatures. Exceptions include calcium hydroxide and methylcellulose. Also, the stability of the drug at the elevated temperatures must be considered.

2. *Viscosity.* As the viscosity increases, dissolution decreases. Therefore, it is best to dissolve drugs in pure solvents such as water or alcohol and then add the more viscous solvents such as glycerin, syrup, or gels.

3. *Radius and surface area.* The surface area of the solid mass increases as the particle size is reduced. Therefore, reducing the overall surface area of the solid mass will increase the rate of dissolution. This can be done by triturating the solid in a mortar with a pestle, or by sonicating the solution while the solute is dissolving.

4. *Thickness of unstirred layer.* Stirring the solution will reduce the thickness of the layer and increase the rate of dissolution. Stirring plates with magnetic stirring bars are extremely useful for this purpose. Blenders and electric mixers also save time and produce acceptable products.

5. *C_s.* The solubility of the drug is a given property of the drug. But salt forms of most drugs have greater solubilities than the base form of the drug, and therefore will generally dissolve faster.

6. *Chemical states.* Various chemical states of drugs such as amorphous state, crystallinity, hydration, and polymorphism all have demonstrated a significant effect on the dissolution rate. As a general rule, different chemical states are expected to affect the dissolution rate; however, whether the rate increases or decreases depends on each individual solute and solvent combination.

Pharmaceutical Buffers

Buffer systems resist changes in pH when limited amounts of strong acids or bases are added to a solution. Buffer systems usually are composed of a weak acid or base and its salt. The pH of a buffer system can be calculated using the Henderson-Hasselbach equation:

$$pH = pKa + \log \frac{[salt]}{[acid]} \text{ (for a weak acid and its salt)}$$

$$pH = pKw - pKb + \log \frac{[base]}{[salt]}$$

(for a weak base and its salt)

where [salt], [acid], and [base] are the molar concentrations of salt, acid, and base.

Buffer capacity is a measure of the efficiency of a buffer in resisting changes in pH. Conventionally, the buffer capacity (β) is expressed as the amount of strong acid or base, in gram equivalents, that must be added to 1 liter of the solution to change its pH by 1 pH unit. The buffer capacity is calculated as:

$$\beta = \frac{\Delta B}{\Delta pH}$$

where ΔB equals the gram equivalent of strong acid/base needed to change the pH of 1 liter of buffer solution, and ΔpH is the pH change caused by the addition of the strong acid/base. Buffer systems have their greatest buffer capacity when the pH of the solution is equal to the pKa of the acid or base. The effectiveness of a buffer system is generally in the pH range of pKa $\pm$ 1.

The buffer capacity depends essentially on two factors:

1. Ratio of the salt to the acid or base. The buffer capacity is optimal when the ratio is 1:1.

2. Total buffer concentration.

The relationship between the buffer capacity (β) and a buffer concentration C is given by the van Slyke equation:

$$\beta = 2.3 \, C \, \frac{Ka[H_3O^+]}{(Ka + [H_3O^+])^2}$$

where

C   = the total buffer concentration (i.e., the sum of the molar concentrations of acid and salt)

Ka   = the dissociation constant for the acid or base

$[H_3O^+]$ = the hydronium ion concentration of the solution

The *maximum buffer capacity* occurs when pH equals pKa or when the hydronium ion concentration $[H_3O^+]$ equals the dissociation constant Ka. If in the van Slyke equation Ka is replaced with $[H_3O^+]$ in the numerator and the denominator, the equation of β_{max} is derived:

$$\beta_{max} = 2.3 \, C \, \frac{[H_3O^+]^2}{(2[H_3O^+])^2} = 2.3 \, C \, \frac{1}{4} = 0.576 \, C$$

where C is the total concentration of the buffer components.

EXAMPLE: Calculate the maximum buffer capacity of the phosphate buffer above with a total concentration of 0.025 M/L.

$$\beta_{max} = 0.576 \times 0.025 \text{ M/L} = 0.014$$

Several steps are involved in preparing a buffer system for a formulation:

1. Determine the optimal pH for the formulation based on physical and chemical stability, therapeutic activity, and the patient's comfort and safety.
2. Select a weak acid with a pKa near the desired pH (must be nontoxic and physically/chemically compatible with other ingredients).
3. Calculate the ratio of salt to acid required to produce the desired pH (Henderson-Hasselbach equation).
4. Determine the desired buffer capacity of the formulation.
5. Calculate the total buffer concentration required to produce this buffer capacity (van Slyke equation).
6. Determine the pH and the buffer capacity of the completed buffer solution by using a reliable pH meter or pH paper.

EXAMPLE: Using acetic acid and sodium acetate, prepare 500 ml of a buffer solution at pH 4.5 with a buffer capacity of 0.05 M/L.

The following information is readily obtained from standard references:

acetic acid mol. wt. = 60

acetic acid Ka = 1.75×10^{-5}; pKa = 4.76

density (glacial acetic acid) = 1.05 g/ml

sodium acetate mol. wt. = 82.0

Salt-to-acid ratio:

$$pH = pKa + \log \frac{[salt]}{[acid]}$$

$$4.5 = 4.76 + \log \frac{[salt]}{[acid]}$$

$$\frac{[salt]}{[acid]} = \text{antilog } (4.5 - 4.76) = 0.55$$

$$[salt] = 0.55 \text{ [acid]}$$

Total buffer concentration:

$$\beta = 2.3 \, C \, \frac{Ka[H_3O^+]}{(Ka + [H_3O^+])^2}$$

$$[H_3O^+] = \text{antilog } (-pH) = \text{antilog } (-4.5) = 3.16 \times 10^{-5}$$

$$0.05 = 2.3 \, C \, \frac{(1.75 \times 10^{-5})(3.16 \times 10^{-5})}{[(1.75 \times 10^{-5}) + (3.16 \times 10^{-5})]^2}$$

$$0.05 = 0.53 \, C$$

$$C = 0.095 \text{ M}$$

Final calculations:

C = [salt] + [acid]

C = 0.55 [acid] + [acid] = 1.55 [acid] = 0.095 M

[acid] = 0.095 M ÷ 1.55 = 0.061 M or 0.061 mole/L; so in 500 ml, 0.061 mole/L × 0.5 L × 60 g/mole = 1.85 g acetic acid

so glacial acetic acid = 1.85 g/1.05 g/ml = 1.76 ml

[salt] = 0.55 [acid] = 0.55 × 0.061 M = 0.034 M or 0.034 mole/L; so in 500 ml, 0.034 mole/L × 0.5 L × 82 g/mole = 1.38 g sodium acetate

EXAMPLE: Using dibasic potassium phosphate (K_2HPO_4) and monobasic potassium phosphate (KH_2PO_4), prepare 500 ml of a buffer solution at pH 7.4 with a buffer capacity of 0.05 M/L. Using a pH meter, measure the pH of 100 ml of the solution. Titrate 100 ml of the solution with an approximate 1.0 N NaOH until the pH increases by one unit, and determine whether the buffer capacity is as calculated. Note that the exact normality of the NaOH solution is recorded on the stock bottle.

From standard references, the following information is obtained:

KH_2PO_4 mol. wt. = 136.09

KH_2PO_4 Ka = 6.2×10^{-8}; pKa = 7.21

K_2HPO_4 mol. wt. = 174.18

Salt-to-acid ratio:

$$pH = pKa + \log \frac{[salt]}{[acid]}$$

$$7.4 = 7.21 + \log \frac{[K_2HPO_4]}{[KH_2PO_4]}$$

$$\frac{[K_2HPO_4]}{[KH_2PO_4]} = \text{antilog } (7.4 - 7.21) = 1.55$$

$$[K_2HPO_4] = 1.55 \, [KH_2PO_4]$$

Total buffer concentration:

$$\beta = 2.3 \, C \, \frac{Ka[H_3O^+]}{(Ka + [H_3O^+])^2}$$

$$\text{so } C = \frac{\beta(Ka + [H_3O^+])^2}{2.3 \, Ka[H_3O^+]}$$

$$[H_3O^+] = \text{antilog } (-pH) = \text{antilog } (-7.4) = 3.98 \times 10^{-8}$$

$$C = \frac{0.05(6.2 \times 10^{-8} + 3.98 \times 10^{-8})^2}{2.3(6.2 \times 10^{-8})(3.98 \times 10^{-8})} = \frac{5.18 \times 10^{-16}}{5.68 \times 10^{-15}}$$

$$C = 0.09 \text{ M}$$

Final calculations:

$$C = [K_2HPO_4] + [KH_2PO_4]$$

$$C = 1.55 [KH_2PO_4] + [KH_2PO_4] = 2.55 [KH_2PO_4]$$
$$= 0.09 \text{ M}$$

$$[KH_2PO_4] = 0.09M \div 2.55 = 0.035 \text{ M}$$

$$0.035 \text{ moles/L} \times 0.5 \text{ L} = 0.0175 \text{ moles} \times$$
$$136.09 \text{ g/mole} = 2.4 \text{ g } KH_2PO_4$$

$$[K_2HPO_4] = 1.55 [KH_2PO_4] = 1.55 \times 0.035 \text{ M} =$$
$$0.054 \text{ M}$$

$$0.054 \text{ moles/L} \times 0.5 \text{ L} = 0.027 \text{ moles} \times$$
$$174.18 \text{ g/mole} = 4.8 \text{ g } K_2HPO_4$$

In the results of the experiment, the pH before any addition of NaOH was 7.4. The exact normality of the NaOH stock solution was 1.010N. It required 3.1 ml of 1.010N NaOH to raise the pH of 100 ml of buffer solution to pH 8.4.

The number of equivalents of NaOH added is calculated in two steps:

1. Determine the number of grams of NaOH contained in the 3.1 ml of 1.010N NaOH solution (NaOH mol. wt. = 40.0). A simple ratio will show that if 40.4 grams of NaOH is contained in 1,000 ml of a 1.010 N solution, then 0.125 grams is contained in 3.1 ml of that solution:

$$\frac{X \text{ g}}{3.1 \text{ ml}} = \frac{1.010 \times 40.0 \text{ g}}{1000 \text{ ml}}$$

$$X = 0.125 \text{ g}$$

2. Another ratio calculation will show that 0.125 grams of NaOH equals 0.0031 Eq (eq. wt. of NaOH is also 40.0 because the valence is 1).

$$\frac{40.0 \text{ g}}{1 \text{ Eq}} = \frac{0.125 \text{ g}}{X \text{ Eq}}$$

$$X = 0.0031 \text{ Eq}$$

So 0.0031 Eq of NaOH increased the pH of 100 ml of buffer solution one pH unit. Because buffer capacity is defined as the number of Eq needed to increase the pH of 1,000 ml of solution, the experimentally determined buffer capacity is 0.031Eq/L.

The experimentally determined β is different from the theoretical buffer capacity used in the calculations.

Differences in these values can be caused by the kind and concentration of the buffer components, the pH region involved, and the kind of acid/base used to determine β.

Many different buffer solutions are used in pharmacy and pharmaceutical practice to buffer a solution. The USP 29/NF24 lists several buffer mixtures used to provide a wide working range of pH values between pH 1.2 and 10.0. These standard buffer solutions are:[2]

- potassium chloride and hydrochloric acid (pH 1.2 – 2.2)
- potassium biphthalate and hydrochloric acid (pH 2.2 – 4.0)
- potassium biphthalate and sodium hydroxide (pH 4.2 – 5.8)
- monobasic potassium phosphate and sodium hydroxide (pH 5.8 – 8.0)
- boric acid with potassium chloride and sodium hydroxide (pH 8.0 – 10.0)
- acetic acid and sodium acetate (pH 4.1 – 5.5).

Iso-osmoticity and Isotonicity

If a semipermeable membrane (one that is permeable only to solvent molecules) is used to separate solutions of different solute concentrations, a phenomenon known as *osmosis* occurs. The solvent molecules cross the membrane from lower to higher concentration to establish a concentration equilibrium. The pressure driving this movement, called *osmotic pressure*, is governed by the number of "particles" of solute in solution. If the solute is a nonelectrolyte, the number of particles is determined solely by the solute concentration. If the solute is an electrolyte, the number of particles is governed by both the concentration and the degree of dissociation of the electrolyte.

Solutions containing the same concentration of particles, and thus exerting equal osmotic pressures, are called *iso-osmotic*. A 0.9% solution of sodium chloride (normal saline) is iso-osmotic with blood. Although the term *isotonic*, which means equal tone, is sometimes used interchangeably with the term *iso-osmotic*, the two are different. Red blood cell membranes are not perfect semipermeable membranes; they allow passage of some solutes such as alcohol, boric acid, ammonium chloride, glycerin, ascorbic acid, and lactic acid. Therefore, a 2% solution of boric acid, which is physically iso-osmotic (containing the same number of particles) with blood will not be isotonic (exerting an equal pressure or tone) with blood. Practically speaking, this differentiation is rarely of clinical significance, and isotonicity values calculated on the basis of the number of particles in solution usually are sufficient.

The importance of using isotonic or iso-osmotic solutions is to assure that there is no tissue damage or pain when the formulation is administered. Solutions that contain fewer particles and exert a lower osmotic pressure than normal saline are called *hypotonic* and tend to produce painful swelling, as water will pass from the administration site into the tissues. Solutions exerting higher osmotic pressures, called *hypertonic,* can produce painful shrinking of tissues as water passes from the tissues in an attempt to dilute the hypertonic solution.

Methods

Three methods are used to adjust the isotonicity of compounded solutions. The most widely used method is the sodium chloride (NaCl) equivalent method.[3] The NaCl equivalent (E) is the amount of NaCl that has the same osmotic effect (based on the number of particles) as 1 g of the drug. Tables of sodium chloride equivalents for various drugs are available in standard references.

Sodium Chloride Equivalent Method

EXAMPLE: Calculate the amount of NaCl required to make the following ophthalmic solution isotonic.

Atropine Sulfate	2%
NaCl	qs
Aqua. dist. q.s. ad.	30 ml

1. Determine the amount of NaCl to make 30 ml of an isotonic solution:

   0.9 g of sodium chloride in 100 ml of water will make an isotonic solution. A simple ratio shows that 0.27 g of sodium chloride is needed to make 30 ml of water isotonic.

   $$\frac{0.9 \text{ g}}{100 \text{ ml}} = \frac{X}{30 \text{ ml}} \qquad X = 0.27 \text{ g}$$

2. Calculate the contribution of atropine sulfate to the osmotic pressure of the solution:

Atropine sulfate, when dissolved in the solution, will contribute "particles" to the solution, and therefore will affect the osmotic pressure of the solution. To determine this contribution, the sodium chloride equivalent for atropine sulfate is taken from standard references: E = 0.13 for atropine sulfate.

   30 ml × 2 g/100 ml = 0.6 g atropine sulfate will be present in the formulation

   0.6 g × 0.13 = 0.078 g will be the sodium chloride equivalent contribution of the atropine sulfate

3. Determine the amount of NaCl to add to the formulation:

Because the atropine sulfate will contribute an equivalent of 0.078 g, the sodium chloride needed to make the

final solution isotonic is calculated by subtracting the answer in step 2 from step 1.

   0.27 g − 0.078 g = 0.192 g

Other substances may be used in addition to, or in place of, NaCl to render solutions isotonic. This is done by taking the process one step further and calculating the amount of the substance that is equivalent to the amount of NaCl calculated in step 3.

Boric acid often is used to adjust isotonicity in ophthalmic solutions because of its buffering and anti-infective properties. If E for boric acid is 0.50, the amount of boric acid needed to replace the NaCl in step 3 can be calculated:

$$\frac{0.192 \text{ g NaCl}}{X \text{ g boric acid}} = \frac{0.50 \text{ g NaCl equiv.}}{1 \text{ g boric acid}}$$

or X = 0.38 g

or, more simply: 0.192 g/0.50 = 0.38 g

Thus, 0.38 g boric acid would be required to render the ophthalmic solution isotonic.

EXAMPLE: Use the NaCl equivalent method and appropriate compounding techniques to prepare the following isotonic ophthalmic solution:

Procaine HCl	1.5 %
Benzalkonium Chloride	1:10,000
Boric Acid	q.s.
Aqua. dist.	q.s. ad 60 ml

From a standard reference, E = 0.21 for procaine HCl, E = 0.16 for benzalkonium chloride, and E = 0.50 for boric acid.

1. Procaine HCl needed = 1.5 g/100 ml × 60 ml = 0.9 g

2. NaCl equivalent from procaine HCl = 0.9 g × 0.21 = 0.189 g

3. Benzalkonium chloride needed

   1:10,000 = 1 g/10,000 g = 1 g/10,000 ml for water

   $$\frac{1 \text{ g}}{10,000 \text{ ml}} = \frac{X \text{ g}}{60 \text{ ml}}$$

   X = 0.006 g

4. NaCl equivalent from benzalkonium chloride = 0.006 g × 0.16 = 0.001 g

5. NaCl and/or equivalent needed to make 60 ml isotonic solution

60 ml × 0.9% NaCl = 0.54 g

6. NaCl still needed = 0.54 g − 0.189 g − 0.001 g = 0.35 g

7. Boric acid needed = 0.35 g NaCl ÷ 0.50 = 0.70 g

or

$$\frac{0.35 \text{ g NaCl}}{X \text{ g boric acid}} = \frac{0.5 \text{ g NaCl}}{1.0 \text{ g boric acid}}$$

X = 0.70 g

Compounding procedure:

1. Weigh 0.9 g procaine HCl and 0.70 g boric acid.

2. Measure 6 ml of a benzalkonium chloride 1:1,000 solution.

3. Dissolve solids in distilled sufficient water (< 60 ml) to effect solution; add benzalkonium chloride 1:1,000 solution.

4. Transfer to graduated cylinder and q.s. to 60 ml with distilled water.

5. Filtration sterilize the solution and package in a sterile final container.

Cryoscopic Method

In this method, the freezing point decrease of a 1% drug solution is used in the calculations, based on the assumption that the freezing point decrease is proportional to the percentage content of the solute in the solution. ΔT_f is specifically the freezing point depression caused for a 1% solution of the solute.

EXAMPLE:

		ΔT_f
Lidocaine hydrochloride	0.25 g	0.13°C
Purified water q.s.	50 ml	
Make isotonic with sodium chloride q.s.		0.52°C

Because it is assumed that a direct proportionality exists between solute concentration and freezing point depression, and keeping in mind that the decrease caused by 1% of lidocaine hydrochloride is 0.13°C, the following proportion may be used to calculate the freezing point depression of 50 ml of water (X) produced by 0.25 g of lidocaine hydrochloride:

$$\frac{\% \text{ of solute}}{\text{degrees depressed}} = \frac{0.5\%}{\text{freezing point depression of water in solution}}$$

$$\frac{1\%}{0.13°C} = \frac{0.5\%}{X}$$

X = 0.065°C

Lidocaine hydrochloride will depress the freezing point of water in this solution by 0.065°C.

Isotonic sodium chloride (0.9%) decreases the freezing point of water by 0.52°C, and in the above solution the sodium chloride will have to lower the freezing point by 0.52°C − 0.065°C = 0.455°C. The percentage of sodium chloride (X) to give this freezing point depression can be calculated from the following ratio:

$$\frac{0.9\%}{0.52°C} = \frac{X}{0.455°C}$$

X = 0.788%

50 ml of a 0.788% NaCl solution will require 0.394 g of sodium chloride

The calculations demonstrated above can be simplified by including them in the following expression:

$$X = \frac{(0.52°C - A)}{B}$$

where

X = number of grams of the adjusting solute for each 100 ml of solution

A = freezing point depression of water produced by the presence of drug(s)

B = freezing point depression of water produced by 1% sodium chloride

0.52°C = freezing point depression of isotonic solution

Using the above simplified equation, the amount of the solute needed to make the solution isotonic is:

B = 0.58°C is the freezing point depression of 1% NaCl

A = 0.52°C × 0.13 freezing point depression of water due to lidocaine

$$X = \frac{0.52°C - (0.52°C \times 0.13)}{0.58°C}$$

Therefore, 0.779 g sodium chloride for 100 ml of solution is needed, or 0.390 g for 50 ml.

Isotonic Solution V Values

The V value of a drug is the volume of water to be added to a specified weight of drug to prepare an isotonic solution.[4] The V values are given in tables constructed for 0.3 g or 1.0 g of drug. The 0.3 g tables are useful in preparing 30 ml of a 1% solution, a commonly prescribed concentration. The basic principle underlying the use of V values is to prepare an isotonic solution of the prescribed drug and then dilute this solution to a final volume with a suitable isotonic vehicle.

The V value for a drug that does not appear in a table of V values can be calculated if the sodium chloride equivalent for 1% drug is known. Generally, tables of sodium chloride equivalents are much more extensive than V value tables.

EXAMPLE: Calculate the V value for anileridine HCl (E = 0.19) when 0.3 g of drug is to be used.

$$\frac{100 \text{ ml of solution}}{0.9 \text{ g NaCl}} \times \frac{0.19 \text{ g NaCl}}{1 \text{ g drug}} \times 0.3 \text{ g drug}$$

$$= 6.33 \text{ ml}$$

V = 6.33 ml water added to 0.3 g of anileridine will make an isotonic solution.

Table 8.9 shows the volume in water (in ml) to be added to 300 mg (0.3 g) of drug to produce an isotonic solution of the drug in water. Then as mentioned, a suitable isotonic solution is added to make a final volume.

NOTES

1. Thompson, J. E. Solutions (chapter 26) in *A Practical Guide to Contemporary Pharmacy Practice*, 2nd edition. Lippincott Williams & Wilkins, Baltimore, MD, 2004, pp. 26.1–26.40.
2. Solutions: The United States Pharmacopeia 29/National Formulary 24, The United States Pharmacopeial Convention, Inc., Rockville, MD, 2005, p. 3167.
3. Allen, L.V. Jr. Featured Excipient: Tonicity-Adjusting Agents. *International Journal of Pharmaceutical Compounding* 4:218–220, 2000.
4. Poon, C. Y. Tonicity, Osmoticity, Osmolality, and Osmolarity (chapter 18) in *Remington: The Science and Practice of Pharmacy*, 21st edition. Lippincott Williams & Wilkins, Philadelphia, PA, 2006, pp. 250–265.

ADDITIONAL READING

Allen, L.V., Jr. Solutions (chapter 15) in *The Art, Science, and Technology of Pharmaceutical Compounding*, 2nd edition. American Pharmaceutical Association, Washington, D.C., 2002, pp. 231–248.

TABLE 8.9: V VALUES OF DRUGS

Drug (0.3 g)	Water Needed for Isotonicity (mL)	Drug (0.3 g)	Water Needed for Isotonicity (mL)
Alcohol	21.7	Phenobarbital sodium	8.0
Ammonium chloride	37.3	Physostigmine salicylate	5.3
Amobarbital sodium	8.3	Pilocarpine hydrochloride	8.0
Amphetamine phosphate	11.3	Pilocarpine nitrate	7.7
Amphetamine sulfate	7.3	Piperocaine hydrochloride	7.0
Antipyrine	5.7	Polymyxin B sulfate	3.0
Apomorphine hydrochloride	4.7	Potassium chloride	25.3
Ascorbic acid	6.0	Potassium nitrate	18.7
Atropine methylbromide	4.7	Potassium phosphate, monobasic	14.7
Atropine sulfate	4.3	Procainamide hydrochloride	7.3
Bacitracin	1.7	Procaine hydrochloride	7.0
Barbital sodium	10.0	Scopolamine hydrobromide	4.0
Bismuth potassium tartrate	3.0	Scopolamine methylnitrate	5.3
Boric acid	16.7	Secobarbital sodium	8.0
Butacaine sulfate	6.7	Silver nitrate	11.0
Caffeine and sodium benzoate	8.7	Silver protein, mild	5.7
Calcium chloride	17.0	Sodium acetate	15.3
Calcium chloride (6 H_2O)	11.7	Sodium bicarbonate	21.7
Chlorobutanol (hydrated)	8.0	Sodium biphosphate, anhydrous	15.3
Chlortetracycline sulfate	4.3	Sodium biphosphate	13.3
Cocaine hydrochloride	5.3	Sodium bisulfite	20.3
Cupric sulfate	6.0	Sodium borate	14.0
Dextrose, anhydrous	6.0	Sodium iodide	13.0
Dibucaine hydrochloride	4.3	Sodium metabisulfite	22.3
Dihydrostreptomycin sulfate	2.0	Sodium nitrate	22.7
Epheprine hydrochloride	10.0	Sodium phosphate	9.7
Epinephrine sulfate	7.7	Sodium proionate	20.3
Epinephrine bitartrate	6.0	Sodium sulfite, exsiccated	21.7
Epinephrine hydrochloride	9.7	Sodium thiosulfate	10.3
Ethylmorphine hydrochloride	5.3	Streptomycin sulfate	2.3
Fluorescein sodium	10.3	Sulfacetamide sodium	7.7
Glycerin	11.7	Sulfadiazine sodium	8.0
Holocaine hydrochloride	6.7	Sulfamerazine sodium	7.7
Homatropine hydrobromide	5.7	Sulfapyridine sodium	7.7
Homatropine methylbromide	6.3	Sulfathiazole sodium	7.3
Hyoscyamine sulfate	4.7	Tetracaine hydrochloride	6.0
Neomycin sulfate	3.7	Tetracycline hydrochloride	4.7
Oxytetracycline hydrochloride	4.3	Viomycin sulfate	2.7
Penicillin G, potassium	6.0	Zinc chloride	20.3
Penicillin G, sodium	6.0	Zinc sulfate	5.0
Pentobarbital sodium	8.3		

Adapted from "Tonicity, Osmoticity, Osmolality, and Osmolarity" (chapter 18), by C. Y. Poon, in Remington: The Science and Practice of Pharmacy, *21st edition (Philadelphia, PA: Lippincott Williams & Wilkins, 2006), pp. 250–265.*

CHAPTER NINE

Compounded Oral Solutions

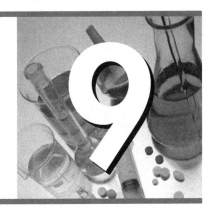

SOLUTIONS ARE THE MOST COMMONLY COMPOUNDED formulations. A solution is a clear liquid (but not necessarily colorless) in which a drug is completely dissolved. Solutions are homogenous, one-phase systems in which the solute is dispersed throughout the solvent in molecular or ionic-sized particles. Solutes include active drug components, flavoring or coloring agents, preservatives, viscosity agents, antioxidants, and buffering salts.

Water is the most common solvent for oral solutions. Other solvents seem to be desirable for use in oral solutions based on their physical properties, but their irritation or toxicity profile limits their usefulness. For example:

- Aromatic hydrocarbons can cause paralysis of the central nervous system and are irritating to the skin.
- Methyl alcohol is toxic.
- Butyl and amyl alcohols are irritating.
- Volatile ethers can paralyze the central nervous system and are irritating to mucous membranes.
- Ketones are mildly irritating.
- Low molecular-weight esters are irritating.

Thus, only a few solvents, such as glycerin, alcohol, and propylene glycol, are indicated for internal use.

Formulations and Routes of Administration and Formulations

For topical use, acetone, isopropanol, polyethylene glycols, saturated aliphatic hydrocarbons, ether, glyceryl esters of aliphatic acids, and various oils may be added to the list of acceptable solvents. Formulations used in the various routes of administration are given in Table 9.1.

The concentration of a drug in a solution can be expressed in many ways, including:

- Molarity (M)
- Normality (N)
- Molality(m)
- Osmolarity (Osmol/L)
- Units of potency/unit volume (I.U.)
- Weight/Unit Volume (g/L, mg/ml, etc.)
- Percentage strength (w/v, v/v, w/w, mg%, μg%, mcg%, etc.)

TABLE 9.1: FORMULATIONS USED IN VARIOUS ROUTES OF ADMINISTRATION

Enteral Route	Dosage Form	Parenteral Route	Dosage Form
Oral	Tablets Capsules Bulk Powders Solutions Suspensions Elixirs Syrups Emulsions	Intraocular	Solutions Suspensions Ointments Inserts
		Intranasal	Solutions Suspensions Sprays Aerosols
Buccal	Tablets Solutions		Inhalers Powders
Sublingual	Tablets Lozenges	Inhalation	Solutions Aerosols Powders
Rectal	Solutions Ointments Suppositories	Intravenous Intramuscular Intradermal }	Solutions Suspensions Emulsions
Parenteral Route	**Dosage Form**		
Subcutaneous	Solutions Suspensions Emulsions Implants	Dermal	Solutions Tinctures Collodions Liniments Suspensions Ointments Creams Gels Lotions Pastes Plasters Powders Aerosols Transdermal patches
Vaginal	Solutions Ointments Creams Aerosol foams Powders Suppositories Tablets IUDs		

- Ratio strength (1:1)
- Parts per million (ppm)
- Equivalent Weight (Eq, mEq)

Classification of Oral Solutions

Solutions intended for topical and parenteral administration are discussed in other chapters of the book. The discussion in the remainder of this chapter will concentrate on solutions intended for oral administration. Oral solutions are administered by the patient by placing a volume of the formulation in their mouth

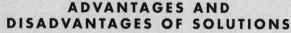

ADVANTAGES AND DISADVANTAGES OF SOLUTIONS

Advantages

- They enable completely homogenous doses.
- They are immediately available for absorption (i.e., short onset time).
- They can be used by most routes of administration.
- They can be taken or administered to patients who cannot swallow tablets or capsules.
- The doses can be easily adjusted.
- They are easy to administer.
- Their taste can be easily masked.

Disadvantages

- Drugs and chemicals are less stable when in solution than when in dry form.
- Some drugs are not soluble in solvents that are acceptable for therapeutic use.
- Drugs with objectionable taste require special additives or techniques to mask the taste when in solution.
- Solutions are difficult to handle, package, transport, and store because of their bulk and weight.
- Solutions in bulk containers require dosage measurement by the patient or caregiver.

and swallowing the contents. They are classified as aqueous, hydroalcoholic, and other non-aqueous solutions.

Aqueous Solutions

Aqueous solutions are the most prevalent of the oral solutions. A simple aqueous solution is made by dissolving a drug in water along with any necessary flavorings, preservatives, or buffering salts. Distilled or purified water always should be used when preparing compounded aqueous solutions. Additional chemical substances that can be dissolved in a solution include:

sweeteners	suspending agents
colorants	antioxidants
isotonicity adjustment agents	chelating agents
viscosity enhancing agents	emulsifying agents

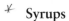 Syrups

A syrup is a concentrated or nearly saturated solution of sucrose in water and typically contains less than 10% alcohol. Syrups containing flavoring agents are known as *flavoring syrups* (e.g., Cherry Syrup, Acacia Syrup). *Medicinal syrups* are those that contain drugs (e.g., Guaifenesin Syrup). Syrups find widespread acceptance with patients because most are sweet and have a pleasing texture. Syrups can be the dosage formulation for a drug, or they can be used as an diluent in compounding a formulation.

When a reduction in calories or glucogenic properties is desired, syrups may be prepared from sugars other than sucrose (e.g., glucose, fructose), non-sugar polyols (e.g., sorbitol, glycerin, propylene glycol, mannitol), or other non-nutritive artificial sweeteners (e.g., aspartame, saccharin). The non-nutritive sweeteners do not produce the same viscosity as is obtained with sugars and polyols, so viscosity enhancers such as methylcellulose are added.

The polyols, though less sweet than sucrose, do produce favorable viscosity and in some solutions act as co-solvents and preservatives. A 70% sorbitol solution is commercially available for use as such a vehicle.

The two primary methods to make syrups are with or without heat. Using heat is faster, but it is not applicable to syrups with thermolabile or volatile ingredients. When using heat, the temperature must be controlled carefully to avoid the inversion of sucrose, which makes the syrup darker in color and more likely to ferment. When making syrups without heat, agitation is the energy source that effects solution. The sucrose should be placed in a vessel about twice as large as the final volume of the product to provide room for agitation.

Aromatic Waters

Aromatic waters are clear, saturated aqueous solutions of volatile oils or other aromatic substances (e.g., Peppermint Water, Stronger Rose Water). Used as flavoring or perfuming solutions, aromatic waters are made by dissolving the volatile substance in water. Many times a dispersant (usually 1–3 g of talc per 100 ml of solution) is used. The volatile substance is first mixed with talc, then the water is added and the mixture is agitated periodically over a period of time. Finally, the aromatic water is collected by filtration. The talc increases the surface area of the volatile substance that is exposed to the water, to facilitate saturation of the solution with the volatile substance.

Talc also is used as a clarification agent to remove excess volatile oil from a solution. When used in this manner, the aromatic water is made and then added to the talc. The mixture is agitated briefly, then filtered. The talc will remove the excess oil, which removes the haziness from the aromatic water.

Hydroalcoholic Solutions

Many oral solutions and almost all syrups are aqueous based, but a group of solutions termed hydroalcoholic contain both alcohol and water. This group of formulations includes elixirs, tinctures, spirits, collodions, liniments, extracts, and fluidextracts. The concentration of alcohol varies widely depending on the type of solution. Some elixirs have very little alcohol (5%–10%), while the spirits and fluidextracts have much larger concentrations of alcohol (approximately 60%–100%). Hydroalcoholic solutions have the advantage that they generally can dissolve more oil soluble drugs (or the free acid or free base form) compared to aqueous solutions, and they have some preservation capacity because of the presence of alcohol.

Elixirs

Elixirs are clear, sweetened, hydroalcoholic liquids intended for oral use. Because they are hydroalcoholic

AROMATIC ELIXIR	
Orange Oil	2.4 ml
Lemon Oil	0.6 ml
Coriander Oil	0.24 ml
Anise Oil	0.06 ml
Syrup	375 ml
Talc	30 g
Alcohol	
Purified Water aa qs	1,000 ml

solutions, they can be used to dissolve either alcohol soluble or water soluble drugs. Elixirs usually are less sweet and less viscous than syrups and tend to be less effective in masking taste. Their alcohol content ranges from 5% to 40% (10–80 proof), although a few commercial elixirs contain no alcohol. The concentration of alcohol typically is determined by the amount required to maintain the active drug in solution.

When compounding elixirs, the alcohol soluble constituents are dissolved in the alcohol portion and the water soluble constituents are dissolved in the water portion, then the aqueous solution is added to the alcohol solution with constant stirring. Adhering to this procedure will maintain the alcohol concentration as high as possible while the two portions are mixed. Adding aqueous solutions to elixirs sometimes causes turbidity as the alcohol concentration is diluted. Alcohol soluble drugs will precipitate out of the lower alcohol concentration.

Iso-Alcoholic Elixir is an elixir made by combining two other elixirs—Low Alcoholic Elixir and High Alcohol Elixir. Table 9.2 gives the alcohol strength of Iso-Alcoholic Elixir when different ratios of the other two elixirs are used. Table 9.3 gives formulas for Low and High Alcoholic Elixirs.

Several vehicles for oral solutions are available to the compounding pharmacist. Listed in Table 9.4 are official USP vehicles, nonofficial vehicles, and some common commercially available branded vehicles.

Spirits

Spirits, or essences, are alcoholic or hydroalcoholic solutions of volatile substances (usually volatile oils) with

TABLE 9.3: FORMULAS FOR LOW ALCOHOLIC AND HIGH ALCOHOLIC ELIXIRS

Low Alcoholic Elixir		High Alcoholic Elixir	
Compound Orange Spirit	10 ml	Compound Orange Spirit	4 ml
Alcohol	100 ml	Saccharin	3 g
Glycerin	200 ml	Glycerin	200 ml
Sucrose	320 g	Alcohol qs	1,000 ml
H₂O qs	1,000 ml		

TABLE 9.4: SOME VEHICLES FOR ORAL SOLUTIONS

Vehicle	pH	Alcohol Content (%)
Official USP/NF Vehicles		
Aromatic elixir	5.5–6.0	21–23
Benzaldehyde compound elixir	6.0	3–5
Peppermint water		0
Sorbitol solution		0
Suspension structured vehicle		
Suspension structured vehicle-SF		0
Xanthan gum solution		0
Nonofficial Vehicles		
Acacia syrup	5.0	0
Aromatic eriodictyon syrup	6.0–8.0	6–8
Cherry syrup	3.5–4.0	1–2
Citric acid syrup		< 1
Cocoa syrup		0
Glycyrrhiza elixir		21–23
Glycyrrhiza syrup	6.0–6.5	5–6
Hydriodic acid syrup		0
High alcoholic elixir	5.0	73–78
Low alcoholic elixir	5.0	8–10
Orange flower water		0
Orange syrup	2.5–3.0	2–5
Raspberry syrup	3.0	1–2
Sarsaparilla compound syrup	5.0	0
Syrup USP	6.5–7.0	0
Tolu syrup	5.5	2–4
Wild cherry syrup	4.5	1–2
Commercial Branded Vehicles		
Coca-Cola syrup	1.6–1.7	0
Ora-Sweet	4.0–4.5	0
Ora-Sweet SF	4.0–4.4	0
Syrpalta	4.5	0

TABLE 9.2: ALCOHOL STRENGTH OF ISO-ALCOHOLIC ELIXIR FOR COMBINATIONS OF LOW ALCOHOLIC AND HIGH ALCOHOLIC ELIXIRS

Low Alcoholic Elixir	High Alcoholic Elixir	Makes Iso-Alcoholic Elixir
Undiluted	None	0–10%
4 volumes	1 volume	10–20%
3 volumes	1 volume	20–30%
2 volumes	1 volume	30–40%
1 volume	1 volume	40–50%
1 volume	2 volumes	50–60%
1 volume	3 volumes	60–70%
None	Undiluted	70% or more

"Pharmaceutical Necessities," by E. A. Swinyard and E. A. Lowenthal, (chapter 6) in Remington's Pharmaceutical Sciences, 15th edition (Easton, PA: Mack Publishing Co., 1975), p. 1240.

Adapted from "Featured Excipient: Oral Liquid Vehicles," by L. V. Allen, Jr., International Journal of Pharmaceutical Compounding 5:65–67, 2001.

alcohol content ranging from 62% to 85% (124–170 proof). They are used most frequently as flavoring agents, such as Peppermint Spirit. Although some spirits are used for their medicinal effect, most are used as stock solutions as a convenient means of obtaining a proper amount of a flavoring oil. Because spirits have a high alcohol content, their addition to aqueous solutions will cause turbidity as alcohol soluble drugs or oils precipitate out of the diluted alcohol concentration.

COMPOUND ORANGE SPIRIT

Orange Oil	200 ml
Lemon Oil	50 ml
Coriander Oil	20 ml
Anise Oil	5 ml
Alcohol qs	1,000 ml

Tinctures

Tinctures are unsweetened alcoholic or hydroalcoholic solutions of nonvolatile substances prepared from vegetable or chemical substances. The concentration of solute varies up to 50%. Examples are Vanilla Tincture and Tincture of Iodine. Tinctures of potent drugs have 10 g of the drug in each 100 ml of the tincture; they are 10% tinctures. With a few exceptions, non-potent tinctures have 20 g of the drug per 100 ml of tincture.

Tinctures are prepared by percolation or maceration.

1. *Percolation* is the procedure of choice when the raw materials are moderately coarse powders or vegetable matter. The materials are packed loosely in a percolator (a narrow, cone-shaped vessel, open at both ends), and an alcohol or hydroalcoholic extracting solvent called the *menstruum* is poured through the material. The materials are dampened with the menstruum and allowed to stand for a short time before packing the percolator. This allows time for the materials to swell. If they were packed without the initial wetting, they would swell in the percolator so tightly that the menstruum flow would be blocked.

The menstruum then is added to cover the material, and the lower opening is closed just when the menstruum is about to drip from the percolator. This permits the air between the materials to escape as the menstruum descends through the percolator. The menstruum remains in contact with the material for a prescribed time, which allows the menstruum time to become saturated with the extracted drug.

Then the menstruum is allowed to flow out or percolate at a definite rate. Normally the percolate collected is assayed and the final volume is adjusted to the proper strength. The choice of menstruum depends on the solubility, stability, and ease of extraction of the desired drug substance. Other inactive constituents also are extracted, but if the materials are not objectionable, they are left in the solution.

2. *Maceration* is the method of choice for fine powders and plant exudates. The powder, or exudate, is soaked with the menstruum in a closed container, which prevents the loss of volatile constituents and the menstruum. The mixture is agitated frequently so the menstruum at the bottom of the container does not become saturated with the drug and become incapable of extracting any more drug from the powder.

Circulatory maceration is an efficient modification that eliminates the need for agitation. When heat is employed in maceration, the process is known as *digestion*. When maceration (or digestion) is complete, the mixture is filtered and the residue is washed with sufficient menstruum to bring the tincture to final volume.

Other Hydroalcoholic Solutions

Other hydroalcoholic solutions include:

- *Fluidextracts*—alcoholic solutions of vegetable drugs that contain 1 g of the drug in 1 ml of the extract. These are made by percolation.
- *Collodions*—liquid preparations containing nitrocellulose pyroxylin in a mixture of alcohol and ethyl ether. They are used as topical protectives or as a topical drug vehicle and are made "flexible" by the addition of castor oil. Examples are Flexible Collodion and Salicylic Acid Collodion.
- *Liniments*—solutions of various substances in oil, alcoholic solutions of soap, or emulsions intended for topical application, such as Ben Gay.

Other Non-Aqueous Solutions

Glycerins, or *glycerites,* are solutions composed of no less than 50% glycerin by weight and are extremely viscous. They are rarely used in practice, generally limited to use in topical products such as Glycerin Otic Solution. Oleaginous solutions are solutions of vegetable oils (e.g., corn, cottonseed, olive, peanut, sesame) or mineral oil. Table 9.5 lists several oleaginous solvents that could be used in non-aqueous solutions.

TABLE 9.5: OLEAGINOUS SOLVENTS USED IN NON-AQUEOUS SOLUTIONS

Substance	Specific Gravity	Substance	Specific Gravity
Alkyl (C_{12}–C_{15}) benzoate	0.915–0.935	Mineral oil, light	0.818–0.880
Almond oil	0.910–0.915	Octyldodecane	—
Corn oil	0.914–0.921	Olive oil	0.910–0.915
Cottonseed oil	0.915–0.921	Peanut oil	0.912–0.920
Ethyl oleate	0.866–0.874	Safflower oil	—
Isopropyl myristate	0.846–0.854	Sesame oil	0.916–0.921
Isopropyl palmitate	0.850–0.855	Soybean oil	0.916–0.922
Mineral oil	0.845–0.905	Squalane	0.807–0.810

Adapted from "Featured Excipient: Oleaginous Vehicles," by L. V. Allen, Jr., International Journal of Pharmaceutical Compounding 4:470–472, 2000.

Preservation of Oral Solutions

Oral solutions can support microbial growth, especially if sucrose is present—which is the case in many aqueous solutions. Therefore, preservation of these solutions becomes an item of consideration for the compounding pharmacist. One method of preserving a solution is simply to added a known preservative in the correct concentration. Because the formulation is a solution, the preservative must be soluble in the formulation. Common preservatives used in oral solutions and their concentrations are given in Table 9.6.

If the absolute alcoholic content is high enough in the formulation, the alcohol can act as the preservative without the need to add more preservatives. A minimum of 15% absolute alcohol is regarded as adequate to preserve products with a pH of 5, and 18% has been considered adequate for neutral or slightly alkaline preparations. Clearly, products such as tinctures, spirits, and some elixirs have alcohol concentrations that far exceed these values and require no other preservative.

Syrup USP, sometimes referred to as "Simple Syrup," is protected from bacterial contamination by virtue of its high solute concentration; it contains 850 grams of sucrose and 450 ml of water in each liter (85% w/v or 65% w/w). Although highly concentrated, the solution is not saturated. Because 1 gram of sucrose dissolves in 0.5 ml water, only 425 ml of water would be required to dissolve the 850 grams of sucrose. The slight excess of water (25 ml) enhances the stability of syrup over a range of temperatures by allowing for refrigeration without crystallization.

Thus, 65% w/w is the minimum amount of sucrose that will preserve the neutral pH syrup. If the pharmacist wants to formulate a syrup containing less sucrose, the quantity of alcohol to add as a preservative may be estimated by considering the "free water" equivalent in the syrup. To calculate the free water equivalent, the volume occupied by sucrose, the volume preserved by sucrose, and the volume occupied or preserved by other additives must be subtracted from the total volume of the syrup. In Syrup USP, 850 g of sucrose occupies an apparent volume of 550 ml, so each gram of sucrose will occupy 550/850, or 0.647 ml. If the 850 g of sucrose preserves 450 ml of water, each gram of sucrose will preserve 450/850 or 0.53 ml of water.

EXAMPLE: How much Alcohol USP is required to preserve 1L of a syrup containing 500 g sucrose?

Volume preserved by sucrose = 500 g × 0.53 ml/g = 265 ml

Volume occupied by sucrose = 500 g × 0.647 ml/g = 324 ml

Free water equivalent = 1,000 ml − 265 ml − 324 ml = 411 ml

Volume of absolute alcohol required to preserve free water equivalent = 411 ml × 18% = 74 ml

74 ml absolute alcohol ÷ 95% = 78 ml Alcohol USP

If other dissolved solids are present, their volume is subtracted from the free water volume. If glycerin is present, its volume is doubled and this figure is subtracted from the free water volume. If propylene glycol is present, it is considered equivalent to Alcohol USP.

Liquid Aliquot Method

A liquid aliquot technique can be used when a formulation calls for an amount of drug that is less than what can be weighed on the prescription balance with a 5% error (the least weighable quantity, L.W.Q.).

EXAMPLE: Prepare 100 ml of a solution containing 0.2 mg/ml clonidine.

In this formulation, 100 ml × 0.2 mg/ml = 20 mg of clonidine is needed. On a Class A prescription balance, 20 mg is less than the least weighable quantity. This problem is solved in the same way as the trituration aliquot method used with powders. A solution (generally aqueous or hydroalcoholic) is made using a weighable quantity of the drug (≥ least weighable quantity). Then an aliquot (or portion) of that solution is taken that will bring the required amount of drug to the final formulation.

Both the total volume of solution and the aliquot volume should be easily and accurately measurable. Some suggest that the volume be a whole number multiple of 5 ml. Consideration has to be given to the concentration of the solution. If the solution is highly concentrated and a small error is made in measuring the aliquot, a large error will occur in the quantity of drug brought to the

TABLE 9.6: CONCENTRATIONS OF PRESERVATIVES USED IN ORAL SOLUTIONS

Preservative	Concentration (%)
Alcohol, absolute	15–20
Benzoic acid	0.1–0.3
Benzyl alcohol	1–2
Methylparaben	0.05–0.25
Potassium sorbate	0.05–0.2
Propylene glycol	15–20
Propylparaben	0.02–0.04
Sodium benzoate	0.1–0.3
Sorbic acid	0.05–0.2

POINTS TO REMEMBER ABOUT PREPARING SOLUTIONS
OR
THINGS THEY DON'T TELL YOU IN THE BOOK

- Do not "QS" with the stirring rod in the graduate.
- Dissolve salts in a minimum amount of water before adding the viscous vehicle.
- Continue constant mixing/stirring when adding two liquids together.
- Observe the minimum measurable quantity in volumetrics and graduates.
- When pouring a cold liquid into a container for dispensing, affix the label first so it will stick; otherwise, moisture may condense on the outside of the container and the label will not adhere to the container.
- Minimize foaming by pouring down the side of the bottle, stirring gently, or by setting a glass rod across the opening of the container.
- Add high viscosity solutions to low viscosity solutions to make mixing easier.
- Watch the alcohol concentration and pH at all times.
- When filtering, know what is being retained and what is passing through.

final formulation. In these cases, larger volumes should be used for the solution.

The liquid aliquot method can be shown as:

$$\frac{\text{(A) Weight of drug in volume}}{\text{(B) Volume of solution}} = \frac{\text{(C) Weight of drug in aliquot}}{\text{(D) Aliquot volume}}$$

1. Select a suitable solvent based on drug solubility and stability, route of administration, and potential toxicity—usually water or alcohol.

2. Select the aliquot volume (D) in which the desired amount of drug (C) will be contained. This establishes the concentration of the solution to be prepared. This volume must be large enough to fully solubilize the drug but small enough so it does not exceed the total volume of the prescription. Clonidine solubility in water is 1 g/13 ml, so if 5 ml is selected as the aliquot volume, the concentration in that solution will be 20 mg/5 ml, or 4 mg/ml. Therefore, solubility will not be a problem in this aqueous solution.

3. Select the weight of drug in volume (A) to be equal to or greater than the least weighable quantity. Whenever practical, use the L.W.Q. quantity to minimize waste. Select 120 mg, as that is the L.W.Q. for a Class A prescription balance.

4. Calculate the volume of solution (B) to be prepared.

$$\frac{120 \text{ mg clonidine}}{\text{X ml solution}} = \frac{20 \text{ mg clonidine}}{5 \text{ ml aliquot}}$$

X = 30 ml

5. Prepare the solution that will contain 120 mg of clonidine in 30 ml of water. Remove a 5 ml aliquot from this solution, transfer the 5 ml to a final container, then add the appropriate vehicle to bring the formulation to its final volume.

Packaging

Because solutions are used for many different purposes and routes of administration, packaging materials to accommodate this wide diversity are required. They vary from simple prescription bottles, to sprays and nebulizers, to roll-on applicators, to parenteral containers such as vials and bags.

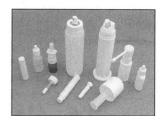

Observing Formulations for Evidence of Instability

The primary concern about oral solutions without preservatives is the potential for excessive microbial contamination and growth. Beyond use dating for aqueous solutions without preservatives is 14 days if stored at cold temperature.[1] Storage at cold temperature should retard bacterial growth. Microbial growth may be accompanied by discoloration, turbidity, or gas formation.

Another sign of solution instability is precipitation in a solution. Tinctures, fluidextracts, and similar preparations usually are dark in color because they are concentrated, and thus they should be scrutinized carefully for evidence of precipitation.[2]

NOTES

1. <795> Pharmaceutical Compounding—Nonsterile Preparations: The United States Pharmacopeia 29/National Formulary 24, The United States Pharmacopeial Convention, Inc., Rockville, MD, 2005, pp. 2731–2735.

2. <1191> Stability Considerations in Dispensing Practice: The United States Pharmacopeia 29/National Formulary 24, The United States Pharmacopeial Convention, Inc., Rockville, MD, 2005, pp. 3029–3031.

ADDITIONAL READING

Thompson, J. E. Solutions (chapter 26) in *A Practical Guide to Contemporary Pharmacy Practice*, 2nd edition. Lippincott Williams & Wilkins, Baltimore, MD, 2004, pp. 26.1–26.25.

CHAPTER TEN

Flavoring, Sweetening, and Coloring Oral Formulations

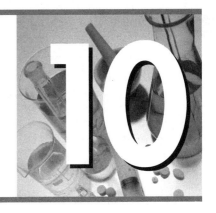

THE ELEMENTS OF FLAVORING, SWEETENING, AND coloring do not provide a therapeutic benefit to a formulation that is administered orally, but they do provide a psychological and medical benefit by increasing patient compliance. Most drugs have disagreeable tastes, and a formulation that is disagreeable in appearance and texture, as well as taste, will not encourage patient compliance. If the formulation can be made more attractive and palatable, and therefore more acceptable to the patient, compliance will be improved. The elements of flavoring, sweetening, and coloring are highly individualized and can be best determined for each patient through trial and patient feedback.

Flavoring

The human tongue contains about 10,000 taste buds, which distinguish salty, bitter, sour, and sweet tastes. The "taste sensation," however, is a complex combination of taste, smell, texture, appearance, and temperature. Most patients want

- immediate flavor identity
- rapid development of full flavor
- acceptable feel in the mouth
- brief aftertaste
- no undesirable sensations.

Tastes also are somewhat age-related. Children generally prefer sweet, fruity, and candy-like tastes and do not like bitter tastes. Adults tend to tolerate a reasonable level of bitterness or less sweet, tart, fruity flavors. For infants under 3–6 months of age, flavoring agents usually are unnecessary and are not recommended.

The length of time a flavor is needed in the mouth depends on the formulation used. For example, drugs in solution stimulate the taste buds immediately on contact, but the solution generally is in the mouth only a few seconds. Therefore, the flavoring time can be quite brief. Drugs in other dosage formulations (e.g., lozenges, lollipops, mouth washes) will have a much longer residence time in the mouth, so the flavor will have to be present over a longer time. Also, if the patient will be taking a medication over a longer period of time, milder flavors

are best, or rotating through a variety of flavors might be needed to avoid "flavor fatigue."

In addition to the active drug, formulation components may produce characteristic tastes or odors. As examples, alcohol has a biting taste and glycerin has a sweet taste. The preservative methylparaben has a floral, gauze-pad like aroma. Propylparaben—another preservative often used in conjunction with methylparaben—produces a numbing feel in the mouth. Menthol and mannitol impart a cooling sensation.

Definitions

Flavorings are mixtures obtained from natural and/or synthetic aromatic substances designed to impart a flavor, modify a flavor, or mask an undesirable flavor. Flavors are isolated by techniques such as

- steam distillation (mint and herbal oils)
- solvent extraction (vanilla and oleoresins)
- expression (citrus oils)
- supercritical fluid extraction.

Reactions also are used to obtain flavors—for example, the reaction of a sugar and an amino acid. Examples of flavors obtained by this method include chicken, cabbage, caramel, and fried potatoes.

Flavors can be obtained as oil soluble or water soluble liquids and as dry powders, of which most are diluted in carriers. Oil soluble carriers include soybean and other edible oils. Water soluble carriers include water, ethanol, propylene glycol, glycerin, and emulsifiers. Dry carriers include maltodextrins, corn syrup solids, modified starches, gum arabic, salt, sugars, and whey protein.

Three important definitions are associated with flavors:[1]

Natural Flavor:
Essential oil, oleoresin, essence or extractive, protein hydrolysate, distillate, or any product of roasting, heating or enzymolysis, which contains the flavoring constituents derived from a spice, fruit or fruit juice, vegetable or vegetable juice, edible yeast, herb, bark, bud, root, leaf or similar plant material, meat, seafood, poultry, eggs, dairy products, or fermentation products thereof whose significant function in food is flavoring rather than nutritional. [CFR 101.22(a)(3)]

Artificial Flavor:

> Any substance used to impart flavor that is not derived from a spice, fruit or fruit juice, vegetable or vegetable juice, edible yeast, herb, bark, bud, root, leaf or similar plant material, meat, fish, poultry, eggs, dairy products, or fermentation products thereof. [CFR 101.22(a)(1)]

Spice:

> Any aromatic vegetable substance in whole, broken or ground form, except those substances which have been traditionally regarded as foods, such as onions, garlic and celery; whose significant function in food is seasoning rather than nutritional; that is true to name; and from which no portion of any volatile oil or other flavoring principle has been removed. [CFR 101.22(a)(2)]

Some commonly used commercial designations are given in Table 10.1.

Choosing a Flavor

The chemical structure of a drug and its taste have some correlations. Low molecular weight salts tend to taste salty, whereas higher molecular weight salts tend toward bitterness. Nitrogen containing compounds, such as the alkaloids, tend to be quite bitter. Organic compounds containing hydroxyl groups are apt to become increasingly sweet as the number of OH groups increase. Organic esters, alcohols, and aldehydes are known for their pleasant taste and cooling sensation produced by their volatility.

Discovering the flavoring agent best suited to masking an unpleasant taste is often an empirical matter, but past experience is a good place to start. For basic tastes, the flavors in Table 10.2 have been found to work well.

In Table 10.3, suggested flavors are grouped by drug class.

TABLE 10.1: COMMON COMMERCIAL FLAVOR DESIGNATIONS

Flavor Designation	Components
Natural AA Flavor	All components derived from AA
	Exact composition is not known
AA Flavor—Natural and Artificial	At least one component derived from AA
	No definition of natural-to-artificial ratio
AA Flavor—with Other Natural Flavors (WONF)	All components natural
	At least one component derived from AA
Natural Flavor—AA Type	All components natural
	No components derived from AA
AA Flavor—Artificial Flavor	All components are artificial
Conceptual Flavors	May contain artificial flavors
	No reference point
	May only have to declare in ingredient declaration
Note: AA would be the flavor name, e.g., Cherry	

Adapted from "Flavors, Sweeteners, and Color," by L. V. Allen, Jr., (chapter 7) in The Art, Science, and Technology of Pharmaceutical Compounding, 2nd edition (Washington, DC, American Pharmaceutical Association, 2002), pp. 93–103.

TABLE 10.2: TASTES TO MASK AND SUGGESTED FLAVORINGS

Taste To Mask	Flavor
Salty	Cinnamon, raspberry, orange, maple, butterscotch, glycyrrhiza (licorice)
Sweet	Fruit, berry, vanilla
Bitter	Cocoa, chocolate, mint, cherry, walnut, glycyrrhiza (licorice), raspberry, tutti fruitti
Sour/Acid	Fruit, citrus, cherry
Oily	Wintergreen, peppermint oil, lemon, anise
Metallic	Mint, marshmallow

TABLE 10.3: DRUG CLASSES AND SUGGESTED FLAVORINGS

Drug Class	Flavor
Antibiotics	Cherry, maple, pineapple, orange, coconut-custard, strawberry-vanilla, banana-pineapple
Antihistamines	Apricot, cherry, cinnamon, grape, honey, lime, peach-orange, root beer
Barbiturates	Banana-pineapple, banana-vanilla, cinnamon-peppermint, grenadine-strawberry, lime, root beer
Decongestants and expectorants	Anise, apricot, butterscotch, cherry, grenadine-peach, strawberry, lemon, maple, orange, coriander, tangerine
Electrolyte and geriatric solutions	Cherry, grape, lemon-lime, raspberry, lime, root beer, strawberry

Commercial vendors market "flavoring systems" based on these suggested flavorings. Generally, the system involves a manual that contains the list of commonly formulated drugs. Each drug is accompanied by a list of suggested flavors that can be used for that formulation. The system also supplies flavoring agents in established concentrations so the recommendations in the manual are easy to apply to a formulation.

If pharmacists are willing to experiment with different flavors on their own, "model formulations" and starting percentages of flavors have been suggested (see Table 10.4).

Once a flavor has been selected, flavor intensifiers, such as monosodium glutamate, can be added as a flavor enhancer. Citrus enhancers include citric, maleic, and tartaric acids. Vanilla has long been used in the food industry as a flavor enhancer, as it seems to intensify and stimulate other flavors to a quicker taste response without altering their basic taste or adding its own taste.[2]

Techniques To Formulate More Appealing Solutions

In general, water miscible flavors are added to aqueous formulations and oil flavors are added to nonaqueous or fixed oil formulations. If an oil flavoring is to be added to an aqueous formulation, dissolve the oil flavoring agent in a small amount of glycerin, alcohol, sorbitol,

TABLE 10.4: FLAVORS, STARTING PERCENTAGES, AND MODEL FORMULATIONS

Type of Flavor	Starting Percentage of Flavor	Model Formulation
Water Soluble Flavors	0.2% of artificial flavor 1%–2% for natural flavor	Sweetened water containing 8%–10% sugar in water If using a fruit flavor, add 0.2%–0.3% citric acid to the above Sugar syrup, high-fructose corn syrup, corn syrup
Oil Soluble Flavors	0.1% of artificial flavor 0.2% for natural flavor	Powdered sugar and melted shortening mixed 1:1 Vegetable oil: mix flavor and taste: especially good for butter and nutty tastes
Powdered Flavor	0.1% of artificial flavor 0.75% for natural flavor	Fruit flavors: Sugar 98% and citric acid 2% If not using a fruit flavor, sugar

Adapted from "Flavors, Sweeteners, and Color," by L.V. Allen, Jr., (chapter 7) in The Art, Science, and Technology of Pharmaceutical Compounding, 2nd edition, (Washington, D.C., American Pharmaceutical Association, 2002), pp. 93–103.

or propylene glycol before adding it to the formulation. Some example fixed oils are cod liver oil, sweet oil, peanut oil, corn oil, mineral oil, sesame oil, and sweet almond oil.

Five techniques or methods of flavoring have been offered:[3]

1. *Blending* is the use of a flavor that blends with the drug taste. For example, drugs with acidic taste can be blended with citrus fruit flavors. Bitter tastes can be improved by adding a salty, sweet, or sour flavor.

2. *Overshadowing* (masking, overpowering) involves using a flavor with a stronger intensity and longer residence time in the mouth. Examples are wintergreen oil and glycyrrhiza.

3. *Physical* methods:
   - Render a drug tasteless by using an insoluble form of the drug; if the drug is not in solution, it may have no taste.
   - Make an o/w emulsion of an oily drug, and flavor/sweeten the external (aqueous) phase.
   - Dissolve the drug in an oil, and then make an o/w emulsion.
   - Use effervescent additives for salty-tasting drugs.
   - Use a high viscosity fluid such as a syrup; it keeps the sweet flavor in the mouth longer.

4. *Chemical* methods can overcome bad tastes by adsorbing, complexing, or making a prodrug of the drug, which eliminates the undesirable taste.

5. *Physiological* techniques:
   - Use anesthetizing agents such as menthol, peppermint, sodium phenolate, and spearmint.

- Use additives that cause a cooling sensation (e.g., mannitol, menthol).
- Use an effervescent formulation.
- Refrigerate the formulation; this reduces the intensity of the undesirable taste and anesthetizes the taste buds.

Stability

Not all drugs are stable in the presence of flavoring materials. Flavors are complex mixtures made up of many chemicals. For example, natural cherry flavor contains more than 70 components; artificial cherry flavor, more than 20; natural banana flavor has more than 150 components, artificial banana, more than 17; natural grape flavor has about 225 components, and artificial grape flavor has more than 18. Because each component is a chemical, it potentially may affect the stability of the active drug in the formulation. Flavors can degrade as a result of exposure to light, temperature, headspace oxygen, water, enzymes, contaminants, and other product components.

Role of Aroma and Texture

Although altering taste perception by masking unpleasant tastes with a flavoring agent is the major factor in producing palatable products, other factors contribute as well. *Aroma* (odor) is a strong determinant of taste perception. Many people are more sensitive to odors than to tastes, and the level of odor required by elderly people may have to be much higher than for young people.

The *scent* of any oral solution should be pleasant and should correlate with the flavor. The aroma of some volatile substances is caused by the warmth and moisture inside the mouth, so increasing the concentration of the volatile compound will produce a more pronounced odor.

Product *texture* also plays a role in taste perception and acceptance by patients. Viscosity seems to play an important role here. The characteristic viscosity of syrups seems to have a positive effect on patients' acceptance, whereas less viscous solutions may be perceived as "watered down" and more viscous solutions as unpleasant (slimy, gooey).

Most patients do not like gritty or chalky preparations. These types of formulations often are suspensions. The grittiness can be minimized by reducing the particle size. When preparing an oral solution from tablets or a saturated solution, filtering the solution will remove any insoluble tablet excipients or undissolved drug and reduce the grittiness. Viscosity is another important factor in suspension formulations.

There is also the challenge of minimizing the taste of a dosage form that remains in the mouth for an extended time, such as troches, lollipops, and gels. For the patient to accept them, these dosage forms also must have a smooth surface and texture that is not disagreeably sticky.

Sweetening

To increase desirability, sweeteners are

* colorless
* odorless
* soluble in water at the concentrations needed for sweetening
* pleasant tasting
* free from aftertaste
* stable over a wide pH range.

Several sweeteners have been used in oral solutions. Simple Syrup, 70% sorbitol solution, sodium saccharin (0.05%), Nutrasweet (0.1%), and dextrose have many of these desired properties. Table 10.5 gives sweetness levels of some common sweeteners as compared to sucrose.

TABLE 10.5: SWEETNESS LEVELS OF SELECTED SWEETENERS

Sweetener	Approximate Sweetness Compared to Sucrose (Times as Sweet)
Acesulfame potassium	200
Aspartame	200
Maltitol solution	75%
Mannitol	70%
Sorbitol	50%–60%
Saccharin	500
Sodium saccharin	500
Stevia	250–300
Xylitol	100% (same as sucrose)

When experimenting with the sweetness of a formulation that contains both a sweetening agent and a flavoring agent, modify the sweetener concentration before the flavoring agent concentration. All flavoring agents are bitter and require sweetening to make them more pleasing to the taste. If a desirable sweetness cannot be found by changing the sweetener concentration first, then experiment with changing the flavoring agent concentration.

Coloring Agents

Colors are substances added to a formulation for the sole purpose of imparting color. They are added to promote the patient's acceptance of a formulation via visual appeal. Coloring agents are not required in every formulation; and they are contraindicated in all sterile solutions. Clear, water-like oral solutions, however, may be perceived

to be inert or lacking potency. Dark colors such as dark purple, navy, black, and brown may be rejected because they are often associated with poisons. More pleasant, fruity colors generally are preferred and should be coordinated with flavors and scents (e.g., yellow with lemon, red with cherry). Flesh-toned colors should be added to topical preparations so the product is less visible on the skin.

Occasionally manufacturers resort to "visual distraction" as a means of enhancing palatability. For example, a particularly bitter drug might be formulated in a blue, peach-flavored, mint-scented vehicle. While the brain tries to reconcile the contradictions of a minty blue peach, the bitter substance has been swallowed. This approach probably is useless with young children who have not yet developed an expectation of color/aroma/taste correlation.

Colors used in pharmaceutical preparations are either natural colors or synthetic dyes. Natural colors include red ferric oxide, titanium oxide, and carbon black. The synthetic dyes are certified by the FDA and are:[4,5]

* FD&C dyes, used in foods, drugs, and cosmetics
* D&C dyes, used in drugs and cosmetics
* External D&C dyes, used in externally applied drugs and cosmetics.

From a practical standpoint, the pharmacist may consider the food colorings available in grocery stores to be safe and appropriate to use. These come in red, blue, yellow, or green aqueous solutions and are ideally suited to coloring aqueous solutions. Blends may be used to produce nearly any color.

Concentrations of dyes needed for coloring solutions are small—0.0005%–0.001%. Tints can be generated with concentrations of 0.0001%. It is probably prudent to make a stock solution of the dye and use a dropper or 1 ml syringe to measure the desired quantity. Also, physicochemical reactions with other formulation ingredients must be considered when choosing a colorant. Many dyes are salts of sulfonic acids and may be incompatible with large cationic compounds such as alkaloids. The pharmacist also should consider how pH changes or light exposure alters the color or stability of the product.

NOTES

1. Section IX, Compounding Supporting Information in USP Pharmacists' Pharmacopeia. The United States Pharmacopeial Convention, Inc., Rockville, MD, 2005, pp. 749–823.

2. Allen, L.V., Jr. Featured Excipient: Flavor Enhancing Agents. *International Journal of Pharmaceutical Compounding* 7:48–50, 2003.

3. Allen, L.V., Jr. Flavors, Sweeteners, and Color (chapter 7) in *The Art, Science, and Technology of Pharmaceutical Compounding*, 2nd edition. American Pharmaceutical Association, Washington, DC, 2002, pp. 93–103.

4. Rudnic, E. M., and Schwartz, J. B. Oral Solid Dosage Forms (chapter 45) in *Remington: The Science and Practice of Pharmacy*, 21st edition. Lippincott Williams & Wilkins, Philadelphia, PA, 2005, pp. 889–928.

5. Reilly, W. J., Jr. Pharmaceutical Necessities (chapter 55) *Remington: The Science and Practice of Pharmacy*, 21st edition. Lippincott Williams & Wilkins, Philadelphia, PA, 2005, pp. 1058–1092.

ADDITIONAL READING

Allen, L.V., Jr. Featured Excipient: Sweetening Agents. *International Journal of Pharmaceutical Compounding* 3:228–231, 1999.

Johnston, M., McElhiney, L. F., Pavlic, B., and Luke, R. Medication Flavoring (chapter 10) in *The Pharmacy Technician Series: Compounding*. Pearson Education, Upper Saddle River, NJ, 2006, pp. 135–145.

Kloesel, L. G. Sugar Substitutes. *International Journal of Pharmaceutical Compounding* 4:86–87, 2000.

Kloesel, L. G. Flavoring: Compounding a Treat. *International Journal of Pharmaceutical Compounding* 5:13–16, 2001.

CHAPTER ELEVEN

Colloids and Gels

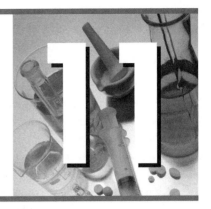

IN THE PREVIOUS CHAPTERS, SOLUTION FORMULATIONS were discussed. Solutions are liquids with molecular-size particles dissolved in a solvent. This chapter begins the discussion of *dispersed systems,* which contain an undissolved or immiscible drug distributed throughout a vehicle. Depending on the physicochemical properties of the *dispersed particles* and the *dispersion medium,* a dispersed system could be a colloid, gel, suspension, emulsion, lotion, cream, ointment, suppository, troche, or medication stick.

One of the important factors determining which type of dispersed system a formulation will be is the size of the dispersed particles. Of the dispersed systems that can be compounded, colloids and gels have the smallest-size particles. Colloids and gels will be discussed in this chapter. Other chapters in the book detail the other dispersed systems.

Colloids

Colloids are dispersed systems with particles ranging from 1 micron to 100 microns, although some texts will give the upper limit as 500 microns. Colloidal particles usually are larger than atoms, ions, or molecules, and generally consist of a single, large molecule of high molecular weight or aggregates of smaller molecules.

Several proteins and natural and organic polymers form colloidal dispersions (e.g., polysaccharides, polypeptides). Starch and cellulose are used as additives in many pharmaceutical formulations. Other polymers are used as coatings of solid dosage forms to protect drugs that are susceptible to moisture and degradation in the acidic environment of the stomach. Colloidal electrolytes are added to suspensions and emulsions to increase the stability and solubility of certain drugs. Colloids also are used as carriers for radiolabeled pharmaceuticals.

Colloids have more than one shape; they occur as globules, rods, flakes, threads, and branched rods and threads.[1] The shape and size of a colloid are important to properties such as flow, sedimentation, and osmotic pressure.

Some medicinal products have a greater therapeutic effect when they are formulated as colloids. Colloidal silver chloride, silver iodide, and silver protein are non-irritating bactericides, but these salts are irritating if they are not in a colloidal size. Colloidal copper and platinum are used in cancer chemotherapy, and colloidal gold is a diagnostic agent. Platinum has a strong catalytic effect only when it is in colloidal form, because it acts by adsorbing the reactants onto its surface.

Classification of Colloidal Systems

The dispersed phase of a colloidal dispersion may be classified as being either *lyophilic* (solvent-loving) or *lyophobic* (solvent-hating). If the solvent is water, these classifications are termed *hydrophilic* (water-loving) and *hydrophobic* (water-hating).

Molecules of a *hydrophilic colloid* have an affinity for water molecules in the dispersion medium and become hydrated when they are dispersed in water. Hydrated colloids swell and increase the viscosity of the system, thereby improving stability by reducing the interaction between particles and their tendency to settle. They also may possess a net surface electrical charge. The charge sign depends on the chemical properties of the colloid and the pH of the system. The presence of a surface charge repels other charged particles and thus reduces the likelihood that particles will adhere to one another and settle. Examples of hydrophilic colloids used in pharmacy are acacia, methylcellulose, and proteins, such as gelatin and albumin. Examples of other *lyophilic colloids* are rubber, cellulose, and polystyrene.

A *hydrophobic colloid* has little or no affinity for water molecules in the dispersion medium and produces no change in system viscosity. The particles may carry a charge, however, because of the adsorption of electrolyte ions from the medium. Hydrophobic colloids maintain their dispersion in the medium as a result of mutual repulsion of like charges and Brownian movement.

Charged particles may be neutralized by adding ions of the opposite charge to the dispersion medium. The neutralized particles, which have high surface free energy, cling together, resulting in a larger particle aggregate that can precipitate. Most important is the influence of the charge type and valence of the ions added to the medium. Their effect is summed up in the Schulze-Hardy Rule:

1. The effectiveness of an electrolyte in the medium is determined primarily by the nature of the ion opposite in charge to the colloidal particles; and

2. As the valence of this ion increases, the effectiveness of the electrolyte increases markedly. Thus, for a negatively charged hydrophobic colloid such as arsenous sulfide, aluminum chloride is about 10 times more effective than magnesium chloride, and 500 times more effective than sodium chloride in causing the colloid to precipitate.

Other examples of substances that form hydrophobic colloids in water are silver iodide, hydrated ferric oxide, sulfur, and gold.

Surface active agents sometimes are termed *association colloids*. These molecules consist of one region that is attracted to aqueous media and another region that is attracted to nonaqueous media. Their size is subcolloidal. They partition at/into surfaces and interfaces, and when the interfaces are saturated, they enter the bulk of the solvent phase and form *micelles*—aggregates of 50 or more single molecules. The size of a micelle is about the same size as a colloid particle.

The concentration at which micelles are formed is called the *critical micelle concentration* (CMC). Below the CMC, the surfactant remains at the surfaces and interfaces of particles as monomers. As the surfactant concentration increases, a saturation point is reached at the surface/interface with the monomers. Any further increase in the concentration causes the surfactants to aggregate in the dispersion medium as micelles. The surface and interfacial tensions decrease up to the formation of (CMC), and subsequently the tensions remain constant. Figure 11.1 illustrates the typical orientation of surfactants in a micelle.

The micelles formed in water are composed of monomers with the lipophilic portions of the molecules facing the inside of the micelle and the hydrophilic portions turned outward. In a nonaqueous dispersion medium, the micelles have a different orientation; the hydrophilic chains are turned inward and the lipophilic part faces the bulk of the medium.

Properties of Colloids

Among the several properties of colloid dispersions is the scattering of a light beam directed through the medium. This is known as the *Tyndall effect,* and its magnitude is a result of the size and number of particles present. When observed under ambient light, colloidal dispersions may appear translucent, opalescent, or cloudy, depending on the type of colloid and the extent of particle concentration and dispersion. The light-scattering effect of colloids can be used to determine the molecular weight, size, and shape of the colloids. Another property is known as Brownian movement, which results from the bombardment of the colloidal particles by molecules of the dispersion medium. Brownian movement usually is observed when particles are smaller than 5 microns in size.

The presence of a charge on the colloidal particles gives them electrical properties. When exposed to an electrical potential, colloids can be forced to migrate toward the electrode of opposite charge. Known as *electrophoresis*, it may be used to separate a mixture of colloidal substances such as proteins.

Colloids do not pass through a semi-permeable membrane. Thus, when a protein dispersion such as albumin is placed into a cellophane sac and submerged in water, water molecules will enter the sac to dilute the albumin molecules that cannot diffuse out. This principle explains the role of human serum albumin in maintaining the *osmotic pressure* of blood. The principle also is operational in the kidney, where ions and small molecules are filtered out of the blood across the glomerular membrane but the macromolecular serum proteins are retained. Sterilization of injections sometimes is performed by filtration through a synthetic membrane having a mean pore size of 0.22 microns. Colloidal injections may not be sterilized by this method unless the particles are smaller than this mean pore size.

Association colloids have the ability to increase the solubility of insoluble or poorly soluble compounds. If the concentration of the surfactant is at or above the CMC, the insoluble compound can be solubilized in the polar or nonpolar region of the micelle, depending on the properties of the insoluble compound. For example, nonpolar insoluble compounds in aqueous systems containing micelles formed by ionic surfactants will be positioned in the lipophilic center of the micelle. Solubilization of many insoluble drugs has led to increased absorption and bioavailability. Some drugs, however, may remain irreversibly bound to the surfactants in the micellar and may have decreased absorption and bioavailability.

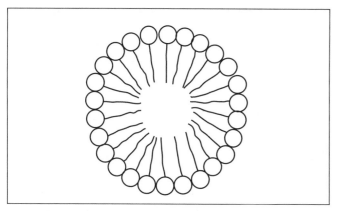

FIGURE 11.1: TYPICAL ORIENTATION OF SURFACTANTS IN A MICELLE

Stability of Colloids

Because a uniform dispersion of particles is important for the diagnostic and therapeutic effectiveness as well as the safe administration of pharmaceutical colloids, stability against settling or co-precipitation is an important consideration. The addition of a hydrophilic colloid to a hydrophobic colloid causes the hydrophilic colloid to adsorb onto and completely surround the hydrophobic particles. The hydrophilic colloid thus shields the hydrophobic system from the destabilizing effects of electrolytes in the medium. The hydrophilic colloid used in this manner is called a *protective colloid*. Stability of such a system is enhanced because to precipitate the hydrophobic colloid, both the protective solvent sheath surrounding it and the electric charge must be removed. Gelatin and methylcellulose derivatives are commonly used as protective colloids.

Sometimes in pharmaceutical formulations buffer salts are added to maintain a pH required for product stability. Occasionally such buffers may contribute to instability by forming insoluble salts with metallic ions. This problem may develop especially with phosphate buffers because most heavy metal phosphates are insoluble. If an insoluble phosphate salt precipitates from a colloidal dispersion, it may co-precipitate the colloidal particles along with it. To prevent this phenomenon, chelating agents may be used that will complex the metal ions preferentially, and thus prevent them from reacting with the phosphate. Another method to prevent this instability would be to substitute non-phosphate buffers for phosphate buffers when feasible.

Gels

Gels are considered colloidal dispersion because they contain particles of colloidal dimension. A gel, however, is composed of small inorganic particles or large organic molecules in which the particles restrict movement of the dispersing medium by forming an interlacing three-dimensional network of particles or solvated macromolecules. Physical or chemical cross-linking may be extensive. A gel may consist of twisted matted strands often wound together by stronger types of van der Waals forces to form crystalline and amorphous regions throughout the system.

Gels are made by using substances called *gelling agents*, which undergo extensive cross-linking or entanglement when dissolved or dispersed in the dispersing medium. This cross-linking increases the viscosity of the dispersing medium and also restricts its movement. If the gel contains small, discrete particles, the gel is called a two-phase system, referred to as a *magma* (e.g., milk of magnesia). Two-phase systems are *thixotropic*; i.e., they are semisolid on standing but liquefy when shaken.

Other examples include Aluminum Hydroxide Gel and Bentonite Magma.

If the gel does not appear to have discrete particles (i.e., no apparent boundary between the dispersed macromolecule and the liquid), it is called a one-phase system. Single phase systems contain linear or branched polymer macromolecules that dissolve in water and have no apparent boundary with the dispensing medium. These macromolecules are classified as natural polymers (e.g., tragacanth), semisynthetic cellulose derivatives (e.g., methylcellulose), or synthetic polymers (e.g., carbomer polymers). Single phase gels made from synthetic or natural macromolecules are called *mucilages*.

Gels are useful as liquid formulations in oral, ophthalmic, nasal, topical, vaginal, and rectal administration. Gels can be clear formulations when all of the particles dissolve completely in the dispersing medium, but this does not occur in all gels and some, therefore, are turbid. Patients prefer gels that appear clear, sparkle, are water washable, water soluble, water absorbing, and greaseless.

Common Gelling Agents

Of the many gelling agents, some of the more common ones are acacia, alginic acid, bentonite, carbomers (Carbopols®), carboxymethyl cellulose, ethylcellulose, gelatin, hydroxyethylcellulose, hydroxypropyl cellulose, magnesium aluminum silicate (Veegum®), methylcellulose, poloxamers (Pluronics®), polyvinyl alcohol, sodium alginate, tragacanth, and xanthan gum. Though each gelling agent has some unique properties, some generalizations can be made.

1. If the gelling agent is added to the dispersing medium too rapidly or haphazardly, the agent tends to "clump." The outer molecules of the gelling agent contact the medium first and hydrate, forming a layer with a gelled surface that is more difficult for the medium to penetrate. The clumps ultimately hydrate, but this takes more time (sometimes several days). Some compounding techniques that can be used to minimize this problem are to

   • sift the powders into the vortex of the rapidly stirring medium;

   • levigate the powder with a water miscible nonsolvent such as absolute alcohol or propylene glycol;

   • use a blender to mix the powder and solvent homogeneously.

2. Some gelling agents are more soluble in cold water than in hot water. Methylcellulose and poloxamers have better solubility in cold water, and bentonite, gelatin, and sodium carboxymethylcellulose are more soluble in hot water. Carbomers, tragacanth, and alginic acid gels are made with tepid water.

3. Some gelling agents (e.g., carbomers) require a "neutralizer" or a pH adjusting chemical to create the gel after the gelling agent has been wetted in the dispersing medium.

4. Most gelling agents require 24 to 48 hours to completely hydrate and reach maximum viscosity and clarity.

5. Gelling agents commonly are used in concentrations of 0.5%–2%, but some may be used up to 10%.

6. Adding the active drug while compounding the gel is easier than trying to add the drug to a gel that already has been formed.

Carbomers

Carbomer is a generic name for a family of polymers known as Carbopol®, first used in the mid-1950s. As a group, they are dry powders with high bulk density and form acidic aqueous solutions (pH around 3.0). They thicken at a higher pH (around 5 or 6). As they thicken, they also swell in aqueous solution as much as 1,000 times their original volume. Their solutions range in viscosity from 0 to 80,000 centipoise (cps). Some examples of this group of gelling agents are given in Table 11.1.

Carbomer polymers are best introduced into water by slowly sprinkling a sieved powder into the vortex created by rapidly stirring the medium. This should prevent clumping. Once all of the powder has been added, the stirring speed should be reduced to decrease the possibility of entrapping air bubbles in the formulation.

As mentioned, when the carbomer is dispersed, the solution will have a low pH. A neutralizer is added to increase the pH and cause the dispersion to thicken and gel. Some neutralizing agents are sodium hydroxide,

potassium hydroxide, and triethanolamine. If the inorganic bases are used to neutralize the solution, a stable water soluble gel is formed. If triethanolamine is used, the gel can tolerate high alcohol concentrations. The viscosity of the gel can be manipulated further by adding propylene glycol and glycerin (to increase viscosity) or by adding electrolytes (to decrease viscosity).

Cellulose Derivates

The cellulose derivatives (methylcellulose, hydroxyethyl cellulose, hydroxypropyl cellulose, hydroxypropylmethyl cellulose, and carboxymethyl cellulose) are commonly used. In addition to their unique properties, they have some commonalties:

• All of the cellulose derivatives except carboxymethyl-cellulose maintain the viscosity of the gel over a wide pH range (3–11). Carboxymethylcellulose can maintain the viscosity between pH 7–9; the viscosity decreases dramatically below pH 4 and above pH 10.

• The addition of salts to the medium reduces the ability of the cellulose derivatives to hydrate. Some derivatives are more sensitive to divalent and trivalent inorganic salts.

Methylcellulose 1500 cps

• Makes thinner gels with high tolerance for added drugs and salts.

• Is compatible with water, alcohol (70%), and propylene glycol (50%).

• Hydrates and swells in hot water. The powder is dispersed with high shear in about 1/3 of the required amount of water at 80°C to 90°C. Once it is dispersed, the rest of the water (as cold water or ice water) is added with moderate stirring.

• Obtains maximum clarity, hydration, and viscosity if the gel is cooled to 0–10°C for about an hour.

Hydroxethyl cellulose

• Makes thinner gels.

• Is compatible with water and alcohol (30%).

• Hydrates and swells in cool water (about 8–12 hours).

• Forms an occlusive dressing when lightly applied to the skin and allowed to dry.

Hydroxypropyl cellulose

• Makes thinner gels with high tolerance for added drugs and salts.

• Is compatible with alcohols and glycols.

• Hydrates and swells in water or hydroalcoholic medium. The powder is sprinkled in portions into water or hydroalcoholic medium without stirring and allowed to thoroughly wet (about 8–12 hours). After

TABLE 11.1: SELECTED CARBOMERS, THEIR VISCOSITY AND PROPERTIES

Polymer Name	Viscosity*	Properties
Carbopol® 910	3,000–7,000	Effective in low concentrations and provides a low viscosity formulation
Carbopol® 934	30,500–39,400	Effective in thick formulations such as emulsions, suspensions, sustained release formulations, transdermals, and topicals Forms clear gels with water
Carbopol® 934P	29,400–39,400	Same properties as 934 but intended for pharmaceutical formulations "P" = highly purified product
Carbopol® 940	40,000–60,000	Effective in thick formulations; very good clarity in water or hydroalcoholic topical gels Forms clear gels with hydroalcoholic systems
Carbopol® 941	4,000–11,000	Produces low viscosity gels, very good clarity
*0.5% solution, pH 7.5		

Adapted from "The Basics of Compounding: Compounding Gels," by L.V. Allen, Jr., International Journal of Pharmaceutical Compounding 3:385–389, 1999.

all of the powder is added and hydrated, the formulation can be stirred or shaken.

- Is a good gelling agent if 15% or more of an organic solvent is needed to dissolve the active drug.

Hydroxypropylmethyl cellulose

- Makes thicker gels but has a lower tolerance for positively charged ions.
- Is compatible with water and alcohol (80%).
- Disperses in cool water.
- Is a good gelling agent for time-released formulations.

Carboxymethyl cellulose

- Generally is used as the sodium salt.
- Makes thicker gels but has lower tolerance than hydroxypropylmethyl cellulose; maximum stability at pH is 7–9.
- Is compatible with water and alcohol.
- Disperse in cold water to hydrate and swell, followed by heating to about 60°C; maximum gelling in 1–2 hours.

Poloxamers

Poloxamers (Pluronic®) are co-polymers of polyoxyethylene and polyoxypropylene. They form reverse thermal gels in concentrations ranging from 15% to 50%. This means they are liquids at cool (refrigerator) temperature but are gels at room or body temperature. Poloxamer co-polymers are white, waxy granules that form clear liquids when dispersed in cold water or cooled to 0°–10°C overnight.

Pluronic® F-127 often is combined with a lecithin and isopropyl palmitate solution to make what is called a "PLO gel." The two components are made and stored separately. When it is time to compound a formulation, water soluble drugs are dissolved in the Pluronic® gel, or oil soluble drugs are dissolved in the lecithin solution. If a small quantity of formulation is to be made, each of the components is put into a syringe and the two syringes are connected by an adapter. The mixture is forced between the two syringes and the shear caused by passing the mixture through the adapter creates the PLO gel.

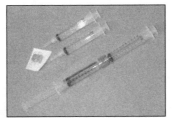

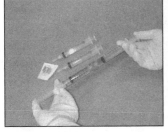

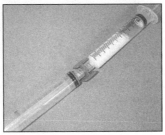

Packaging

Gels generally are stored in tight containers at refrigerated or room temperature. The tight containers can be tubes, jars, squeeze bottles, or pump dispensers. Some gels can be dispensed in applicators or syringes.

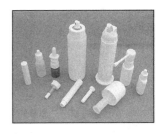

Observing Formulations for Evidence of Instability

Gels should be observed for shrinkage, separation of liquid, discoloration, and microbial contamination.[2] Preservatives are recommended for gels, because they neither inhibit microbial growth nor promote it. Depending on the concentration, some preservatives in the gel may make it cloudy in appearance. This results when the preservative is not being completely dispersed or it has formed aggregates that disperse light (see Table 11.2).

Because carbomer polymers are quite hygroscopic, they should be stored away from moisture. Moisture does not affect the efficacy of the polymers, but the high water content makes them more difficult to weigh accurately and dispense.

TABLE 11.2: COMMON PRESERVATIVES USED IN GELS

Preservative	Concentration (%)	Appearance
Benzalkonium chloride	0.01–0.1	clear – cloudy
Sodium benzoate	0.01–0.1	clear – cloudy
Methylparaben	0.18	clear
Propylparaben	0.02	clear
Thimerosal	0.01–0.1	clear

Adapted from "Gels," by L. V. Allen, Jr., (chapter 19) in The Art, Science, and Technology of Pharmaceutical Compounding, 2nd edition (Washington, DC: American Pharmaceutical Association, 2002), pp. 301–324.

NOTES

1. Martin, A. Colloids (chapter 15) in *Physical Pharmacy*, 4th edition (Philadelphia, PA: Lea & Febiger, 1993), pp. 393–422.

2. Basics of Compounding—Compounding Gels in *USP Pharmacists' Pharmacopeia*. The United States Pharmacopeial Convention, Inc., Rockville, MD, 2005, pp. 764–767.

ADDITIONAL READING

Allen, L.V., Jr. Featured Excipient: The Poloxamers. *International Journal of Pharmaceutical Compounding* 6:58–61, 2002.

CHAPTER TWELVE

Suspensions

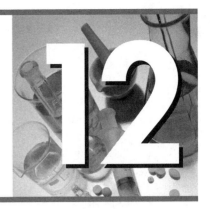

PHARMACEUTICAL *SUSPENSIONS* ARE COARSE DISPERSIONS consisting of a finely divided insoluble solid that is evenly dispersed (suspended) in a liquid (the dispersing medium). Suspensions are intended for oral administration as sweetened, flavored formulations or for topical application, in which case they are referred to as *lotions*. Suspensions also are used as non-sweetened, non-flavored formulations for many parenteral routes of administration (e.g., intraocular, intranasal, intravenous, intramuscular, intradermal, subcutaneous).

Suspensions are used when an oral or topical dosage form is needed and the active drug is not soluble in a solvent or the stability of the drug is poor in solution. *Gels, magmas,* and *mucilages* also contain suspended particles but are different from suspensions in that these dispersions create a three dimensional structure of inter-lacing particles or solvated macromolecules that restrict the movement of the dispersing medium.

Advantages of suspensions are the following:

- Some drugs are insoluble in all therapeutically accept-able solvents and, therefore, must be administered in another dosage form such as a tablet, a capsule, or a suspension. Because of their liquid character, suspen-sions represent an ideal dosage form for patients who have difficulty swallowing tablets or capsules. This factor is of particular importance when administering drugs to children.

- Disagreeable tastes can be masked in a suspension of the drug. Many drugs do not have a taste when they are formulated as the insoluble dispersed phase in a suspension.

- Drugs in suspension are chemically more stable than drugs in solution.

- Oral suspensions can be given for both systemic and local therapeutic effects. If the formulation is to pro-duce a systemic effect, the suspended particles will have to dissolve after administration so the drug can be absorbed into the circulatory system. The dispersed phase in suspensions used for local effects such as adsorption of excess gastrointestinal (GI) fluid (e.g., activated charcoal, kaolin) does not have to dissolve.

The disadvantages of suspensions are the following:

- The primary disadvantage of suspensions is their physical instability, or their tendency to settle over time, leading to a lack of uniformity of dose. This can be minimized by carefully formulating the suspension, and by shaking the suspension before administering each dose.

- The texture may be unpleasant to patients.

Formulating Acceptable Suspensions

A good pharmaceutical suspension must have these desirable properties:

- Should not precipitate rapidly, and if the particles settle at the bottom of the container, they should be redispersed by rapidly shaking the container.

- Should be of the correct viscosity to pour freely from bottles and/or to flow through an administration needle.

- If used in dermatology, the suspension must be suffi-ciently fluid to spread over the skin with no resistance and adhere to the skin after application.

The primary concern in formulating suspensions is that they tend to settle over time, leading to a lack of dose uniformity. The settling properties of a suspension are controlled by:

1. adding *flocculating agents* to enhance particle "dispersability"

2. adding *viscosity enhancers* to reduce the sedimenta-tion rate.

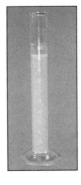

These two parameters have to be balanced. On one hand, the range of particles that might be dispersed has a lower limit of approximately 0.1 micron, but the upper limit (typically 0.5–3 microns) is dependent upon the combination of flocculating agents and viscosity enhancers used. On the other hand, the viscosity of the final product must allow the suspension to be easily poured and swallowed.

Flocculating Agents

Flocculating agents are electrolytes that carry an electrical charge opposite from that of the net charge on the suspended particles. At some critical concentration (experimentally determined), the flocculating agent negates the surface charge on the suspended particles and allows for the formation of *floccules* or clusters of particles. Because the floccules are aggregates of particles, they will settle faster than single particles. Floccules also assume the charge of the flocculating agent, so as they settle, they repel each other because of the surface charge, thereby preventing intimate contact between the floccules. This loose association of floccules keeps the suspension from *caking* and allows it to be easily redispersed when shaken. Floccules in well prepared suspensions are approximately the same size; therefore, a clear boundary is seen in the dispersing medium as the floccules settle.

The rate of sedimentation of a suspended phase depends on several factors that can be controlled by pharmaceutical manipulation. Many of these factors are empirically known:

- Light objects float and dense objects sink.
- Larger particles sink faster than smaller particles.
- Particles settle more slowly in a viscous liquid than in a less viscous liquid.

Assuming that all dispersed particles are of uniform shape and size and that the particles are sufficiently far apart so that the movement of one does not affect the movement of another particle, the rate of sedimentation can be estimated by *Stokes' equation:*

$$V = \frac{d^2(\rho_1-\rho_2)g}{18\eta}$$

where

V	= sedimentation rate (cm/sec)
d	= diameter of the suspended particles (cm)
ρ_1	= density of the suspended particles (g/cm^3)
ρ_2	= density of the dispersing medium (g/cm^3)
g	= acceleration of gravity (980.7 cm/sec^2)
η	= viscosity of the dispersing medium (g/cm sec)

Only dilute suspensions (0.5–2.0 g of solid material per 100 ml of suspension) will follow Stokes' equation. Most pharmaceutical suspensions are more concentrated, and the particles interfere with the movement of one another. But the Stokes' equation shows the pharmacist what factors can be altered in compounding the suspension to optimize the sedimentation process. If the particle diameter is reduced by trituration, the sedimentation rate will be retarded. This probably will be of little practical utility because most powders are supplied as fine particles and trituration will do little to further reduce the particle size. Selecting a micronized powder might be an option for some powders. Passing the solid through a 35–45 mesh sieve might be another option.

Viscosity Enhancers

The difference between the densities of the suspended particles and the dispersing medium can be decreased by increasing the viscosity of the dispersing medium. This is commonly done by adding sucrose, sorbitol, glucose, or glycerin to the dispersing medium. In a real, practical sense, then, the viscosity of the dispersion medium is the only other Stokes' equation variable that the pharmacist can change. Viscosity is increased by adding viscosity enhancers—sometimes called *suspending agents* or *thickening agents*—to thicken the dispersing medium, thereby reducing the sedimentation rate of the floccules.

In selecting viscosity enhancers, care must be taken, as many of these agents carry a net charge in solution, possibly negating the effects of the flocculating agent used. Viscosity enhancers also are used to enhance the stability of emulsions, altering the release rate of drugs at sites of application, and helping dermatological formulations adhere to the skin after application.

Ideally, a suspension should be rheologically *pseudoplastic*—it should have high viscosity at low shear rates (during storage) and low viscosity at high shear rates (during shaking, pouring, or spreading). Therefore, selecting a viscosity enhancer that has the desirable rheological properties allows the formulation to remain fluid long enough to be poured and spread. Table 12.1 shows some of the properties of commonly used viscosity enhancers.

Experimental Determination of an Acceptable Suspension

Several parameters are used to experimentally determine an acceptable suspension. Well flocculated suspensions have approximately equal floccule sizes, so sedimentation should be rapid and uniform. A clear boundary in the suspension should be evident as the suspended particles settle. If a suspension is not well flocculated, the suspended particles vary in size and will settle at different rates—larger particles more rapidly than the smaller ones. No clear boundary between the settling particles and the clear supernatant liquid will be observed, and the supernatant layer will remain turbid much longer.

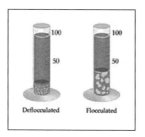

An acceptable suspension also should have a larger sedimentation volume. The floccules are not in intimate contact with one another, so there will be more room between the floccules and the entire settled mass will occupy more volume.

TABLE 12.1 PROPERTIES OF COMMONLY USED VISCOSITY ENHANCERS

Substance	Solubility*		Usual Suspension Concentration (%)	pH of Aqueous Solution (% solution)	Most Effective pH Range
	Water	Alcohol			
Acacia, NF	2.7	PI	5–10	4.5–5.0 (5%)	
Agar, NF	Swells	I	<1		
Alginic acid, NF	Swells	PI		1.5–3.5 (3%)	
Attapulgite, colloidal/activated	PI	PI		7.5–9.0 (5%)	6.0–8.5
Bentonite, NF	PI	PI	0.5–5.0	9.5–10.5 (2%)	>6
Carbomer 910, 934, 934P, 940, 941, 1342, NF	S	S	0.5–1.0	2.5–3.0 (1%)	6–11
Carboxymethylcellulose calcium, NF	I	PI	0.25–5.0	4.5–6.0 (1%)	2–10
Carboxymethylcellulose sodium, NF	S	PI	0.25–5.0	6.5–8.5 (1%)	2–10
Carrageenan, NF	1:100 +				
Cellulose, microcrystalline, NF	PI		0.5–5.0	5–7	
Microcrystalline cellulose and carboxymethylcellulose sodium, NF	S			6–8 (1.2%)	
Dextrin, NF	S	PI			
Gelatin, NF Type A	S	PI		3.8–6.0	
Type B				5.0–7.4	
Guar gum, NF	FS		2.5	5–7 (1%)	4.0–10.5
Hydroxyethyl cellulose, NF	S	PI	1.0–5.0	5.5–8.5 (1%)	2–12
Hydroxypropyl cellulose, NF	2.0	2.5		5–8 (1%)	6–8
Hydroxypropylmethyl cellulose, USP	S	PI	0.5–5.0	5.5–8.0 (1%)	3–11
Magnesium aluminum silicate, NF	PI	PI	0.5–10.0	9–10 (5%)	
Methylcellulose, USP	S	PI		5.5–8.0 (1%)	3–11
Pectin, USP	20.0	PI			
Poloxamer, NF	Varies	Varies	10–40	6.0–7.4 (2.5%)	
Polyethylene oxide, NF			1		
Polyvinyl alcohol, USP	FS		0.5–3.0	5–8 (4%)	
Povidone, USP	FS	FS	2–10	3–7 (5%)	
Propylene glycol alginate NF	S		1–5		3–6
Silicon dioxide, NF colloidal	PI	I	2–10	3.5–4.4 (4%)	1.0–7.5
Sodium alginate, NF	S	PI	1–5	7.2 (1%)	4–10
Tragacanth, NF	PI	PI		5–6 (1%)	4–8
Xanthan gum, NF	S	PI	1–2	6–8 (1%)	3–12

* ml required to dissolve 1 g of material: + hot water

PI = practically insoluble   I = insoluble   S = soluble   FS = freely soluble

Adapted from "Featured Excipient: Viscosity Increasing Agents for Aqueous Systems," by L. V. Allen, Jr., International Journal of Pharmaceutical Compounding 3:479–486, 1999.

Table 12.2 presents experimental data of suspensions containing 4% bismuth subnitrate in varying concentrations of monobasic potassium phosphate. The Sedimentation Rate of each suspension was determined by measuring the time needed to fall successive 10 ml marks in a graduated cylinder, and then graphically determining the slope of the line.

The Final Volume was the volume occupied by settled bismuth subnitrate after 3–4 days. When there was no evidence that sedimentation was complete, the value "zero" was used. The Sedimentation Volume was calculated as the volume occupied by bismuth subnitrate divided by 100 ml (which was the original volume occupied by bismuth subnitrate). The greatest flocculation coincides with the maximum Sedimentation Volume. The Degree of Flocculation is the ratio of the Sedimentation Volume of each cylinder divided by the smallest Sedimentation Volume of all the cylinders.

The Ease of Redispersion was determined by counting the number of inversions necessary to resuspend the settled material off the bottom of the graduated cylinder.

When plotting the Sedimentation Volume and Sedimentation Rate as a function of the logarithmic value of

KH$_2$PO$_4$ (%)	Sedimentation Rate (ml/sec)[1]	Final Volume (ml)[2]	Sedimentation Vol.[3]	Degree of Flocculation[4]	Ease of Redispersion[5]
0.00	Too slow to measure	0	—	—	Caked
0.01	Too slow to measure	0	—	—	10
0.05	1.64	7	0.07	2.3	8
0.10	1.91	6	0.06	2.0	4
0.50	0.98	6	0.06	2.0	3
1.0	1.12	5	0.05	1.7	12
5.0	0.49	3	0.03	1.0	25

1. Sedimentation Rate—calculated from slopes of graphs
2. Final volume—sedimentation volume in graduated cylinder after 24 hours
3. Sedimentation volume = $\dfrac{\text{final volume of sediment}}{\text{original volume of suspension}}$
4. Degree of flocculation = β = $\dfrac{\text{sedimentation volume of suspension}}{\text{sedimentation volume of most deflocculated suspension}}$
5. Number of inversions needed to resuspend sediment off the bottom of the graduated cylinder

the electrolyte concentration, it can been seen that the range of electrolyte concentration between 0.05% and 0.1% produced suspensions with the faster sedimentation rates and larger sedimentation volumes. These electrolyte concentrations also had the highest Degree of Flocculation and showed the greatest ease of redispersion. Therefore, electrolyte concentrations between 0.05% and 0.1% produced the most acceptable suspension.

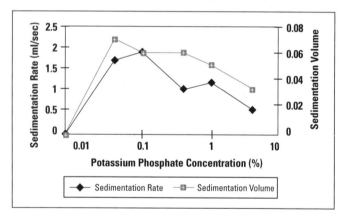

Table 12.3 summarizes the important comparisons between a flocculated and a deflocculated system.

TABLE 12.3: COMPARISON BETWEEN FLOCCULATED AND DEFLOCCULATED SYSTEMS

Variable	Flocculated	Deflocculated
Sedimentation rate (comparative)	Rapid	Slower
Presence of distinct boundary during sedimentation	Distinct boundary	No distinct boundary
Ultimate sediment volume (comparative)	Relatively large	Relatively small
Ease of redispersion	Redisperses easily, little or no caking	Does not redisperse easily; cakes

Wetting Particles

Powders that are going to be incorporated into a suspension have to be "wetted" before they are included in the formulation, to ensure a more uniform dispersion of particles. If the particles have air, grease, dirt, or other contaminates on their surface, they will not be wetted in the suspension and will float on the surface even if they are very dense.

Hydrophilic powders (e.g., ZnO, MgCO$_3$, talc) can be wetted with water or other polar liquids (e.g., alcohol, glycerin) using a mortar and pestle. Hydrophobic powders (e.g., sulfur, charcoal) also are wetted with alcohol or glycerin, or with a nonpolar liquid such as mineral oil. Only the minimal amount of any wetting agent should be used.

Sometimes a surfactant is needed to ensure sufficient wetting. Surfactants lower the interfacial tension between solid particles and a liquid. As the tension is lowered, contaminants on the surface of the particles are removed and wetting is enhanced. Surface active agents that induce wettability are called wetting agents, and their HLB values are between 7 and 9. Table 12.4 shows the solubility of some surfactants used as wetting agents in water and alcohol.

Packaging

Suspensions should be packaged in tight containers that have an opening large enough to pour a viscous liquid easily. Sufficient headspace should be allowed for ease of shaking. The containers should be stored at room temperature or refrigerated, depending on the physico-chemical characteristics of the ingredients. The instruction "Shake well before using" or "Shake well before taking" always should appear on the label. A label also

TABLE 12.4: SOLUBILITY OF SURFACTANTS IN WATER AND ALCOHOL

Surfactant	Solubility	
	Water	Alcohol
Benzalkonium chloride, NF	VS	VS
Benzethonium chloride, USP	S	S
Cetylpyridinium chloride, USP	VS	VS
Docusate sodium, USP	SS	FS
Nonoxynol 9, USP	S	S
Octoxynol 9, NF	M	M
Polaxamer 124, NF	FS	FS
Poloxamers 188, 237, 338, and 407, NF	FS	FS
Polyoxyl 35 castor oil, NF	VS	S
Polyoxyl 40 hydrogenated castor oil, NF	VS	S
Polyoxyl 10 oleyl ether, NF	S	S
Polyoxyl 20 cetostearyl ether, NF	S	S
Polyoxyl 40 stearate, NF	S	S
Polysorbate 20, NF	S	S
Polysorbate 40, NF	S	S
Polysorbate 60, NF	S	
Polysorbate 80, NF	VS	S
Sodium lauryl sulfate, NF	FS	
Sorbitan monolaurate, NF	I	
Sorbital monooleate, NF	I	
Sorbitan monopalmitate, NF	I	
Tyloxapol, USP	M	

VS = very soluble   S = soluble   I = insoluble
FS = freely soluble   SS = sparingly soluble   M = miscible

Adapted from "Featured Excipient: Wetting and/or Solubilizing Agents," by L.V. Allen, Jr., International Journal of Pharmaceutical Compounding 5:310–312, 2001.

should be affixed to specify whether the medications are for internal or external use.

Observing Formulations for Evidence of Instability

The USP/NF chapter <1191> states that the major sign of suspension instability is "a caked solid phase that cannot be resuspended by a reasonable amount of shaking." The presence of caking would mean that the suspension is no longer flocculated. Another sign of instability is the presence of relatively large particles which suggest that there is excessive crystal growth.

Because suspensions are also liquid dosage forms, the concern about excessive microbial contamination and growth would be applicable to these formulations.[1] The reference also reminds pharmacists that "instabilities may be indicated by cloudiness or precipitation in a solution, and that microbial growth may be accompanied by discoloration, turbidity, or gas formation."

NOTES

1. <1191> Stability Considerations in Dispensing Practice: The United States Pharmacopeia 29/National Formulary 24, The United States Pharmacopeial Convention, Inc., Rockville, MD, 2005, pp. 3029–3031.

ADDITIONAL READING

Allen, L.V., Jr. Basics of Compounding: Suspensions. *International Journal of Pharmaceutical Compounding* 5:294–297, 2001.

Allen, L.V., Jr. Quality Control Analytical Methods: Viscosity Measurement. *International Journal of Pharmaceutical Compounding* 7:305–309, 2003.

CHAPTER THIRTEEN

Emulsions

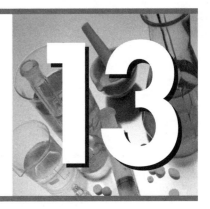

W E HAVE ALL HEARD THAT "OIL AND WATER DON'T mix." Yet, many times the pharmacist is required to prepare a formulation that contains both oleaginous and aqueous components. These two immiscible components can be formulated into an elegant product when "emulsified" using an emulsifying agent. One of the components (aqueous or oleaginous) will be intimately dispensed in the other component in the form of "droplets" or "globules" about 0.1–10 microns in size.

Actually, there is a fourth component, but it is not a chemical. It is energy. Energy must be infused into the system to make the three other ingredients come together and form an emulsion. The energy can be supplied by:

- triturating the ingredients in a mortar with a pestle,
- heating the ingredients,
- shaking the ingredients in a bottle,
- extruding the ingredients through a small orifice of an homogenizer, or
- mechanically blending the ingredients with a high speed mixer or blender.

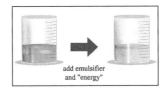

add emulsifier and "energy"

Therefore, an emulsion is a formulation consisting of an emulsifying agent and at least two immiscible liquids, one of which is dispersed throughout the other in the form of small droplets. The dispersed liquid is known as the *internal or discontinuous phase*, whereas the dispersion medium is known as the *external or continuous phase*. When oils, petroleum hydrocarbons, or waxes are the dispersed phase and water or an aqueous solution is the continuous phase, the system is called an *oil-in-water (o/w) emulsion*. An o/w emulsion generally is formed if the aqueous phase constitutes >45% of the total weight and a hydrophilic emulsifier is used. Conversely, when water or aqueous solutions are dispersed in an oleaginous medium, the system is known as a *water-in-oil (w/o) emulsion*. W/O emulsions generally are formed if the aqueous phase constitutes <45% of the total weight and a lipophilic emulsifier is used.

Emulsions are used in many routes of administration. Emulsions that are administered orally are o/w emulsions,

but patients generally object to the oily feel of emulsions in the mouth. Sometimes, though, oral emulsions are the formulation of choice to mask the taste of a bitter drug or when the oral solubility or bioavailability of a drug is to be increased dramatically.

Also, emulsions can be used as lotions and creams, and as ointment bases, and they can be used in parenteral nutrition therapy. More typically, emulsions are used for topical administration. *Lotions* are fluid emulsions for external application (some lotions actually are suspensions rather than emulsions). Lotions most often are applied to intertriginous areas—places where skin rubbing occurs, as between fingers and thighs, under the arms—because they have a lubricating effect. Although "lotion" is not an official term, it is used most often to describe these types of fluid liquids intended for topical use.

Creams are opaque, soft solids, or thick liquids intended for external application, consisting of medicaments dissolved or suspended in a water removable or emollient base. They can be either o/w or w/o. Creams have the added feature that they tend to "vanish" or disappear with rubbing. Lotions often can be prepared from creams (oil/water creams) by diluting the cream with water or an aromatic water such as rose water. The water should be added slowly to the cream, while stirring continuously.

W/O emulsions used as *ointment bases* tend to be immiscible in water, are not water washable, will not absorb water, are occlusive, and may be "greasy." This is primarily because oil is the external phase and oil repels any of the actions of water. These ointment bases are occlusive; the oil will not allow water to evaporate from the surface of the skin. Conversely, o/w emulsions are miscible with water, are water washable, will absorb water, are nonocclusive, and are nongreasy. Here, water is the external phase and will associate readily with any other water molecules that are present.

The consistency of emulsions varies from easily pourable liquids to semisolid creams and ointments. A major contributor to the final consistency of an emulsion is the amount of solidified material contained in the final formulation. Many ointments, creams, and lotions start with an emulsion base, but excess material or other solid components may be present as a micronized solid in the emulsion formulation. Therefore, the final consistency of an emulsion depends upon:

- the ratio of internal phase volume to external phase volume
- the phase in which the solid materials are located
- what the solid materials are.

As an example, *stearic acid creams* (sometimes called vanishing creams) are o/w emulsions and have a semisolid consistency but are only 15% internal phase volume. Other emulsion creams have internal phases that account for 40%–50% of the total volume of the formulation. Any semisolid character with w/o emulsions generally is attributable to a semisolid external phase.

Stability

Emulsions are thermodynamically unstable and tend to separate into two distinct phases over time. The separation can be a mark of instability.

Levels of Instability

The three levels of instability are:

1. *Creaming* occurs when dispersed droplets merge and rise to the top or fall to the bottom of the emulsion. This results in a lack of uniformity of drug distribution and a product that is not appealing to the sight. Creaming in o/w emulsions is characterized most often by the oil globules gathering and rising to the top, because the oil generally is less dense than the water phase. Creaming is easily reversible, and the product can be evenly redistributed by shaking. It is reversible because the dispersed globules still have a protective film around them which prevents coalescence.

2. *Coalescence*, or breaking, is an irreversible process because the film surrounding the individual droplets has been destroyed. Viscosity alterations may help to stabilize the droplets and minimize a tendency to coalescence. Using an optimum phase:volume ratio may also help stabilize the emulsion against coalescence. The phase:volume ratio is the ratio of the internal volume to the total volume of the product.

3. *Phase inversion* is a change in the type of emulsion and is considered a sign of instability, particularly if the inversions occur unintentionally and occur after the product has been formulated.

Increasing the Stability of an Emulsion

The stability of an emulsion can be enhanced in several ways:

a. use the optimum phase:volume ratio,

b. reduce the globule size of the internal phase,

c. increase the viscosity of the external aqueous phase,

d. adjust the densities of both the internal phase and the external phase so the densities are the same.

The maximum phase:volume ratio that can be achieved in an emulsion, assuming perfectly spherical particles, is 74%. But in general, a phase:volume ratio of about 50%, which approximates the loose packing of spherical particles (i.e., a porosity of 48% of the total bulk volume of a powder), results in a reasonably stable emulsion. Changing the phase:volume ratio is not always possible because it is determined by the concentration of the active ingredient and the volume of ingredient needed to either dissolve the active ingredient or form the emulsion base. Another consideration is that as the percentage of the internal phase increases, the viscosity of the formulation also will increase.

Reducing the globule size can be done with a mortar and pestle or a homogenizer. If the droplet size is reduced to less than 5 microns, the stability generally will increase. In some cases, though, the stability is not increased. The distribution of the droplet sizes also plays a part in emulsion stability. If the dispersion consists of nonuniform droplets, the smaller droplets will position themselves between larger ones and may facilitate coalescence.

Increasing the viscosity of the external phase tends to enhance the stability of the emulsion. This is accomplished by adding a substance that is soluble in or miscible with the external phase. For o/w emulsions, hydrocolloids can be used. For w/o emulsions, waxes and viscous oils, as well as fatty alcohols and fatty acids, can be used.

The Stokes' equation is generally applied to the sedimentation rate of particles in suspension. But it does show a variable that can be applied to emulsions. Sedimentation will occur if there is a difference in the densities of the suspended particle and the dispersing medium. Adjusting the density of the internal phase to approximate the external phase density will reduce the tendency of either phase to separate (either settle or rise) from the other phase.

Emulsifying Agents

Emulsions are formed by adding an emulsifier or emulsifying agents. All emulsifying agents concentrate at and are adsorbed onto the oil:water interface to provide a protective barrier around the dispersed droplets. In addition to this protective barrier, emulsifiers stabilize the emulsion by reducing the interfacial tension of the system. Some agents also enhance stability by imparting a charge on the droplet surface, thereby reducing the physical contact between the droplets and decreasing the potential for coalescence.

Emulsifying agents can be classified according to: (1) chemical structure, or (2) mechanism of action. Classes according to chemical structure are:

- synthetic
- natural
- finely dispersed solids
- auxiliary agents.

Classes according to mechanism of action are:

- surface active agents (adsorb at the oil/water interface forming a monomolecular layer),
- hydrophilic colloids (form multimolecular layers at the interface),
- finely divided solid particles (adsorb at the interface and form a layer of particles around the droplets).

Regardless of their classification, all emulsifying agents must be chemically stable in the system, be chemically nonreactive with other emulsion components, and be nontoxic and nonirritating. They also should be reasonably odorless and not cost prohibitive.

Synthetic Emulsifying Agents

The synthetic emulsifying agents are predominately *surfactants*—compounds that move to a liquid:liquid interface, thereby creating a higher concentration at the interface compared to the bulk of the liquid. This reduces the surface/interfacial tension of the system. These agents have both a hydrophilic (e.g., carboxyl, hydroxyl, amino groups) and a lipophilic part (e.g., alkyl chain) in their chemical structure. Surfactants can be classified based on the properties of the hydrophilic part of their structure as anionic, cationic, and nonionic. Examples and uses of these surfactants are shown in Table 13.1.

Anionic surfactants are soaps and detergents. Because soaps are subject to hydrolysis, they are less desirable than the more stable detergents. These surface active agents contain carboxylate, sulfate, and sulfonate groups. The carboxylate surfactants have a tendency to undergo hydrolysis

and decompose. Therefore, the long alkyl sulfates typically are used as surfactants, of which sodium lauryl sulfate is probably the best known. The long alkyl chain sulfonates also are used because the sulfonate ion is less susceptible to hydrolysis. An example is sodium bis-(2-ethylhexyl) sulfosuccinate (Aerosol OT or docusate sodium).

Cationic surfactants, used as bactericidal agents, are long chain amino and quaternary ammonium salts. Cationic and anionic emulsifiers are used in topical o/w emulsions, with cationic agents used less frequently than anionic agents.

Nonionic surfactants are the most frequently used of all the surfactants. They are superior in compatibility, stability, and lack of toxicity because they have a neutral pH and resist the addition of acids and electrolytes. They are divided into those that are more hydrophobic (not water insoluble) and hydrophilic (relatively water soluble). The more hydrophobic group is composed of long chain fatty acids, fatty alcohols, glycerin esters, and fatty acid esters of alcohols and acids. Surfactants in the hydrophilic group have an ether linkage between two alcoholic groups. The most commonly used compounds of this class are the polyoxyethylene sorbitan fatty acid esters.

Natural Emulsifying Agents

Various emulsifiers are natural products derived from plant or animal sources. Most of these emulsifiers form a hydrated lyophilic colloid called a *hydrocolloid*, which forms multimolecular layers around the emulsion droplets. These hydrocolloid-type emulsifiers have little or no effect on interfacial tension, but they do exert a protective colloid effect and reduce the potential for coalescence by

- providing a protective sheath around the droplets,
- imparting a charge to the dispersed droplets (so they repel each other), and
- swelling to increase the viscosity of the system (so droplets are less likely to merge).

The hydrocolloid emulsifiers may be classified as:
- vegetable derivatives: acacia, tragacanth, agar, pectin, carrageenan
- animal derivatives: gelatin, lanolin, cholesterol, lecithin
- semi-synthetic agents: methylcellulose, carboxymethylcellulose
- synthetic agents: Carbopols®.

Vegetable hydrocolloids have the advantages of being inexpensive, easy to handle, and nontoxic. Their disadvantage is that they require relatively large quantities to be effective as emulsifiers and they are subject to microbial growth, so their formulations require a preservative. Vegetable derivatives generally are limited to use as o/w emulsifiers. Once their multimolecular film is

TABLE 13.1: USES AND EXAMPLES OF SURFACTANTS

Classification	Examples	Uses
Anionic	Alkali soaps (sodium or potassium oleate)	Soaps, detergents
	Amine soaps (triethanolamine stearate)	
	Detergents (sodium lauryl sulfate, sodium dioctyl sulfosuccinate, sodium docusate)	
Cationic	Benzalkonium chloride	Bactericidal agents
	Benzethonium chloride	
Nonionic	Sorbitan esters (Spans®)	Neutral pH, resistant to added acids and electrolytes
	Polyoxyethylene derivatives of sorbitan esters (Tweens®)	
	Glyceryl esters	

formed around the droplets, however, they are resistant to coalescence. The stability of o/w emulsions using hydrocolloids is a result largely of the increase in viscosity of the external phase, which reduces movement of the droplets in the internal phase.

The *animal derivatives* generally form w/o emulsions. Lecithin and cholesterol form a monomolecular layer around the emulsion droplet instead of the typical multimolecular layers. Cholesterol is a major constituent of wool alcohols; it gives lanolin the capacity to absorb water and form a w/o emulsion. Lecithin (a phospholipid derived from egg yolk) produces o/w emulsions because of its strong hydrophilic character. Animal derivatives are more likely to cause allergic reactions and are subject to microbial growth and rancidity. Their advantage is in their ability to support the formation of w/o emulsions.

Semi-synthetic agents are stronger emulsifiers, are nontoxic, and are less subject to microbial growth. *Synthetic hydrocolloids* are the strongest emulsifiers, are nontoxic, and do not support microbial growth, but their cost may be prohibitive. These synthetic agents generally are limited to use as o/w emulsifiers.

Finely Divided or Dispersed Solid Particle Emulsifiers

Dispersed solid particle emulsifiers form a particulate layer around the dispersed particles. Most will swell in the dispersion medium to increase viscosity and reduce the interaction between the dispersed droplets. Although most of these agents support the formation of o/w emulsions, some may support w/o emulsions. Members of this class of emulsifiers include bentonite, Veegum®, magnesium hydroxide, aluminum hydroxide, and magnesium trisilicate.

Auxiliary Emulsifying Agents

A variety of fatty acids (e.g., stearic acid), fatty alcohols (e.g., stearyl or cetyl alcohol), and fatty esters (e.g., glyceryl monostearate) stabilize emulsions by thickening the formulation. Because these agents have only weak emulsifying properties, they always are used in combination with other emulsifiers.

The Hydrophile–Lipophile Balance (HLB) System

A system was developed to assist in making systematic decisions about the amounts and types of surfactants needed in stable products. The system, called the HLB (hydrophile–lipophile balance) system, was developed for surfactants. It has an arbitrary scale of 1–18, but some compounds have values greater than 18. HLB numbers are determined experimentally for the different surfactants. If a surfactant has a low HLB number, it means that there are few hydrophilic groups on the

molecule and it will have more of a lipophilic character. For example, the Spans® generally have low HLB numbers and they also are oil soluble. Because of their oil soluble character, Spans® are predominately used to form a w/o emulsion.

The higher HLB numbers indicate that the surfactant has a large number of hydrophilic groups on the molecule and, therefore, should be more hydrophilic in character. The Tweens® have higher HLB numbers, and they also are water soluble. Because of their water soluble character, Tweens® are used generally in o/w emulsions.

Table 13.2 shows the range of HLB values that typically are used in various aspects of compounding formulations. If a surfactant has a HLB value of 7–9, it typically is used as a wetting agent. To prepare emulsions, surfactants with HLB values of 3–8 are expected to form a w/o emulsion, and those with HLB values of 8–16 are expected to form an o/w emulsion.

TABLE 13.2: HLB VALUE OF SURFACTANTS AND THEIR USE

HLB Value	Use
1–3	Antifoaming agents
3–8	Emulsifying agents for w/o emulsions
7–9	Wetting agents
8–16	Emulsifying agents for o/w emulsions
13–16	Detergents
15–20	Solubilizing agents

Using combinations of surfactants sometimes can produce more stable emulsions than using a single surfactant with the same HLB number. The HLB value of a combination of surfactants can be calculated as follows:

$$HLB = \frac{(\text{Quantity of surfactant 1})(\text{HLB surfactant 1}) + (\text{Quantity of surfactant 2})(\text{HLB surfactant 2})}{(\text{Quantity of surfactant 1}) + (\text{Quantity of surfactant 2})}$$

EXAMPLE: What is the HLB value of a surfactant system composed of 20 g Span® 20 (HLB = 8.6) and 5 g Tween® 21 (HLB = 13.3)?

$$HLB = \frac{(20 \text{ g})(8.6) + (5 \text{ g})(13.3)}{(20 \text{ g}) + (5 \text{ g})}$$

The influence of the HLB can be seen in the following simple experiment: Equal volumes of peanut oil and water were placed in a test tube. Combinations of Tween® 20 (polyoxyethylene sorbitan monolaurate) and Span® 85 (sorbitan trioleate) were added to the tubes to give a range of HLB values. The tubes were vortex-mixed, and the time required for the oil:water interface to rise to a predetermined level was measured.

Test Tube #	1	2	3	4	5	6	7	8
Drops Tween® 20	15	12	12	6	6	3	0	0
Drops Span® 85	3	6	9	9	15	18	15	0
Calculated HLB	14.2	11.7	10.3	7.8	6.1	3.9	1.8	0
Separation time	2.3 min	2.3 min	3.0 min	3.5 min	7.2 min	5.7 min	2.5 min	12 secs

Test tube 5 had the most stable emulsion, as it showed the longest separation time. Compare test tube 5 to test tube 8. Note that test tube 8, with no emulsifier activity (HLB = 0), did not even form an emulsion. A list of common surfactants and their HLB values are listed in Table 13.3.

Methods of Compounding Emulsions

Several methods are used to compound emulsions. Each method has an oleaginous and aqueous component and some type of emulsifying agent. Each requires that energy be introduced into the system in some form. This energy is supplied in a variety of ways: trituration, homogenization, agitation, and heat.

Continental (Dry Gum or 4:2:1) Method

The dry gum method is used to prepare the initial or primary emulsion from oil, water, and a vegetable derived hydrocolloid or "gum" type emulsifier (usually acacia). The primary emulsion, or emulsion nucleus, is formed from 4 parts oil, 2 parts water, and 1 part emulsifier. The 4 parts oil and 1 part emulsifier represent their total amounts in the final emulsion.

In a dry mortar, the 1 part emulsifier is triturated with the 4 parts oil until the powder is wetted thoroughly. Then the 2 parts water are added all at once and the mixture is vigorously and continually triturated (usually 3–4 minutes) until the creamy white primary emulsion is

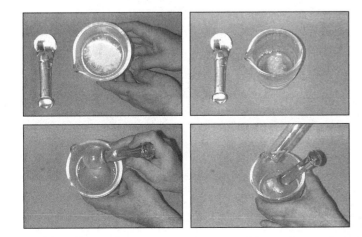

TABLE 13.3: SURFACTANTS AND THEIR HLB VALUES

Commercial Name	Chemical Name	HLB Value
Acacia	Acacia	8.0
Arlacel 83	Sorbitan sesquioleate	3.7
Brij 30	Polyoxyethylene lauryl ether	9.7
Glyceryl monostearate	Glyceryl monostearate	3.8
Methocel 15 cps	Methylcellulose	10.5
Myrj 45	Polyoxyethylene monostearate	11.1
Myrj 49	Polyoxyethylene monostearate	15.0
Myrj 52	Polyoxyl 40 stearate	16.9
PEG 400 monooleate	Polyoxyethylene monooleate	11.4
PEG 400 monostearate	Polyoxyethylene monostearate	11.6
PEG 400 monolaurate	Polyoxyethylene monolaurate	13.1
Pharmagel B	Gelatin	9.8
Potassium oleate	Potassium oleate	20.0
Sodium lauryl sulfate	Sodium lauryl sulfate	40.0
Sodium oleate	Sodium oleate	18.0
Span 20	Sorbitan monolaurate	8.6
Span 40	Sorbitan monopalmitate	6.7
Span 60	Sorbitan monostearate	4.7
Span 65	Sorbitan tristearate	2.1
Span 80	Sorbitan monooleate	4.3
Span 85	Sorbitan trioleate	1.8
Tragacanth	Tragacanth	13.2
Triethanolamine oleate	Triethanolamine oleate	12.0
Tween 20	Polyoxyethylene sorbitan monolaurate	16.7
Tween 21	Polyoxyethylene sorbitan monolaurate	13.3
Tween 40	Polyoxyethylene sorbitan monopalmitate	15.6
Tween 60	Polyoxyethylene sorbitan monostearate	14.9
Tween 61	Polyoxyethylene sorbitan monostearate	9.6
Tween 65	Polyoxyethylene sorbitan tristearate	10.5
Tween 80	Polyoxyethylene sorbitan monooleate	15.0
Tween 81	Polyoxyethylene sorbitan monooleate	10.0
Tween 85	Polyoxyethylene sorbitan trioleate	11.0
	Diethylene glycol monolaurate	6.1
	Ethylene glycol distearate	1.5
	Pluronic F – 68	17.0
	Propylene glycol monostearate	3.4
	Sucrose dioleate	7.1

Adapted from "Emulsions," by L. V. Allen, Jr., (chapter 17) in The Art, Science, and Technology of Pharmaceutical Compounding, 2nd edition (Washington, DC: American Pharmaceutical Association, 2002), pp. 263–276.

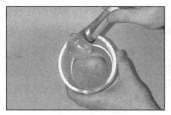

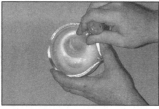

formed and produces a crackling sound as it is triturated. Light, rapid trituration is the most effective way to produce an emulsion by this method.

English (Wet Gum) Method

In the wet gum method, the proportions of oil, water, and emulsifier can be the same (4:2:1), but the order of mixing is different. The 1 part emulsifier is triturated with 2 parts water to form a wetted mixture. The 4 parts oil is added slowly, in portions, while triturating. After all the oil is added, the mixture is triturated for several minutes to form the primary emulsion. Light, rapid trituration is also required to produce an emulsion by this method. Generally, the English method is more difficult to perform successfully, especially with more viscous oils, but it may result in a more stable emulsion.

The ratio of oil:water:emulsifier has been found to be different depending on the oil being used to form the primary emulsion when acacia or tragacanth are the emulsifiers (gums). Table 13.4 gives suggested ratios for the three components in the primary emulsion when different oils are used.

Bottle (Forbes) Method

The Forbes method, which is a variation of the dry gum method, may be used to prepare emulsions of volatile oils or oleaginous substances of very low viscosities. This method is not suitable for highly viscous oils, as they cannot be agitated sufficiently in a bottle. One part acacia (or another gum) is placed in a dry bottle and the 4 parts oil are added. The bottle is capped and thoroughly shaken rapidly with short strokes. To this, the required volume of water is added all at once and the mixture is shaken thoroughly until the primary emulsion is formed. It is important to minimize the initial amount of time the

gum and oil are mixed, as the gum will tend to imbibe the oil and will become more waterproof.

This method also is effective in preparing an olive oil and lime water (calcium hydroxide solution) emulsion that is self-emulsifying. In this case, equal parts of lime water and olive oil are added to the bottle and shaken. No emulsifying agent is added because calcium oleate is formed "in situ" following a chemical reaction between the components and it serves as the emulsifier for the system.

Beaker Method

The methods described above use vegetable-derived hydrocolloid (i.e., gum type) emulsifiers. Those methods are not suitable when using non-gum or synthetic type emulsifiers. They also are not the method of choice when compounding a lotion or a cream. In these cases the beaker method is the method of choice to compound the emulsion.

The ingredients in the formulation are divided into water soluble and oil soluble components. All oil soluble components are dissolved in one beaker, and all water soluble components are dissolved in a separate beaker. Both beakers are heated to approximately 70°C using a low-temperature hotplate or steam bath. The aqueous phase should be heated to a few degrees higher temperature than the oleaginous phase because the aqueous phase will cool faster than the oleaginous phase when removed from the heat, which may cause some of the higher melting point ingredients to solidify prematurely. The two beakers are removed from the heat, and the internal phase is added slowly to the external phase while continually stirring. The product is allowed to cool to room temperature while being stirred constantly with a stirring rod or spatula.

Auxiliary Methods

Instead of any of the preceding methods, a pharmacist can prepare an excellent emulsion using an electric mixer or blender or a hand homogenizer (which forces the emulsion through a very small orifice, thereby reducing the droplet size to about 5 microns). The ingredients are added together and then blended by the equipment. An emulsion also can be prepared by one of the methods described above, and then the formulation is blended using one of these pieces of equipment. The formulation usually is improved in both stability (because the droplet size is reduced) and appearance.

TABLE 13.4: SUGGESTED RATIOS FOR THE DIFFERENT OILS

Type of Oil	Oil:Water:Emulsifier Ratio	
	Acacia	Tragacanth
Fixed oils	4:2:1	40:20:1
Mineral oil	3:2:1	30:20:1
Linseed oil	2:2:1	20:20:1
Volatile oils	2:2:1	20:20:1

Adapted from "Emulsions," by L. V. Allen, Jr., (chapter 17) in The Art, Science, and Technology of Pharmaceutical Compounding, 2nd edition (Washington, DC: American Pharmaceutical Association, 2002), pp. 263–276.

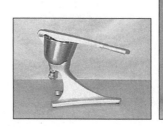

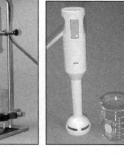

Adding Ingredients to an Emulsion

Ingredients can be added to the primary emulsion or to commercially prepared emulsions.

Adding Ingredients to a Primary Emulsion

Once a primary emulsion is formed, additional ingredients can be added to the formulation. Solid substances (active ingredients, preservatives, colors) generally are dissolved and added as a solution to the primary emulsion. Any volatile ingredients (flavors, odors, or active drugs) should be added once the product has cooled if heat was used to effect emulsification. Oil soluble substances may be incorporated directly into the primary emulsion in small amounts. Any substance that might

reduce the physical stability of the emulsion, such as alcohol (which may precipitate the gum), should be added as near to the end of the process as possible, to avoid breaking the emulsion. When all agents have been incorporated, the emulsion should be brought to final volume and then homogenized or blended to ensure uniform distribution of ingredients.

Viscosity enhancers can be added to a primary emulsion to increase the stability of the formulation. The enhancers should be soluble in or miscible with the external phase of the emulsion. For o/w emulsions, hydrocolloids are suitable viscosity enhancers. For w/o emulsions, viscous oils, fatty alcohols, or fatty acids can be added. Table 13.5 gives properties of common viscosity enhancers.

TABLE 13.5: PROPERTIES OF COMMONLY USED VISCOSITY ENHANCERS

Substance	Solubility*		Usual Suspension Concentration (%)	pH of Aqueous Solution (% solution)	Most Effective pH Range
	Water	Alcohol			
Acacia, NF	2.7	PI	5–10	4.5–5.0 (5%)	
Agar, NF	Swells	I	<1		
Alginic acid, NF	Swells	PI		1.5–3.5 (3%)	
Attapulgite, colloidal/activated	PI	PI		7.5–9.0 (5%)	6.0–8.5
Bentonite, NF	PI	PI	0.5–5.0	9.5–10.5 (2%)	> 6
Carbomer 910, 934, 934P, 940, 941, 1342, NF	S	S	0.5–1.0	2.5–3.0 (1%)	6–11
Carboxymethylcellulose calcium, NF	I	PI	0.25–5.0	4.5–6.0 (1%)	2–10
Carboxymethylcellulose sodium, NF	S	PI	0.25–5.0	6.5–8.5 (1%)	2–10
Carrageenan, NF	1:100 +				
Cellulose, microcrystalline, NF	PI		0.5–5.0	5–7	
Microcrystalline cellulose and carboxymethylcellulose sodium, NF	S			6–8 (1.2%)	
Dextrin, NF	S	PI			
Gelatin, NF Type A	S	PI		3.8–6.0	
Type B	S	PI		5.0–7.4	
Guar gum, NF	FS		2.5	5–7 (1%)	4.0–10.5
Hydroxyethyl cellulose, NF	S	PI	1.0–5.0	5.5–8.5 (1%)	2–12
Hydroxypropyl cellulose, NF	2.0	2.5		5–8 (1%)	6–8
Hydroxypropylmethyl cellulose, USP	S	PI	0.5–5.0	5.5–8.0 (1%)	3–11
Magnesium aluminum silicate, NF	PI	PI	0.5–10.0	9–10 (5%)	
Methylcellulose, USP	S	PI		5.5–8.0 (1%)	3–11
Pectin, USP	20.0	PI			
Poloxamer, NF	Varies	Varies	10–40	6.0–7.4 (2.5%)	
Polyethylene oxide, NF			1		
Polyvinyl alcohol, USP	FS		0.5–3.0	5–8 (4%)	
Povidone, USP	FS	FS	2–10	3–7 (5%)	
Propylene glycol alginate NF	S		1–5		3–6
Silicon dioxide, NF colloidal	PI	I	2–10	3.5–4.4 (4%)	1.0–7.5
Sodium alginate, NF	S	PI	1–5	7.2 (1%)	4–10
Tragacanth, NF	PI	PI		5–6 (1%)	4–8
Xanthan gum, NF	S	PI	1–2	6–8 (1%)	3–12

* ml required to dissolve 1 g of material, + hot water   PI = practically insoluble   I = insoluble   S = soluble   FS = freely soluble

Adapted from "Featured Excipient: Viscosity Increasing Agents for Aqueous Systems" by L. V. Allen, Jr., International Journal Pharmaceutical Compounding 3:479–486, 1999.

Adding Ingredients to a Commercially Prepared Emulsion

Many times, pharmacists have to incorporate additional ingredients into emulsions that are commercially manufactured. With w/o emulsions, oils and insoluble powders can be incorporated directly into the external phase, using a pill tile and spatula or low heat. If heat is used, the preparation should not be held at a high temperature very long, as some water may be lost, resulting in a change in volume of the product.

In many commercial w/o emulsions, sufficient emulsifying agent is already present in the preparation to accommodate the added oils or powders. If a large amount of insoluble powder is being added, however, a levigating agent may be necessary. If a levigating agent is to be used with the insoluble powders, it should be miscible with the oil phase; mineral oil would be a suitable agent. If the insoluble powder has a different salt form that is oil soluble, consideration should be given to using that salt form.

Adding aqueous soluble materials to a w/o emulsion is more difficult. Excess emulsifier must be present in the emulsion to accommodate the additional water. Some commercial emulsions do have the necessary excess emulsifier. For those that do not, additional emulsifier may have to be added. The ingredients should be dissolved in the aqueous solution before adding, which may require using a different salt form of the drug or ingredient. An aqueous solution can be added to the emulsion using a pill tile and spatula, but some ingredients will require heat to affect their incorporation.

With o/w emulsions, the converse of the considerations for w/o emulsions must be taken. Good levigating agents for aqueous insoluble substances should be water miscible, so glycerin, propylene glycol, polyethylene glycol (PEG) 300 or 400, or alcohol would be acceptable. If the insoluble substance has a different salt form that is aqueous soluble, consideration should be given to using that salt form. If heat is used while incorporating an ingredient into an o/w vehicle, it is important to work quickly, as water may be lost from the product rapidly. If this occurs, the product becomes stiff and waxy and loses its elegant character.

Incorporating ingredients into the aqueous external phase of the emulsion using a pill tile and spatula is relatively easy. It is more difficult to incorporate oil soluble ingredients into the o/w formulation. If heat is used, it is important to work quickly so water does not evaporate from the product.

Table 13.6 lists some commercial o/w and w/o emulsions.

Flavoring Emulsions

An appropriate flavoring agent must be selected with consideration to the external phase of an o/w emulsion. For example, if a flavoring oil is used and most of the oil

TABLE 13.6: COMMERCIALLY AVAILABLE EMULSIONS

O/W Emulsions	W/O Emulsions
Acid mantle cream	Aquabase
Allercream skin lotion	Aquaphor
Almay emulsion base	Cold cream
Aquaphilic	C-Solve lotion
Cetaphil	E-Solve lotion
Dermabase cream	Eucerin
Dermovan cream	Hydrocream
HEB cream base	Lanolin, anhydrous
Hydrophilic ointment USP	Lanolin, hydrous
Keri lotion	Hydrophilic petrolatum USP
Lanaphilic ointment	Nivea cream
Multibase	Nutraderm lotion
Neutrogena lotion	Polysorb hydrate cream
pHorsix	Rose water ointment USP
Lubriderm cream	
Neobase	
Unibase	
Vanicream	
Velvacol cream	
VanPen	

partitions into the internal phase, the strength of the flavor in the external phase will be reduced. To reduce such partitioning, flavoring oils can be mixed with small quantities of emulsifier, then added to the emulsion. As a rule, use three to five times as much emulsifier as flavoring oil to ensure that the oil will be solubilized. The flavoring oil also can be mixed with a water miscible solvent such as ethanol or glycerin before adding it to the emulsion.

Determining Type of Emulsion

As mentioned earlier in the chapter, o/w emulsions generally are formed if the aqueous phase constitutes >45% of the total weight and w/o emulsions are formed if the aqueous phase constitutes <45% of the total weight. These are somewhat nebulous guidelines because the emulsifier used also plays a role in determining the type of emulsion. The pharmacist would have to know the type of emulsion if additional ingredients are to be added to a formulation. Three simple tests that can be performed: the dilution test, the dye test, and the drop test.

Dilution Test

To perform the dilution test, dilute a portion of the formulation with an equal volume of water. An o/w

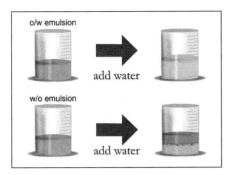

emulsion will form a stable, diluted emulsion. A w/o emulsion will break and separate into layers.

Dye Test

In the dye test, add a water soluble dye to a sample of the emulsion, and mix. If this produces a uniform color, the product is an o/w emulsion (i.e., the dye is distributed through the external phase). A globular distribution indicates that water is the internal phase and that the formulation is a w/o emulsion. If an oil soluble dye is used, the converse will be seen. Using a low power microscope or some other magnification device may be needed to clearly see the results.

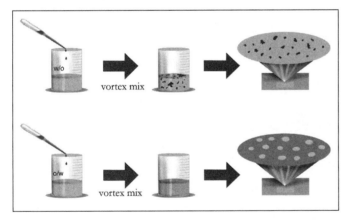

Drop Test

In the drop test, put a drop of the formulation on the surface of water. If the drop spreads out, the emulsion probably is an o/w emulsion because the external phase is miscible with water. If the drop stays as a drop or "balls up," it probably is a w/o emulsion.

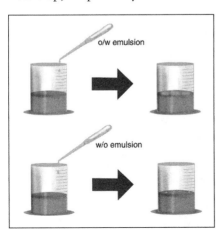

Packaging

Tight containers should be used to minimize the loss of water through evaporation. If the formulation is a liquid, it should be placed in a container with enough room to allow for shaking. Oral liquids also require a bottle with a large opening to allow easy pouring. Squeeze bottles are convenient for topical lotions. Tubes or pump containers can be used for more viscous creams. Ointment jars or tubes are convenient for packaging thicker creams and ointments.

Observing Formulations for Evidence of Instability

Evidences of instability have been mentioned previously in this chapter. For emulsions, the breaking of an emulsion (i.e., separation of an oil phase that is not easily dispersed) is a characteristic sign of instability. A similar type of instability is also an indication of an instability in a lotion or cream, since they are often emulsions.[1] Other evidences of instability are crystal growth, shrinking due to evaporation of water, and gross microbial contamination.

Preservatives

All emulsions require an antimicrobial agent because the aqueous phase will support the growth of microorganisms. The presence of a preservative is particularly critical in o/w emulsions where contamination of the external phase occurs readily.[2] Microbiological growth may produce changes in an emulsion's appearance, and cause discoloration, the development of gases and odors, and changes in the formulation's viscosity. Microorganisms can also decompose nonionic and anionic surfactants and other additives such as glycerin, gums, and hydrocolloids. It is recommended that the preservative be fungistatic as well as bacteriostatic because fungi and yeasts are prevalent in emulsions. Recommended preservatives include methylparaben, propylparaben, benzoic acid, and benzalkonium chloride.

Antioxidants

Oils are subject to rancidification, which produces a formulation with an unpleasant odor and taste. Antioxidants should be added to the formulation to inhibit this type of instability. Some appropriate antioxidants are ascorbic acid, butylated hydroxyanisole, butylated hydroxytoluene, and l-tocopherol.

NOTES

1. <1191> Stability Considerations in Dispensing Practice: The United States Pharmacopeia 29/National Formulary 24, The United States Pharmacopeial Convention, Inc., Rockville, MD, 2005, pp. 3029–3031.

2. <1151> Pharmaceutical Dosage Forms: The United States Pharmacopeia 29/National Formulary 24, The United States Pharmacopeial Convention, Inc., Rockville, MD, 2005, pp. 2996–3006.

ADDITIONAL READING

Al-Achi, A., Mosley, A., Patlolla, S, Acacia and Mineral Oil Emulsion NF. *International Journal of Pharmaceutical Compounding* 10:44, 2006.

Allen, L. V., Jr., Featured Excipient: Topical Oil-in-Water Cream Bases. *International Journal of Pharmaceutical Compounding* 6:303–304, 2002.

Allen, L. V., Jr. The Basics of Compounding: Featured Excipient: Ointment Vehicles. *International Journal of Pharmaceutical Compounding* 5:145–146, 2005.

Semisolid Dosage Forms

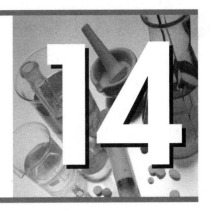

A SEMISOLID DOSAGE FORM HAS A SOFT SOLID CONSIS-tency. Several dosage forms are semisolids, and within each dosage form type the final consistency of the formulation can vary greatly. As examples, a cream formulation can be a thick liquid designed to be applied to the skin, whereas a suppository must be more rigid because it will be inserted into an orifice. With creams, some are pourable and some are ointment-like. Types of semisolid dosage forms that may be compounded include

- medication sticks
- lozenges
- suppositories
- lotions
- creams
- ointments
- pastes
- plasters.

Lozenges, sticks, and suppositories require that a mold be used in their preparation. Lozenges are oral dosage forms that are placed in the oral cavity, either under the tongue or between the cheek and gum, and usually are meant to disintegrate over several minutes. Medication sticks are used to topically apply local anesthetics, sunscreens, antivirals, antibiotics, and cosmetics (lip balm). Suppositories are used to administer medication by way of the rectum, the vagina, or the urethral tract. Suppositories will melt or dissolve at body temperature, and deliver the active drug either locally or systemically. Lotions, creams, ointments, and pastes are dermatological formulations applied to the skin for either local or systemic effect.

Preparation of Semisolids

Most compounded semisolids have the following two predominant components:

1. a fluid base that is most often an emulsion but also can be a suspension; and
2. an amount of solid material that is dispersed within the fluid base.

The final consistency of the formulation depends on the relative amounts of these two components and any excess solid material. The final texture of the formulation also depends on the ingredients used.

Because semisolids are dispersions, the ingredients must be blended together in some fashion. Some formulations are incorporated together using mechanical equipment. For example, urea can be incorporated into white petrolatum in a variety of ways such as (a) spatulation, (b) using a mortar and pestle, or (c) using an ointment mill. In the majority of formulations, however, heat will be used to facilitate the preparation.

The pharmacist must recognize that heating semisolid ingredients to make the formulation has two different outcomes:

1. In one instance, the heat is used to simply liquefy some of the formulation ingredients. After these have been melted, additional ingredients are added to the melt. The mixture then is allowed to cool and the semisolid becomes a uniform dispersion of all of the ingredients.

2. In the other instance, heat again melts some of the ingredients but the melted ingredients undergo a series of chemical reactions that will play a role in the final consistency of the formulation.

Most of these reactions involve ingredients that are, or have a large content of, fatty acids and alkyl alcohols. As the formulation ingredients are heated, the acids and alcohols readily form long chain esters, many of which will have emulsifying properties. Thus, these reactions create emulsifying agents "in situ" and form an emulsion type base for the formulation. Depending on which ingredients are present (i.e., acid, alcohol, emulsifying agent), the emulsion base can have very different properties.

Consider the following medication stick formulation.

Hydrocortisone	2%
Cetyl ester wax	28%
White wax	28%
Mineral oil	18%
Acacia	6%

White wax is a 70%–75% mixture of C_{18} hydroxy acids and esters made from straight chain monohydric alcohols with even-numbered carbon chains from C_{24} to C_{36} esterified with straight chain acids with even-numbered carbon atoms up to C_{36}. Cetyl ester wax is a mixture of esters made of saturated fatty alcohols (C_{14}–C_{18}) and saturated fatty acids (C_{14}–C_{18}). Mineral oil is refined liquid saturated aliphatic (C_{14}–C_{18}) and cyclic hydrocarbons obtained from petroleum.[1]

The white wax is melted first, and then the heat is reduced. White wax supplies a mixture of esters and C_{18} hydroxy acids. White wax possibly contains other alcohols and acids because only 70%–75% of the wax consists of esters and hydroxy acids. Cetyl esters wax is melted next, adding more esters and free alcohols and acids to the mixture. The heat is removed, and the mineral oil is added to the warmed mixture. Mineral oil supplies aliphatic hydrocarbons to the mixture, which will be involved in the final texture of the stick but also adds more reactants. Acacia and the active drug are added last, blended into the other ingredients, and the formulation is poured into a stick applicator device just before it congeals.

As mentioned above, the amount of excess solid material in a semisolid formulation plays a major role in determining the final texture and stiffness of the formulation. The unreacted material may be some of the original material that did not undergo reaction, or may be other ingredients added to the formulation that were not intended to undergo reaction. For example, if some of the ingredients are expected to undergo reaction but their stoichiometric amount is in excess, extra unreacted solid will be incorporated into the final formulation.

Heating the Ingredients

Most ingredients used in compounding semisolids will melt at or under 70°–75°C. When heat is used to melt ingredients, a water bath or a special low temperature hotplate is used. These two heating devices provide adequate control over the heating and ensure that the ingredients are not overheated. Special low temperature hotplates (full range is 25°C to 120°C) are not a standard laboratory type hotplate, as standard laboratory hotplates heat at 125°C to 150°C at their lowest setting. If available, a steam bath can be used to heat ingredients; it has a maximum temperature, which is 100°C, of boiling water.

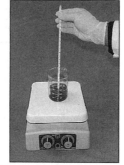

- When heating is part of a compounding procedure, apply heat only to melt the specified ingredients. Do not constantly apply heat unless instructed to do so. Continually applying heat can lead to the destruction of ingredients and change the final consistency of the formulation.

- If more than one ingredient is to be melted, melt the compound with the highest melting point first. Then turn down the heat and melt the ingredient with the second highest melting point. Continue this stepwise process for all ingredients that have to be melted. This will ensure that the ingredients were exposed to minimum heat, which will enhance the stability of the final formulation.

- When both an oil and an aqueous portion are being heated to make a semisolid, heat the aqueous portion a few degrees higher than the oil portion prior to mixing. The aqueous phase tends to cool faster than the oil phase and may cause premature solidification of some ingredients. Use the lowest temperature possible, however, and keep the heating time as brief as possible to minimize the quantity of water lost through evaporation.

Cooling the Formulation

Once all of the ingredients have been added to the melt, the mixture is allowed to congeal at its own rate. This cooling process should not be interrupted or augmented by *shock cooling* the formulation. Shock cooling is most often accomplished by putting the formulation in a refrigerator or a freezer but also can be done by placing a heated melt in a vessel of cold water.

As mentioned above, compounding semisolids often involves chemical reactions catalyzed by heat. These reactions continue even though the temperature is decreasing in the cooling formulation. The reactions would be expected to slow down as the temperature decreases, but they do not stop immediately when the heat is removed. The cooling process must be allowed to occur at its own rate to ensure that the final formulation has the properties and characteristics expected. Shock cooling a formulation will stop the chemical reactions prematurely, which will change the properties of the final formulation.

It is not unusual for a semisolid formulation to change texture and consistency over a period of hours after it has been compounded. No information is available about how much time is necessary for a given formulation to reach its final state. Therefore, any unfamiliar formulation should be observed repeatedly to determine the time and properties of the final state. As a possible estimate, 3 to 4 hours seems to be a reasonable time for all of the chemical reactions to stop in a cooling formulation.

As an example, a coal tar lotion formulation is:

Coal tar solution	12 ml
Salicylic acid	6 g
Tween 80	1 ml
Cetyl alcohol	6 g
Stearyl alcohol	6 g

| Sodium lauryl sulfate | 6 g |
| Glycerin (5%) in propylene glycol | qs 120 ml |

When the formulation is first prepared, it is a dark brown liquid. After 1½ hours, the formulation changes in both color and consistency. The color becomes golden (typical of coal tar ointments) and the consistency stiffens to form a lotion or fluid cream.

Another example is cold cream:

Cetyl esters wax	125 g
White wax	120 g
Mineral oil	560 g
Sodium borate	5 g
Purified water	190 ml

When this formulation is prepared initially, it does not have any luster or sheen, but overnight, the appearance and texture of the ointment does change to a almost luminescent cream.

When transferring a heated formulation to a package:

- Do not pour a heated semisolid formulation into an ointment jar and let it cool. The jar will be a different temperature than the heated formulation and will act as a shock cooling reservoir. As a result, the formulation will have a "layered" appearance created by the different parts of the formulation cooling at different rates.

- Transfer the semisolid from the compounding vessel to the packaging device when the formulation is just a few degrees above the congealing temperature. At this stage, the formulation should be a thick, viscous fluid.

Practical Considerations

Knowing when to transfer the semisolid to the final container is important. If the congealing temperature is known and the temperature can be measured with a thermometer, the temperature can be directly measured and the semisolid transferred to the final container when just a few degrees above the congealing point. Thermometers can be used to measure the temperature of semisolids in a vessel, but most thermometers must be immersed to the mark etched on the glass to obtain an accurate temperature reading. In working with small batches, the mixture may not come up to the mark. Therefore, using the thermometer to determine the mixture temperature is not appropriate.

A practical method to determine when to transfer the semisolid material to a mold or final container is to touch the heated vessel to the back of the hand. If the temperature is uncomfortably hot, the material should be assumed to be too hot to pour. If the vessel has just become comfortably hot, however, the semisolid can be poured into the mold or final container.

If adding volatile ingredients such as oils, flavors, or drugs to a heated semisolid formulation, they should be added just before the semisolid is transferred to the final container. The melt will still be fluid enough for quantitative transfer but not hot enough to evaporate the ingredients.

Powders

Powders should be in a very fine state of subdivision prior to incorporation into the semisolid formulation. This can be accomplished using a mortar and pestle, a mechanical grinder, or a levigating agent and a pill tile and spatula. This will reduce the gritty texture of a formulation and avoid additional injury or irritation to damaged skin, which would impede the healing process. Also, a more finely divided powder will increase the drug's surface area, thereby increasing the potential availability for therapeutic activity.

If a soluble powder is being incorporated with the aid of a solubilizing agent, solvents that have low vapor pressure (e.g., water, glycerin, propylene glycol) should be used. Generally, volatile solvents are not used because if the solvent evaporates during incorporation, the drug crystallizes out, and the crystals cause irritation when applied to the skin. The solubilized powder should be incorporated into a formulation using the technique of *geometric dilution*.

Additional Considerations

- Between 2 and 4 grams of a semisolid will be lost during the compounding process. The semisolid is lost as it adheres to beakers, ointment tiles, or becomes overfill for molds. To compensate for this loss, add 10% or 3 grams more material than prescribed.

- If semisolid ingredients are to be heated as part of the compounding process, use the smallest beaker that will contain all of the material. The sides of beakers are colder than the bottom, so when heated materials are poured out of a beaker, the material congeals quickly on the sides. The larger the beaker, the more material will be lost on the sides of the beaker.

- When melting ingredients, add the ingredients to the heating vessel and let the ingredients melt at their own rate without stirring them with a glass rod or magnetic stirring bar. The stirring will place some of the mixture on the sides of the vessel, which will remove it from the heating source. It is important to remember that hotplates heat only the bottom of a vessel, not the sides. If the ingredients are disturbed repeatedly, a large amount of material can be lost from the formulation and may also result in a nonuniform distribution of ingredients in the final formulation.

- If a large amount of material is lost on the sides of a beaker, put the beaker in a water bath or use a steam bath to heat the sides of the beaker. Generally, the material will liquefy quickly and fall back into the rest of the material.

- Most semisolids are dispersions of ingredients, and materials can settle quickly. When pouring heated ingredients into molds or final containers, stir the formulation once more just prior to pouring the ingredients, and then pour rapidly. A slow rate of pouring will allow more congealing on the sides of the beaker, and more time for ingredients to settle in the heating vessel. These factors would lead to an increased loss of materials and a nonuniform dispersion of ingredients.

NOTES

1. Rowe, R. C., Sheskey, P. J., and Weller, P. J., editors. *Handbook of Pharmaceutical Excipients*, 4th edition. Pharmaceutical Press and American Pharmaceutical Association, Grayslake, IL and Washington, DC, 2003, pp. 687–688, 681–682, 395–397.

CHAPTER FIFTEEN

Dermatological Formulations: Ointments and Pastes

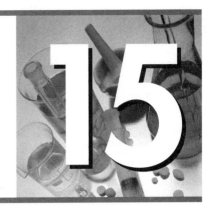

ERMATOLOGICAL FORMULATIONS ARE AMONG THE most frequently compounded products because of their wide range of potential uses. The formulations include solutions (collodions, liniments, aqueous and oleaginous solutions), suspensions and gels, emulsions, lotions, creams, ointments, and pastes. Dermatological formulations that typically are manufactured and not commonly compounded include aerosols and devices such as transdermal patches, tapes, and gauzes.

Dermatological formulations generally are used for one of the following purposes:

- to protect the skin or mucous membranes from chemical or physical irritants in the environment, permitting the skin to rejuvenate and heal;
- to provide emollient (skin softening) effect by hydrating the skin;
- to provide a topical vehicle for medications for local (anti-infective, anti-pruritic, astringent, keratolytic) or transdermal/systemic effect (e.g., nitroglycerin).

Protective formulations contain materials that will protect the skin from various external factors such as moisture, air, sun, and chemicals. These formulations may be either a base or a base containing active ingredients. For example, sunscreen agents that prevent the infiltration of ultraviolet rays may be included in various types of dermatological products.

Emollients are preparations that soften the skin surface. They contain fatty components such as mineral oil, petrolatum, or paraffins. Oleaginous compounds also may maintain soft skin by forming an occlusive layer on the skin surface, thereby reducing or retarding the evaporation of water.

A *dermatological* vehicle is a formulation that releases an active drug to the application site. The release (diffusion) of the drug depends on the type of vehicle as well as the solubility (hydrophilicity/lipophilicity) of the drug in that vehicle. The extent to which a drug is absorbed into the skin is influenced by several factors, including the area to which the ointment is applied, the condition of the skin (whether intact, denuded, or diseased), the method of application, and the total amount of drug released from the vehicle.

This chapter deals with two dermatological formulations: ointments and pastes. Pastes contain more solid material than ointments do. Lotions and creams are common dermatological formulations and are discussed in the chapters on suspensions and emulsions. *Lotions,* which can be either suspensions or emulsions, are fluid liquids that typically are used for their lubricating effect. *Creams* are emulsions that possess a fluid consistency and typically are opaque, thick liquids or soft solids used for their emollient properties.

Structure of the Skin

Regardless of the formulation, all dermatological formulations are applied to the skin. The skin is the largest and heaviest organ in the body, accounting for about 17% of a person's weight. Its major function is to protect the underlying organ systems from trauma, temperature, humidity, harmful penetrations, moisture, radiation, and microorganisms. It is composed of three layers of stratified tissue: epidermis, dermis, and subcutaneous. The skin is 3–5 millimeters thick, depending on the part of the body. The thickest parts of the skin are the palms of the hands and the soles of the feet, and the thinnest parts are the eyelids and genitals.

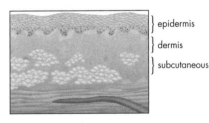

The *epidermis* is approximately 75 to 150 microns thick except in the palms and soles of the feet, where it is 400–600 microns. The outermost part of the epidermis contains sebum, sweat, and several layers of dead cells called the *stratum corneum*. The innermost part of the epidermis is a layer of living cells called the *stratum germinatuvum*. In normal skin, the stratum germinatuvum continually produces viable cells, which progress toward the skin surface. As the cells progress, they die and displace the cells in the stratum corneum, which are sloughed off to the environment. As the cells die, they become flattened and lose their nuclei, and the organized cell contents are replaced with keratin fibrils. The turnover time from germination to sloughing is about 21 days.

The *dermis* contains blood capillaries, nerve fibers, hair follicles, and sweat and sebaceous glands. Sweat glands yield their product through ducts ending on the skin surface. Oil glands and hair follicles from the dermis also terminate on the skin surface. The *subcutaneous* layer consists of connective tissue and adipose tissues. Its primary role is to protect the body from mechanical impacts.

The stratum corneum is the barrier to drug penetration through the skin. Approximately 10 microns thick, it can swell to approximately three times its original thickness and absorb about five times its weight in water. When the stratum corneum hydrates, it becomes more permeable. Therefore, occlusive dressings often are used to hydrate the stratum corneum and increase the penetration of certain drugs. Dermatoses such as eczema and psoriasis also can hydrate the stratum corneum and increase the absorption of some drugs.

⚡ Local and Systemic Effects of Dermatological Formulations

Dermatological formulations can produce a *local drug effect* either on or in the skin. The formulations serve as protectants, lubricants, emollients, or drying agents in addition to any therapeutic benefit from incorporated active drugs. Examples of topical injuries that are treated via the local activity of dermatological formulations include minor skin infections, itching, burns, diaper rash, insect stings and bites, athlete's foot, corns, calluses, warts, dandruff, acne, psoriasis, and eczema.

Also, dermatological formulations can be used to provide *systemic drug delivery*, called *percutaneous absorption*. The formulation is placed on the skin, and the drug penetrates the epidermis into the dermis and subcutaneous tissues, where it is absorbed into the systemic circulation. Some dermatological formulations provide continual percutaneous absorption. The transdermal patch is the primary example of this type of formulation. The extent of percutaneous absorption is the result of three competing processes:

1. the potential of the drug to cross the stratum corneum,
2. the potential of the drug to leave the formulation, and
3. the influence of the formulation on the stratum corneum.

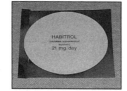

Although percutaneous absorption of drugs is a complex process, several generalizations are possible:

- More drug is absorbed when the formulation is applied to a larger surface area.

TABLE 15.1: CHEMICAL CLASSIFICATION OF PENETRATION ENHANCERS

Chemical Classification	Examples
Alcohols	Methanol, ethanol, propanol, octanol
Fatty alcohols	Myristyl alcohol, cetyl alcohol, stearyl alcohol
Fatty acids	Myristic acid, stearic acid, oleic acid
Fatty acid esters	Isopropyl myristate, isopropyl palmitate
Polyols	Propylene glycol, polyethylene glycol, glycerol
Anionic surfactants	Sodium lauryl sulfate
Cationic surfactants	Benzalkonium chloride, cetylpyridinium chloride
Amphoteric surfactants	Lecithins
Nonionic surfactants	Spans®, Tweens®, poloxamers, Miglyol®

Adapted from "Compounding Dermatological Products," by L. V. Allen, Jr., International Journal of Pharmaceutical Compounding 2:260–264, 1998.

- Formulations or dressings that increase hydration of the skin generally enhance percutaneous absorption.
- The greater the amount of rubbing in or inunction of the formulation, the greater is the absorption.
- The longer the formulation remains in contact with the skin, the greater is the absorption.

The major disadvantage of the dermal route of administration is that the amount of drug that can be absorbed into or through the skin is about 2 mg/day. This may become a significant limitation if the route is being used for percutaneous absorption. To overcome this potential limitation, several chemicals are used as ⚡ *penetration enhancers*, which promote the percutaneous absorption of drugs. These enhancers improve the solubility of the active drug in the stratum corneum and facilitate the drug's diffusion into the systemic circulation. Table 15.1 gives examples of some penetration enhancers used in dermatological formulations. Other common enhancers include DMSO (dimethyl sulfoxide), urea, triethanolamide, and DMF (dimethyl formamide).

Percutaneous absorption also can be increased using mechanical methods. *Phonophoresis* uses ultrasonic vibrations to increase the absorption of drugs such as lidocaine, tetracycline, and penicillin into and through the skin. Another technique is *iontophoresis*, in which local anesthetics and analgesic are transported into the skin with the aid of an electrical field. It also is used to enhance the percutaneous absorption of large molecular peptides and proteins.[1,2,3]

Ointment Bases

The five classes or types of ointment bases are differentiated on the basis of their physical composition as:

1. oleaginous bases

2. absorption bases
3. w/o emulsion bases
4. o/w emulsion bases
5. water soluble or water miscible bases.

Ointments—mixtures of drugs in an ointment base—typically are used on dry, scaly lesions because of their protective and emollient properties, and they stay on the skin for an extended time, which aids in drug absorption. A specific ointment base is chosen for its inherent properties and/or for its potential to serve as a drug delivery vehicle. If an ointment base is chosen as a drug delivery vehicle, it must release the active drug in a reproducible manner. The release (diffusion) rate of a drug from an ointment base is dependent on the properties of the base, as well as the solubility of the drug in the base. Generally, oleaginous (hydrophobic) bases release drugs slowly and more unpredictably because water cannot penetrate the base sufficiently to dissolve the drug. Water miscible or hydrophilic bases tend to release drugs more rapidly and more predictably because water can penetrate into the base.

A common laboratory experiment incorporates a drug into different bases and measures the release rate of the drug into a continuously stirred beaker filled with solution. The data from one such experiment are shown in Table 15.2.

It is easy to see the marked differences in the release rate depending on the type of base. Of course, a different drug with different hydrophilic/lipophilic characteristics would yield different release rate values, but the generalizations seem to hold for a wide range of compounds with the wide range of different properties. Once the drug has been released from the base, percutaneous penetration is influenced by several factors, including the area to which the ointment is applied, the condition of the skin (whether intact, denuded, or diseased), and the location and method of application.

Each type of ointment base has different physical characteristics and therapeutic uses based upon the nature of its components. Table 15.3 summarizes the properties of the five types of ointment bases, including the composition, common uses, and examples.

TABLE 15.2: RELEASE RATE OF SALICYLIC ACID FROM VARIOUS OINTMENT BASES

Type of Ointment Base	Release Rate of 6% Salicylic Acid
Oleaginous base	$31\ \mu g/min^{1/2}$
Absorption base	$46\ \mu g/min^{1/2}$
W/O Emulsion base	$122\ \mu g/min^{1/2}$
O/W Emulsion base	$798\ \mu g/min^{1/2}$
Water miscible base	$3,496\ \mu g/min^{1/2}$

TABLE 15.3: PROPERTIES OF OINTMENT BASES

Property	Oleaginous Bases	Absorption Bases	Water/Oil Emulsion Bases	Oil/Water Emulsion Bases	Water Miscible Bases
Composition	oleaginous compounds	oleaginous base + w/o surfactant	oleaginous base + water (<45% w/w) + w/o surfactant (HLB $\leq$ 8)	oleaginous base + water (>45% w/w) + o/w surfactant (HLB $\geq$ 9)	polyethylene glycols (PEGs)
Water content	anhydrous	anhydrous	hydrous	hydrous	anhydrous, hydrous
Affinity for water	hydrophobic	hydrophilic	hydrophilic	hydrophilic	hydrophilic
Spreadability	difficult	difficult	moderate to easy	easy	moderate to easy
Washability	nonwashable	nonwashable	non- or poorly washable	washable	washable
Greasiness	greasy	greasy	greasy	nongreasy	nongreasy
Drug incorporation potential	solids or oils (oil solubles only)	solids, oils, and aqueous solutions (small amounts)	solids, oils, and aqueous solutions (small amounts)	solid and aqueous solutions (small amounts)	solid and aqueous solutions
Drug release potential	poor	poor, but > oleaginous	fair to good	fair to good	good
Occlusiveness	yes	yes	sometimes	no	no
Uses	protectants, emollients (+/−), vehicles for hydrolyzable drugs	protectants, emollients (+/−), vehicles for aqueous solutions, solids, and non-hydrolyzable drugs	emollients, cleansing creams, vehicles for solid, liquid, or non-hydrolyzable drugs	emollients, vehicles for solid, liquid, or non-hydrolyzable drugs	drug vehicles
Examples	White Petrolatum, White Ointment	Hydrophilic Petrolatum, Anhydrous Lanolin, Aquabase™, Aquaphor®, Polysorb®	Cold Cream type, Hydrous Lanolin, Rose Water Ointment, Hydrocream™, Eucerin®, Nivea®	Hydrophilic Ointment, Dermabase™, Velvachol®	PEG Ointment, Polybase™

Ingredients and Compounding Procedures

The ingredients and compounding procedure for several of the ointment bases shown in Table 15.3 are listed below.

White Ointment

White Wax	5%
White Petrolatum	95%

Procedure for preparation:

1. Melt the white wax on a hotplate.

2. When the wax has completely melted, add the white petrolatum and allow the entire mixture to remain on the hotplate until liquefied.

3. Following liquification, remove from heat and stir the mixture until it begins to congeal.

Hydrophilic Petrolatum

Cholesterol	3%
Stearyl Alcohol	3%
White Wax	8%
White Petrolatum	86%

Procedure for preparation:

1. Melt the stearyl alcohol, white wax, and white petrolatum together on a hotplate.

2. Add the cholesterol to the mixture while still on the hotplate, and stir until completely dissolved.

3. Following dissolution, remove from heat and stir the mixture until congealed.

Cold Cream Type

White Wax	12.0%
Spermaceti	12.5%
Mineral Oil	56.0%
Sodium Borate	0.5%
Purified Water	19.0%

Procedure for preparation:

1. Melt the white wax and spermaceti together on a hotplate in one container.

2. Add the mineral oil to this mixture and bring the temperature to 70°C.

3. Dissolve the sodium borate in water.

4. Heat the sodium borate solution to 75°C in another container.

5. When both phases have reached the desired temperature, remove both phases from the hotplate and add the aqueous phase slowly and with constant stirring to the oil phase.

6. When the addition is completed, stir the mixture briskly and continuously until congealed.

Hydrophilic Ointment

Methylparaben	0.025%
Propylparaben	0.015%
Sodium Lauryl Sulfate	1.0%
Propylene Glycol	12.0%
Stearyl Alcohol	25.0%
White Petrolatum	25.0%
Purified Water	37.0%

Procedure for preparation:

1. Melt the stearyl alcohol and white petrolatum on a hotplate in one container.

2. Heat this mixture to 70°C.

3. Dissolve remaining ingredients in water and heat the solution to 75°C in another container.

4. When both phases have reached the desired temperature, add the aqueous phase slowly and with constant stirring to the oil phase while still applying heat.

5. When the addition is complete, remove from heat and stir the mixture briskly and continuously until it congeals.

Water Miscible Type

Polyethylene Glycol 400	60%
Polyethylene Glycol 3350	40%

Procedure for preparation:

1. Melt the PEGs on a hotplate.

2. Heat the mixture to about 65°C.

3. When the desired temperature is attained, remove the mixture from heat and stir until congealed.

Incorporating a Drug Into an Ointment Base

Insoluble powders that are to be incorporated into an ointment base should be in the *finest possible state of subdivision* because these formulations often are applied to sensitive, diseased, or denuded skin areas. Using the finest subdivision will prevent a gritty texture and allow the final formulation to be smooth to the touch. The powder form should be used instead of a crystalline form. The powder may have to be triturated in a mortar and pestle before being incorporated into an ointment base. *Pulverization by intervention* also can also be used, in which the powder is dissolved in a small volume of solvent, and the solvent allowed to evaporate. The powder recrystallizes as very fine particles.

Levigating agents also can be used to reduce the particle size of the powder. When choosing a levigating agent, the one that is selected should be miscible with the ointment base or the part of the ointment base where the drug will reside. For oleaginous, absorption, and w/o emulsion bases, mineral oil is a reasonable levigating agent. Other levigating agents might be castor oil, cottonseed oil, olive oil, or Tween® 80. For o/w emulsion and water soluble bases, glycerin is a good choice. Other possible levigating agents include propylene glycol and polyethylene glycol 400.

Sometimes a small portion of melted ointment base can serve as the levigating agent, using the minimum amount of levigating agent necessary to wet the powders. For some powders, 10 to 15 drops of the agent is a sufficient amount. Other powders require 1 to 2 ml of levigating agent. Levigating agents generally are not used when preparing pastes because the volume of levigating agent required to wet the high percentage of solid in the paste is too large.

Some powders can be incorporated into ointment bases by first dissolving the solid in a solvent or oil that can be taken up by the ointment base. In this technique, use solvents that have low vapor pressures so they will not easily evaporate. Solvents that easily evaporate may crystallize the drug out in the base and cause skin irritation upon application. Table 15.4 shows the relative amounts of water, alcohol, and lipophilic solvents that can be incorporated into the different types of ointment bases.

To incorporate a powder into an ointment base using any of the procedures given above, use an ointment slab (or tile) and large metal spatulas. Ointment slabs—either ground glass plates or porcelain—provide a hard, nonabsorbable surface for mixing. *Ointment pads* have the advantage that clean-up is quicker, but the ointment can soak into the parchment paper. Further, the paper can absorb liquids and may tear when using

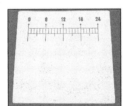
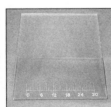

sticky or thick ointments. Large metal spatulas are used instead of smaller metal spatulas because they have the proper combination of flexibility and strength for adequate shearing and mixing. Black rubber or plastic spatulas are not used in ointment compounding.

If preparing a large quantity of ointment, a mixing device of some type might be used instead of the ointment slab and spatulas. Two options are an ointment mill and an electric mortar and pestle. Ointment mills produce very smooth and elegant ointments. The electric mortar and pestle option allows the mixing to be done and the formulation to be dispensed in the same container.

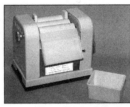
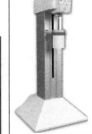

For small scale homogenizations (approximately 500 ml), hand homogenizers are available.

Comments Specific to Each Ointment Base

Procedures to incorporate drugs into the various types of ointment bases are given below.

Oleaginous Bases

To incorporate an insoluble drug into oleaginous bases, first pulverize the powder on the ointment slab with a spatula or in a mortar and with a pestle. Use a levigating agent to wet the powder, and then incorporate the wetted powder into the ointment base. A good levigating agent is mineral oil, as it is compatible with oleaginous bases. Sometimes, using a small quantity of the base itself as the levigating agent is sufficient.

Generally, the amount of drug to be incorporated into the ointment will be much less than the amount of ointment; i.e., a small amount of drug will be incorporated into a large amount of ointment. The process of *geometric dilution* "dilutes" the drug into the ointment.

TABLE 15.4: WATER, ALCOHOL, AND OIL SOLVENTS THAT CAN BE INCORPORATED INTO OINTMENT BASES

Base Type	Water	Alcohol	Oils
Oleaginous	None	Very limited	Easily, but will decrease viscosity of base
Absorption	Large quantities Aquaphor® absorbs several times its weight	Less volume than water Aquaphor® absorbs equal to its weight	Easily, but will decrease viscosity of base
W/O emulsion	Cold Cream, Rose Water Ointment—very little Eucerin®, more than these but less than Aquaphor®	Varied amounts	Easily, but will decrease viscosity of base
O/W emulsion	Absorbs some, but decreases viscosity of base. Hydrophilic Ointment and Unibase® take up 30% of their weight	Less volume than water	Some will be taken up and emulsified, but larger amounts may require additional Tween® 80
Water miscible	Very limited without loss of viscosity	Base is soluble in alcohol	Incorporate with levigation with a liquid of intermediate chemical properties (glycerin, propylene glycol)

Geometric dilution involves a series of dilution steps. First the drug is incorporated into an amount of ointment of approximately the same size. Then a second amount of ointment approximately equal to the first mixture is added and mixed. This stepwise dilution process is continued until all of the ointment has been used.

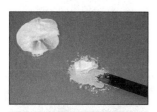

Levigate the powder to reduce the particle size and wet the powder.

Bring a portion of ointment about equal in size to the powder

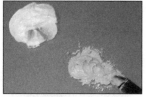

and incorporate the ointment and levigated powder together.

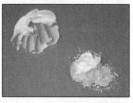

Bring another portion of ointment about equal in size to the first mixture

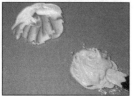

and again incorporate the ointment and the mixture from the first addition.

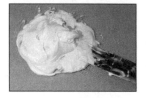

Continue the additional steps until all of the powder has been incorporated into the ointment.

Soluble drugs can be incorporated into oleaginous bases by fusion. The base is liquefied over low heat (not to exceed 70°C), then the drug is added to the molten base. The mixture is allowed to cool, with continual stirring.

Absorption Bases

An absorption base is an oleaginous base containing a w/o emulsifying agent. When water is taken up into the base, it will remain a w/o emulsion. Absorption bases typically can incorporate about 50% of their volume in water.

Incorporating insoluble drugs into these bases can be done mechanically or by fusion. The final destination (internal or external phase of the emulsion) of the drug must be considered when selecting a water soluble levigating agent. If the drug will reside in the internal phase (water phase), the levigating agent should be water soluble, or

water miscible. Water, glycerin, alcohol, or propylene glycol are suitable levigating agents. If the drug will reside in the external phase, mineral oil should be used.

Water soluble ingredients can be added to the water phase of the w/o emulsion. If the drug will dissolve in a small amount of water, the aqueous solution can be added directly to the base using an ointment slab and spatulas. If a larger quantity of water is needed to solubilize the drug or if an aqueous solution is being added to the base, heat may be needed to compound the formulation. It may be necessary to add emulsifier to the emulsion to accommodate the added water. Some commercial emulsions do have the necessary excess emulsifier.

W/O Emulsion Bases

Oils and insoluble powders can be incorporated into the external phase directly, using a ointment slab and spatulas. If a levigating agent is to be used with the insoluble powders, it should be miscible with the oil phase; mineral oil is a suitable agent. If the insoluble powder has a different salt form that is oil soluble, consideration should be given to using that salt form.

The same comments that apply to incorporating water soluble ingredients into absorption bases apply to w/o emulsion bases.

O/W Emulsion Bases

Water soluble powders can be incorporated directly into the external phase using a ointment slab and spatulas. If the powder is insoluble, the levigating agent should be water miscible, so glycerin, propylene glycol, polyethylene glycol (PEG) 300 or 400, or alcohol are acceptable. If the insoluble substance has a different salt form that is aqueous soluble, consideration should be given to using that salt form.

Incorporating oil soluble ingredients into the o/w formulation may be more difficult. A small amount of oil can be incorporated into the base if there is excess emulsifier. Some commercial products do have the necessary excess emulsifier. If a larger portion of oil is to be added, more emulsifier may have to be added. If heat is used to incorporate the oil, it is important to work quickly so water does not evaporate from the product and cause it to become stiff and waxy.

Water Miscible Bases

Water soluble drugs can be dissolved in a small quantity of water and incorporated using a ointment slab and spatulas. Insoluble powders require a water miscible levigating agent such as glycerin, propylene glycol, or polyethylene glycol 400. Oils can be added to these bases by first mixing the oil with glycerin or propylene glycol, then incorporating the mixture into the base. If the quantity of liquid to add to the base is large, heat may be necessary.

Pastes

Pastes contain more solid material than ointments—generally at least 20% solids—so pastes are stiffer than ointments. This increased stiffness reduces the percutaneous absorption potential of any drug incorporated in the paste. Pastes, however, generally are not used for their absorption potential but rather for their protective action and for their ability to absorb serous discharges from skin lesions. They also remain in place longer than ointments. Examples of pastes listed in the USP 29/NF24 are Zinc Oxide Paste, Zinc Oxide and Salicylic Acid Paste, Carboxymethylcellulose Sodium Paste, Magnesium Hydroxide Paste, and Triamcinolone Acetonide Dental Paste.

Pastes generally are prepared using oleaginous bases and heat. Heat improves the workability of pastes and also allows a high percentage of solids to be incorporated into the base. With such a high content of solids, it is imperative that the formulation be stirred thoroughly and continuously during the cooling process to prevent the solids from settling out of the formulation. Levigating agents are not used in pastes because the large volume needed may dilute the base and cause them to liquefy and become less stiff.

Packaging

All of these formulations can be packaged in a variety of devices such as tubes, jars, applicators, syringes, patches, and pump dispensers. The packaging should keep the formulation clean during repeated use, and as free from air exposure and microbial contamination as feasible. All of the packaging devices except the ointment jar meet these criteria. With an ointment jar, a tongue depressor can be used to remove the required quantity of formulation and thereby keep the formulation free from the formulation free from hand contamination. Because of their stiff consistency, pastes usually are packaged in ointment jars.

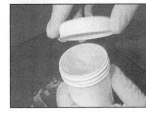

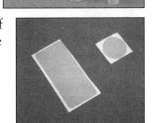

Packing an Ointment Jar

When hand packaging an ointment jar, care should be taken to remove air pockets that form as the ointment is packed. Also, the top of the ointment should be smoothed to give the ointment a "finished" look and to keep the ointment from sticking to the jar lid.

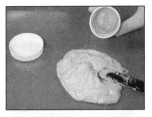

Begin by taking some of the ointment and filling the bottom crevices.

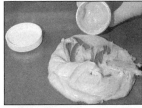

Work the additional ointment along the sides of the jar, rotating the jar while filling it.

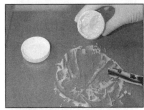

Continue adding ointment.

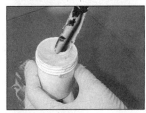

Slightly depress the spatula toward the center, and rotate the jar. This makes a professional looking finish and keeps the ointment from sticking to the lid of the jar.

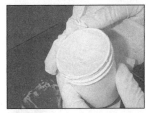

Clean the threads of the jar with a tissue.

Place the lid on the jar.

Filling and Sealing an Ointment Tube

An ointment tube can be filled conveniently using a urethra tip and a plastic bag. A corner of the bag is cut and the tip is secured into position. The bag then is filled with the ointment and squeezed into the open end of an ointment tube. Once the tube is filled, the open end has to be sealed.

Other methods are used to fill ointment tubes. Regardless of the filling method, the tube will have to be sealed before dispensing.

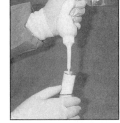

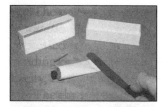

After the ointment tube is filled, use a stainless steel spatula and flatten the last ½ inch of the ointment tube.

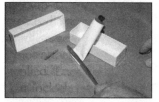

Use the edge of the spatula and make one fold ⅛ inch from the end of the tube. Bend the tube all the way over the spatula.

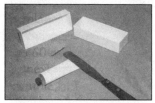

Using the spatula again, make a second fold ¼ inch from the end of the tube.

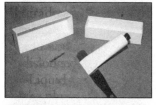

Again, bend the tube all the way over the spatula.

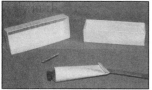

Turn over the ointment tube and make a third fold ⅛ inch from the end of the tube.

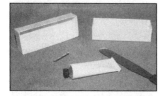

This will create a "T" at the end of the tube.

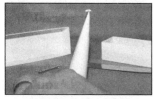

The "T" at the end of the tube (side view).

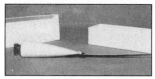

Turn the edges of the "T" down into the tube and place the clip on the tube.

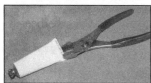

Use pliers or a suitable crimping tool to collapse the clip onto the tube.

Dispense the tube in a telescoping box.

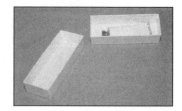

Observing Formulations for Evidence of Instability

Chapter <1191> notes that, "the primary indication of instability is often either discoloration or a noticeable change in consistency or odor." Specifically for ointments, excessive "bleeding" (i.e., separation of excessive amounts of liquid) and formation of granules or grittiness are other possible indicators of instability.[4]

In a more general sense, instability of the various dermatological formulations can be identified by a separation of components, discoloration, development of rancid odor, dryness, crystal growth, shrinkage resulting from water loss, and gross microbial contamination. Anhydrous formulations tend to be relatively more stable than hydrous products and can have a 6 month beyond use dating if any incorporated drug is also stable for that period. For formulations containing water, it is recommended that no more than a 2 week supply be dispensed if no preservative is used.

Ointments are susceptible to contamination by *Pseudomonas aeruginosa* and *Staphylococcus aureus*. Dermatological preparations are not required to be sterile, but the use of preservatives may be justified because of the potential contamination. Preservatives commonly used in ointments are methylparaben and propylparaben, benzoic acid, benzyl alcohol, quaternary ammonium salts (e.g., benzalkonium chloride), thimerosal, and sorbic acid.[5]

NOTES

1. Heim, B. Transdermal Administration of Anti-inflammatory Medications in Sports Injuries: Use of Iontophoresis and Phonophoresis to Enhance Delivery. *International Journal of Pharmaceutical Compounding* 10:14–18, 2006.

2. Allen, L. V., Jr. Basics of Compounding: Phonophoresis. *International Journal of Pharmaceutical Compounding* 6:362–365, 2002.

3. Allen, L. V., Jr. Basics of Compounding: Iontophoresis, Part II. *International Journal of Pharmaceutical Compounding* 6:288–292, 2002.

4. <1191> Pharmacy Compounding. The United States Pharmacopeia 29/National Formulary 24, The United States Pharmacopeial Convention, Inc., Rockville, MD, 2005, pp. 3029–3031.

5. Allen, L. V., Jr. Featured Excipient: Preservatives. *International Journal of Pharmaceutical Compounding* 3:142–143, 1999.

CHAPTER SIXTEEN

Lozenges and Medication Sticks

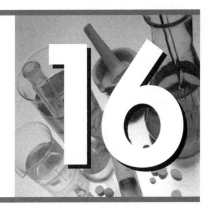

T HE LOZENGE IS INTENDED FOR BUCCAL OR SUBLINQUAL administration, and the medication stick is used for the topical application of drugs. But both dosage forms are semisolids. The principles discussed in Chapter 14, Semisolid Dosage Forms, apply to these two formulations.

Lozenges

"Lozenges are semisolid preparations that are intended to dissolve or disintegrate slowly in the mouth. They contain one or more medicaments usually in a flavored, sweetened base."[1] Lozenges are most often used for localized effects in the mouth. They also can be used for systemic effect if the drug is well absorbed through the buccal lining or is swallowed.

The name *troche* is applied to compressed lozenges, but in lay language *lozenge* and *troche* are used interchangeably. Troches can be used for hospice patients and chemotherapy patients who have severe nausea. Formulas can be modified for both geriatric and pediatric patients. More traditional drugs found in troches include phenol, sodium phenolate, benzocaine, and cetylpyridinium chloride. Newer drugs include analgesics, anesthetics, antiseptics, antimicrobials, antitussives, antinauseants, and decongestants.

Lozenges have the following advantages:

- They are easy to administer to pediatric and geriatric patients.
- The formulas are easy to change and can be patient and dosing specific.
- The drug stays in contact with the oral cavity for an extended time.

One disadvantage of using a "gummy type" lozenge with children is that they may perceive it as candy and not as a serious dosage form.

Lozenges can be made by molding or by compression. Commercial troches are made by compression, using mucilages or natural gums to effect adhesion. These troches are harder than ordinary tablets so they will dissolve or disintegrate slowly. Compounded lozenges can be prepared by molding mixtures of ingredients containing

- sugars to form a hard lozenge,

- polyethylene glycol (PEG) to form a soft lozenge, and
- gelatin to form a chewable lozenge.

Hard Lozenges

Hard lozenges might be considered semisolid syrups of sugars. These dosage forms are made by heating sugars and other ingredients together to about 160°C, then pouring the mixture into a mold. The molds can shape the mixture to look like a sucker or a lollipop. Hard lozenges will not disintegrate in the mouth but will erode or dissolve over 5–10 minutes.

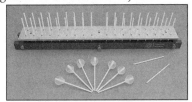

Hard lozenges are similar to hard candy. In fact, many hard lozenge formulas are modifications of hard candy formulas. The dosage form requires a low moisture content (0.5%–1.5%), so water is evaporated by boiling the sugar mixture during the compounding process. All formulation instructions must be followed carefully, with particular attention to temperatures. The success of forming the amorphous crystalline product depends on it. For example, if a formula states that the syrup should not be stirred until it reaches a certain temperature, or if it states that the syrup must reach a certain temperature, these instructions must be followed precisely.

The primary disadvantage of hard lozenges is apparent: heat labile drugs cannot be used in these formulations because of the high temperatures required for preparation. Another problem is that hard lozenges become grainy. The speed at which this happens depends on the sugar used and its concentration in the formulation. The best compromise seems to be 55%–65% sucrose and about 35%–45% corn syrup.

The final pH of the product has to be considered. If acidic flavoring agents (citric, tartaric, fumaric acid) are to be used, the final pH may be quite low (around 3). The pH of hard candies is around 5 or 6, so the pH of the hard lozenge will have to be raised to obtain this pH. Calcium carbonate, sodium bicarbonate, and magnesium trisilicate can be added to the formulation for this purpose.

Soft Lozenges

Soft lozenges are easily compounded and can be colored and flavored. They usually are taken to dissolve in the mouth over 10–15 minutes, but some soft lozenges are to be chewed. These typically are made of ingredients such as polyethylene glycol (PEG) 1000 or 1450, chocolate, or a sugar-acacia base. Because of their soft texture, these lozenges can be hand-rolled and then cut into pieces that contain the correct amount of active ingredient. A more accurate and convenient dispensing method is to pour the warm mass into a plastic troche mold, where a specific amount of drug can be assured.

Filling a Soft Lozenge Mold

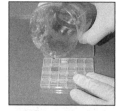

Begin filling in an interior cavity.

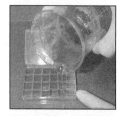

Continue by filling the surrounding cavities.

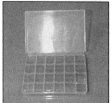

Continue to fill the mold in a systematic manner.

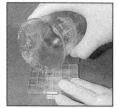

Complete pouring the mold. Overfill each cavity if necessary.

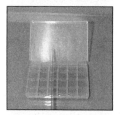

With a spatula, skim the top of the filled mold first one direction…

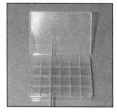

…and then back again.

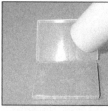

A low heat gun can produce a smooth appearance.

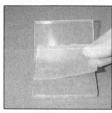

A piece of wax paper keeps the troches from sticking to the top of the mold.

1. When using a troche mold, start the pour in the B2 position and continue to fill all of the cavities in one pouring. PEGs contract as they cool, so the cavities of the troche mold should be overfilled. Chocolate does not shrink as it cools, so overfilling is not necessary.

2. Before the material has solidified in the mold, use the edge of a spatula to level and even out the poured mass.

3. Once the material has cooled in the troche mold, use a warm spatula or light heating with a hot air blow dryer to impart a smooth appearance.

4. Package with a piece of wax paper to keep the troches from sticking to the top of the plastic mold.

Some soft lozenge formulations contain acacia and silica gel. Acacia is used to add texture and smoothness to the lozenge, and silica gel is used as a suspending agent to keep materials from settling to the bottom of the mold cavity during the cooling process. Because mixtures typically are heated to about 50°C during preparation, other ingredients such as sweeteners (e.g., sodium saccharin) should be heat stable.

Chewable Lozenges

Chewable lozenges are intended to be chewed and swallowed and are popular with the pediatric population, as they are "gummy type" lozenges. Most formulations are based on the glycerinated gelatin suppository formula, which consists of glycerin, gelatin, and water. These lozenges often are intensely fruit-flavored and may have a slightly acidic taste to cover the acrid taste of the glycerin. Experimentation will be needed to achieve a satisfactory flavored and sweetened formulation.

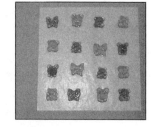

Calibration Procedure

Lozenge molds must be calibrated just like any other mold (e.g., suppository, tablet triturates). The mold will have to be calibrated for each lozenge base. The reader should refer to the mold calibration procedure in Chapter 17, Suppositories, to understand the rationale for the following steps in the lozenge mold calibration procedure:

1. Determine the average weight of a lozenge using only the base materials.

2. Calculate the density factor of substances that will be added to the lozenge base. Any substances added to the base will occupy a specific volume, so the amount of base required in the formulation will have to be adjusted. As an approximation if a density factor is not available, solid ingredients will displace most lozenge bases from 70%–90%. Liquid ingredients will displace 100% of the base.

Flavoring and Sweetening

Flavoring and sweetening soft lozenges to achieve a satisfactory taste will require some experimentation on the pharmacist's part. Flavors can be obtained from sources such as food extracts, syrup flavor concentrates, and volatile oils. Sweeteners, either alone or in combination, will have to be added. A mixture of 9 parts Nutrasweet® and 1 part saccharin might be a suitable starting point for developing a suitable sweetener.

A rule of how to determine the amount of flavoring agent that should be added to a lozenge is as follows: Prepare the lozenges without any drug present, and flavor these blank lozenges to taste. Then, when the drug is added to the formulation, start with about 5 to 10 times the amount of flavoring used in the blank lozenges. In general, 0.05 ml–0.65 ml of flavor per 24 troches will mask most chemical tastes. If the flavoring agent to be added is immiscible in the base, an intermediate solvent might be added to dissolve the flavoring agent before incorporating the solvent into the base. A few drops of glycerin should be sufficient in a ratio of 1 part glycerin to 3–5 parts flavoring.

A gelatin soft lozenge would be a good base for lozenges used to enhance buccal or sublingual absorption because it dissolves more slowly than the polyethylene glycol bases. More drug would be absorbed from the buccal cavity and less would be swallowed and lost to the gastrointestinal (GI) tract. But the long contact time would limit gelatin's usefulness if the drug is extremely bitter or if the taste is hard to mask. The polyethylene glycol bases are more palatable for the patient and should be used if buccal or sublingual absorption is a therapeutic goal.

Sample formulations of the different types of lozenges are given in Table 16.1.

Medication Sticks

Sticks are an easily transportable and convenient dosage form for administering topical medications. They can be compounded in different sizes and shapes for application to different areas of the body. They can be applied directly to the affected site of the body for local activity, or they can be applied to specific epidermal sites if systemic activity is desired. Epidermal penetration enhancers can be added to the formulation to promote this latter use. Local anesthetics, sunscreens, oncology drugs, antivirals, and antibiotics all can be administered by medication sticks.[2]

Soft Sticks

Sticks get their consistency from a combination of waxes, polymers, resins, and in some cases, from drug solids fused into a firm mass. Medication sticks containing waxes, polymers, oils, and gels (or combinations of these) that will soften at body temperature and allow the formulation to be spread evenly over the affected area are called *soft sticks*. These sticks are either clear or opaque, depending on the base used in the formulation. When applied to the skin, they leave no visible residue. Clear soft sticks contain sodium stearate, glycerin, and/or propylene glycol in their base. Opaque soft stick bases might contain petrolatum, cocoa butter, and polyethylene glycol (PEG).

The consistency of soft sticks usually is determined by the blend of high and low melting point ingredients used as the base. This produces a product that will melt or soften at body temperature, spread easily on the application site without crumbling or cracking, and is not excessively greasy. Some common substances used in base formulations and their melting points are given in Table 16.2.

Additional high melting point ingredients can be added to "stiffen" (make more solid) some stick formulations (these same ingredients are also used in ointments, creams, and suppositories for the same purpose). These agents have higher melting points (50°–100°C) and, when blended with lower melting point ingredients, will raise the overall melting point of the formulation. Several stiffening agents that can be used for this purpose are given in Table 16.3.

TABLE 16.1: EXAMPLE LOZENGE FORMULATIONS

Hard Lozenge		Soft Lozenge		Chewable Lozenge	
Drug	1 g	Drug	1 gm	Drug	0.5 gm
Powdered sugar	42 g	PEG 1000	10 gm	Glycerin	70 ml
Corn syrup	16 g	Aspartame	20 packets	Gelatin	18 gm
Water	24 ml	Mint extract	1 ml	Water	12 ml
Mint extract	1.2 ml	Color qs		Flavoring oil	3 to 4 drops
Color qs				Methyl paraben	0.4 gm

TABLE 16.2: MELTING POINTS OF COMMON MEDICATION STICK INGREDIENTS

Ingredient	Melting Point (°C)
Carnauba wax	81–86
Cetostearyl alcohol	48–55
Cetyl alcohol	45–50
Cetyl esters wax	43–47
Cholesterol	147–150
Cocoa butter	30–35
Glyceryl monostearate	55
Hard fat	27–44
Stearic acid	69–70
Stearyl alcohol	55–60
White wax (beeswax, white and yellow)	62–65
Hydrogenated vegetable oil	61–66
PEG 1500	44–48
PEG 3350	54–58
PEG 6000	58–63

Adapted from "Sticks," by L. V. Allen, Jr., (chapter 14) in The Art, Science, and Technology of Pharmaceutical Compounding, 2nd edition (Washington, DC: American Pharmaceutical Association, 2002), pp. 213–229.

TABLE 16.3: MELTING POINTS OF STIFFENING AGENTS

Ingredient	Melting Point (°C)
Castor oil, hydrogenated	85–88
Cetostearyl alcohol	48–55
Cetyl alcohol	45–50
Cetyl esters wax	43–47
Hard fat	27–44
Stearyl alcohol	55–60
White wax (beeswax, white and yellow)	62–65

Adapted from "Featured Excipient: Stiffening Agents," by L. V. Allen, Jr., in International Journal of Pharmaceutical Compounding 4:60–62, 2000.

Additional substances used in stick bases include paraffin, corn oil, cottonseed oil, oleic oil, peanut oil, soybean oil, and PEG 300 and 400. Adding lubricants minimizes the coherence of the waxes and improves spreadability. Vitamins A and E can be added to enhance emollient and skin care effects. Zinc oxide and p-amino benzoic acid (PABA) could be added to the stick as sun blocks.

Hard Sticks

Hard sticks are made of crystalline powders that are either fused together by heat or held together with a binder. The stick must be moistened to be "activated."

When it is wetted, a concentrated solution of the drug forms on the wetted surface of the stick. When the stick is touched to the affected area, the solution is transferred to the skin. The crystalline powder in the stick may leave a white residue on the skin. The prime example of a hard stick is a styptic pencil.

Table 16.4 gives sample formulations of medication sticks.

TABLE 16.4: EXAMPLE FORMULATIONS OF MEDICATION STICKS

Soft Opaque Stick		Soft Clear Stick		Hard Stick	
White beeswax	30 g	Sodium stearate	13%	Ammonium chloride	7 g
Cetyl alcohol	8 g	Methyl salicylate	35%	Aluminum sulfate	27 g
Cocoa butter (or Fattibase™)	6 g	Menthol	15%	Ferric sulfate	40 g
Carnauba wax	1 g	Propylene glycol	25%	Copper sulfate	26 g
Castor oil tasteless	2 ml	Water	12%		
Aquabase™	20 g				
Petrolatum	13.5 g				
Perfume	0.9 ml				
Preservative	0.1 g				
Butyl stearate	5 mg				
Active drug	qs				

Filling Applicators

Applicators are administration devices that hold the medication stick formulation. Two sizes are typically available: a 45 g and a 5 g (lip balm) applicator. After all of the ingredients have been incorporated into a melt, they are poured into the applicator.

Turn the applicator base two full turns upward to raise the bale.

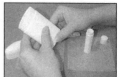

Slightly overfill the applicator with the melted formulation. A hole may appear in the center of the stick as the formulation continues to cool.

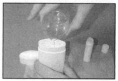

After the stick has stiffened, press a warm spatula on the top of the formulation. This will melt just the surface of the formulation and fill in the hole.

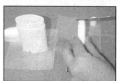

Turn the base of the applicator downward, and place the applicator cap on the device.

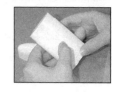

Observing Formulations for Evidence of Instability

The USP Chapter <1191> has no specific recommendations for observing lozenges and sticks for signs of instability.[3] But some guidelines can be obtained from the general comments about semisolids.

> For creams, ointments, and suppositories, the primary indication of instability is often either discoloration or a noticeable change in consistency or odor.

Because many of the ingredients used in lozenges and sticks also are used in creams, ointments, and suppositories, it is reasonable to use changes in color and odor as signs of instabilities.

Hard lozenges and PEG polymers have a tendency to be hygroscopic and to soften when exposed to elevated temperatures. Therefore, these formulations should be stored in tight containers, which also keeps the products from drying out—a specific problem with chewable lozenges. Sticks or lip balms are contained in applicators, and the patient must be advised to replace the applicator

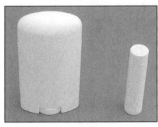

cap after each use. Both lozenges and sticks should be stored in a cool, dry place. Refrigeration may or may not be needed, depending on the active drug incorporated and the type of base used.

A quality assessment procedure for these dosage forms has been published.[4] Attributes such as weight variation, appearance, odor, melting point, and hardness can be observed, and should be evaluated as appropriate for each type of formulation. It also is advisable to prepare an extra batch of a new formulation (new to the pharmacist) for observation over the expected use or life of the formulation.

Because these formulations can be considered "dry" formulations, a beyond use date assignment for that type of formulation is appropriate. The beyond use date would be 25% of the time remaining to the expiration date if the product is prepared using a manufactured product, or 6 months, whichever is earlier.[5]

NOTES

1. <1151> Pharmaceutical Dosage Forms: The United States Pharmacopeia 29/National Formulary 24, The United States Pharmacopeial Convention, Inc., Rockville, MD, 2005, pp. 2996–3006.

2. Allen, L.V., Jr. The Basics of Compounding: Compounding Medication Sticks. *International Journal of Pharmaceutical Compounding* 4:44–47, 2000.

3. <1191> Stability Considerations in Dispensing Practice: The United States Pharmacopeia 29/National Formulary 24, The United States Pharmacopeial Convention, Inc., Rockville, MD, 2005, pp. 3029–3031.

4. Allen, L.V., Jr. Standard Operating Procedure for Performing Physical Quality Assessment of Suppositories, Troches, Lollipops and Sticks. *International Journal of Pharmaceutical Compounding* 3:56–57, 1999.

5. <795> Pharmaceutical Compounding—Nonsterile Preparations: The United States Pharmacopeia 29/National Formulary 24, The United States Pharmacopeial Convention, Inc., Rockville, MD, 2005, pp. 2731–2735.

ADDITIONAL READING

Mason, D., and Fields, S. Lollipops: The Evolution of a Dosage Form. *International Journal of Pharmaceutical Compounding* 6:178–179, 2002.

CHAPTER SEVENTEEN

Suppositories

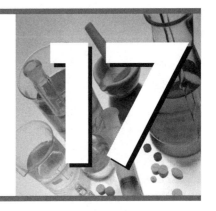

SUPPOSITORIES ARE MEDICATED SEMISOLID FORMULA-tions that are inserted into body cavities. They are made in a variety of shapes and sizes to facilitate insertion into different body cavities and to meet the specific requirements of those routes of administration. Once inside the body cavity, they melt, soften, or dissolve, releasing the active drug. Drugs administered via suppositories provide both local and systemic activity.

Routes of Administration

The routes of administration include rectal, vaginal, and urethral.

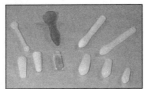

Rectal Route of Administration

The most common rectal formulations are suppositories, solutions, and ointments. Among the many advantages of this route of administration are the following.

- The rectal route of administration is viable when nausea and vomiting are involved, patients are unconscious, or the patients are infants/small children or severely debilitated patients.
- This route has no taste limitations—particularly important with children.
- Hepatic first-pass metabolism may be avoided partially or completely.
- Drugs are not exposed to gastric fluids or gastrointestinal membrane enzymatic activity.

Major disadvantages of this route are the following.
- Absorption may be interrupted by defecation.
- This route has a small surface area (200 to 400 cm²) for passive absorption.
- A small rectal fluid content may cause problems with drug dissolution or absorption.
- Many patients do not prefer suppositories because of their inconvenience.
- Rectal absorption of most drugs frequently is erratic and unpredictable.

- Some suppositories "leak" or are expelled after insertion.

The rectum consists of the terminal portion of the colon, is approximately 15 to 20 cm in length, and generally is smaller in women than in men. When empty of fecal material, the rectum contains only 2 to 3 ml of fluid. The pH of the fluid is approximately 6.8 to 7.4. The rectal content has minimal buffer capacity, and its pH is easily altered by the presence of drugs or other compounds.

The smooth muscle of the colon and rectum has two layers: an outer layer of longitudinal fibers and an inner circular layer. In the resting state the rectum is non-motile. The rectum is lined with a furrowed mucous membrane consisting of both cuboidal and columnar epithelium, as well as mucous-producing Goblet cells. These cells have no villi or microvilli. The main blood supply to the rectum is via the inferior mesenteric artery, which becomes the superior hemorrhoidal artery below the sigmoid arteries.

Venous return occurs through the inferior, middle, and superior rectal hemorrhoidal veins. The superior hemorrhoidal vein empties into the hepatoportal vein, and the lower and middle rectal veins bypass the liver and enter the general circulation. The rectum has two lymphatic networks—one in the mucosa and one in the muscular layer. Both of these drain into the anorectal nodes, located outside the upper rectum, and ultimately into the general circulation.

Most commercially prepared rectal suppositories are torpedo-shaped, with the pointed end tapering to the blunt end. The characteristic suppository shape originally was adopted with the thinking that when suppositories were inserted pointed end first, expulsion would be prevented by the anal sphincter prohibiting the broader part of the suppository from leaving the rectum. That assumption has been challanged by the finding that the ease of insertion, retention, and lack of expulsion are enhanced when the suppository is inserted blunt end first.[1] Here the lack of expulsion is thought to be caused by the reversed vermicular contractions of the external anal sphincter that move the inserted suppository up into the rectum.

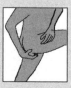

Rectal suppositories are about 20 mm in length and weigh about 2 grams. Infant rectal suppositories are about half the size of adult suppositories. The maximum amount of solid material that can be incorporated into a suppository is about 30% of the blank weight. Therefore, doses greater than 500 mg cannot be delivered with rectal suppositories but can be administered easily in vaginal suppositories.

Drugs are administered via the rectum for a local effect or to achieve a systemic effect. Local effects include soothing the inflamed hemorrhoidal tissues and promoting laxation and evacuation. Rectal administration to achieve systemic activity has been used to treat a variety conditions such as asthma, nausea, motion sickness, anxiety, migraine headaches, and bacterial infections. Drugs are absorbed systemically by passive diffusion, but the absorption is less extensive and slower than after oral administration because the surface area of the rectal mucosa is about 1/10,000 the surface area of the small intestine.

Rectal bioavailability is influenced by various factors including the site of absorption, any absorption enhancers used in formulation, the colonic content, and the suppository base employed in the dosage form. Another factor is the lack of buffer capacity of the rectal fluids. Because the fluid has no effective buffer capacity, the rectal environment will not influence the form in which the drug is absorbed (i.e., unionized or ionized). Bioavailability thus can be predictably changed by using an alternative form of the drug (e.g., a salt form), or other components in the formulation may change the pH of the rectal lumen.

The bioavailability of a specific drug depends on the site of absorption in the rectal mucosa. If the drug is absorbed into the upper rectal (hemorrhoidal) veins that drain into the portal system, the drug may undergo significant first-pass metabolism and have reduced bioavailability. If absorbed through the lower veins that drain into the inferior vena cava, however, the extent of absorption might approximate the absorption of the drug following oral administration. Generally, drugs appear to be absorbed mainly in the lower hemorrhoidal veins; however, exceptions have been reported.

The bioavailability of poorly absorbable drugs can be increased by the use of adjuvants in the rectal formulations. Research has shown that the rectal absorption of small drug molecules, as well as peptides and proteins, can be enhanced by compounds such as sodium salicylate, glyceryl esters of acetoacetic acid, polyacrylic acid, bile salts, fatty acids, and N-acyl derivatives of amino acids. They are thought to promote absorption by temporarily altering the rectal mucosal integrity by interacting with calcium involved in the intercellular structure of the mucosal cells. Adding surfactants seems to enhance absorption under certain circumstances but tends to

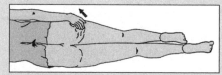

INSERTING RECTAL SUPPOSITORIES

1. If possible, go to the toilet and empty the bowels.
2. Wash your hands carefully with soap and warm water.
3. Remove any foil or plastic wrapping from the suppository.
4. Lubricate the tapered end of the suppository with a small amount of K-Y® Jelly. If the jelly is not available, moisten the suppository with a small amount of water.
5. Either stand with one leg on a chair, or lie on one side with one leg straight and the other leg bent toward your stomach.

6. Separate the buttocks to expose the rectal area.
7. Gently but firmly push the suppository into the rectum until it passes the sphincter (about 1/2 to 1 inch in infants, and 1 inch in adults).
8. Close your legs and sit (or lie) still for about 15 minutes. Avoid emptying bowels for at least 1 hour (unless the suppository is a laxative). Also, avoid excessive movement or exercise for at least one hour.
9. Wash your hands again with soap and warm water after inserting the suppository.

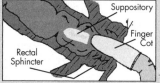

physiologically damage the rectal membrane. Incorporating co-solvents into the delivery system also can promote absorption by altering the vehicle:membrane partitioning behavior.

Greater drug absorption is expected from an evacuated rectum compared to one that is filled with fecal matter. In the absence of fecal matter, the drug will have a better chance of reaching the absorbing surface of the rectum. Other conditions, such as diarrhea and tissue dehydration, also can alter drug absorption.

The suppository base employed has a marked influence on the release of active drug incorporated into it. For example, cocoa butter melts rapidly at body temperature but is immiscible with the rectal fluids. Thus, it fails to release fat soluble drugs readily. Therefore, using the ionized drug form in a cocoa butter base is preferable to maximize bioavailability. Unionized drugs readily partition out of water miscible bases such as glycerinated gelatin and polyethylene glycol, but these bases tend to dissolve slowly, reducing the drug release.

Vaginal Route of Administration

Drugs given in vaginal suppositories are administered most often for local effects. Systemic absorption of drug from the vagina is possible, however, as evidenced by the widespread extemporaneous compounding of progesterone vaginal suppositories. Therefore, this route of administration is a viable alternative to other routes of administration for some drugs.

Among the many advantages of vaginal administration are the following:

- Generally the drug has less absorption variability than oral administration.
- The dose can be retrieved if necessary.
- There is the potential of long term drug administration with various intrauterine devices (IUDs).
- Patient–client compliance is improved.

Some of the disadvantages of vaginal administration are the following:

- Absorption can be variable because the vagina is a physiologically and anatomically dynamic organ and physiological parameters change over time.
- Retention of some delivery systems during menstruation could dispose the patient to toxic shock syndrome.
- This dosage form can interfere with sexual activities.
- The dosage form potentially can be expelled.

The vagina is a fibromuscular tube-shaped organ attached to the uterus and measures about 10 to 15 cm (4 to 6 inches) in length. The vagina is a sheet of smooth muscle consisting of three layers—an outer fibrous layer, a middle muscular layer, and an inner epithelial layer with stratified squamous cells. The surface of the epithelium consists of microridges in either longitudinal or circular patterns, responsible for the vagina's absorptive capacity. A network of vessels supplying blood to the vagina is provided by the uterine and the pudendal arteries that branch from the internal iliac arteries. Blood travels from the vagina through a venous network that ultimately empties into the internal iliac veins.

The vaginal epithelial surface usually is covered with an aqueous film whose volume, pH, and composition vary with age, stage of the menstrual cycle, and location. A pH gradient is evident, with the lower pHs (~ 4) near the anterior fornix and the highest pHs (~ 5) near the cervix. The vaginal mucosa consists of large amounts of glycogen, which forms organic acids upon degradation. These acids help to create the local pH environment in the vagina and retard bacterial growth.

Vaginal formulations include solutions, powders for solutions, ointments, creams, aerosol foams, suppositories, and tablets. Vaginal suppositories are employed as contraceptives, feminine hygiene antiseptics, or bacterial antibiotics, or to restore the vaginal mucosa.

Sometimes called *pessaries*, vaginal suppositories usually are globular, oviform, or cone-shaped and weigh between 3 to 5 grams. Those intended for local activity are employed as contraceptives, as feminine hygiene antiseptics, and as antimicrobial agents against *Trichomonas vaginalis* and *Candida albicans* in particular. Vaginal suppositories intended for systemic activity account for just a few commercial products, which are associated

INSERTING VAGINAL SUPPOSITORIES

1. Wash your hands carefully with soap and warm water.
2. Remove any foil or plastic wrapping from suppository.
3. Place suppository in applicator.
4. Hold the applicator by the end opposite from the suppository.
5. Either lie on the back with your knees bent, or stand with the feet spread a few inches apart and knees bent.
6. Gently insert the applicator into the vagina as far as it will go comfortably. Then push the inside of the applicator, which will place the suppository as far back in the vagina as possible.
7. Remove the applicator from the vagina.
8. Wash your hands again with soap and warm water.

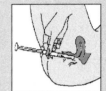

with the vaginal administration of contraceptive steroids and prostaglandins.

Vaginal suppositories are inserted high in the vaginal tract with the aid of a special applicator. Patients should be instructed to dip the suppository quickly in water before insertion. Because suppositories tend to be used at bedtime and can be messy if the formulation is an oleaginous base, the woman should wear a sanitary napkin to protect nightwear and bed linens.

Urethral Route of Administration

Urethral suppositories, sometimes called *bougies*, are not described specifically in the USP/NF by either weight or dimension. Traditionally, these are cylindrical in shape (3–6 mm in diameter) and vary in length according to gender. Female urethral suppositories can be 25–70 mm in length, and male urethral suppositories can be about 50–125 mm in length. The one commercially available urethral suppository actually is marketed as a "pellet" and is 1.4 mm in diameter and 3 or 6 mm in length, depending on its strength. Urethral suppositories may be used as antibacterials and as local preparative anesthetics. They are unusual, however, and are unlikely to be encountered in a compounding practice.

Suppository Bases

The ideal suppository base is nontoxic, nonirritating, inert, compatible with the incorporated drug(s), and easily pliable into the desired shape. The base also should dissolve or melt in the presence of mucous secretions at body temperature, and allow release of the drug. Although no one base satisfies all of those requirements, many bases are used routinely in compounding. Suppository bases may be classified by composition and physical properties as:

- oleaginous (fatty) bases, or
- water soluble or water miscible bases.

Oleaginous Bases

Oleaginous bases have several advantages that make them appealing as suppository material. Among these benefits are their mild and nonirritating action on the rectal mucosa and their tendency to melt in 3 to 7 minutes so the drug can be released quickly from the formulation. All of the oleaginous bases have lower melting points than the water miscible bases and must be kept in controlled room temperature environments or refrigerated in warmer climates.

The classic example of an oleaginous base is cocoa butter (Theobroma Oil). At room temperature, cocoa butter is a hard, amorphous solid, but at body temperature it melts to a bland, nonirritating oil. But good cocoa butter suppositories are difficult to make for several reasons. Two of the most important are the following:

- When the base is melted to incorporate a drug, it must not be heated above 35°C (95°F). Cocoa butter is a polymorphic compound with four structural forms and, if overheated, will form a metastable form that will melt around room temperature (25°C, 77°F). The proper method of melting cocoa butter is to use a hotplate or water bath (just warm water) at about 55°C and melt the base carefully. Correctly melted cocoa butter should have an opalescent, creamy appearance. Cocoa butter that has been overheated will change to a clear, golden liquid and should not be used.

- Certain common ingredients will lower the melting point of cocoa butter suppositories. Chloral hydrate, phenolic compounds (e.g., camphor, menthol, phenol, thymol), and volatile oils tend to lower the melting point. If the melting point is lowered too much, waxes such as spermaceti, cetyl esters wax (about 20%), or beeswax (about 4%) can be added to raise the melting point of the finished suppositories. If too much wax is added, though, the suppositories do not melt at body temperature.

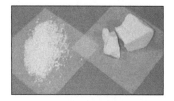

Newer synthetic triglycerides (e.g, Wecobee®, Witepsol®) do not have the formulation difficulties of cocoa butter. They are more expensive, though. Other newer bases composed of mixtures of fatty acids do not have the formulation problems or the expense (e.g., MBK®, FattiBase®). These newer bases have a major advantage over cocoa butter in that they do not exhibit polymorphism. Therefore, controlling melting temperatures is not as critical in the formulation process. Certain names denote a series of bases. In a series, the bases are varied to give a range of melting points. For example, Wecobee® is a series of bases. Wecobee FS, M, R, and S all are made from triglycerides of coconut oil, but FS has a melting point range of 39.4 to 40.5°C, M has a range of 33.3 to 36.0°C, R has a range of 33.9 to 35.0°C, and S has a range of 38.0 to 40.5°C. Other synthetic triglyceride type bases include Dehydag®, Hydrokote®, Suppocire®, and Witepsol®.

Water Soluble/Water Miscible Bases

The water soluble or water miscible bases are those containing glycerinated gelatin or the polyethylene glycol (PEG) polymers. These bases dissolve in rectal mucosal fluids in contrast to the triglycerides, which melt at body temperature. Therefore, the problems of handling, storage, and shipping are simplified.

Glycerinated gelatin is a suitable suppository base for vaginal suppositories. It dissolves slowly in mucous secretions (generally in about 30 to 40 minutes), providing prolonged release of the active drug. It can be used with a wide range of drugs including alkaloids, boric acid, and zinc oxide. Glycerinated gelatin suppositories are made of 70 parts glycerin, 20 parts gelatin, and 10 parts water. They are translucent, are resilient, and have a soft, rubbery consistency.

When making glycerinated gelatin suppositories, the glycerin and water are mixed and heated. The heating should be controlled throughout the preparation process by using a steam bath or a boiling water bath. Then the

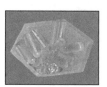

gelatin is added to the glycerin/water mixture slowly and with gentle mixing so air will not be entrapped in the mixture. If air is entrapped, the finished suppositories will contain air bubbles. The resulting mixture is heated an additional 40 to 50 minutes until a clear solution is obtained.

Suppositories made with glycerinated gelatin must be kept in airtight containers in a cool place because they are hygroscopic and will absorb atmospheric moisture. If the suppositories are intended for extended use, a preservative should be added. Generally, methylparaben, propylparaben, or a combination of the two is used as the preservative.

Polyethylene glycol (PEG) polymers possess many desirable properties that make them suitable as a suppository base. They are chemically stable, are miscible with water and mucous secretions, and can be formulated in a wide range of hardnesses and melting points. The different hardnesses and melting points are obtained by using different combinations of PEGs. A major advantage of PEG suppositories is that they

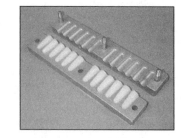

can be formulated with much higher melting points because they dissolve, not melt, in body fluids. Thus, they can be stored safely at room temperature.

Polyethylene glycols are available in various ranges of molecular weight. Those under 1,000 molecular weight are liquids; those with molecular weights over 1,000 are solids. Table 17.1 gives the molecular weight averages, ranges, and melting ranges.

Certain PEGs may be used alone as suppository bases, but combinations of two or more molecular weights typically are used to obtain a desired hardness or dissolution time. Several example formulations are listed in Table 17.2. Polybase® is a commercially available base that is a combination of PEGs.

TABLE 17.1: POLYETHYLENE GLYCOLS: MOLECULAR WEIGHT AVERAGES, WEIGHT RANGES, AND MELTING RANGES

Molecular Weight Average	Molecular Weight Range	Melting Range (°C)
300	285–315	–15 to –8
400	380–420	4–8
600	570–630	20–25
1000	950–1050	37–40
1450	1300–1600	43–46
3350	3000–3700	54–58
4600	4400–4800	57–61
8000	7000–9000	60–63

TABLE 17.2: EXAMPLE FORMULATIONS OF PEG SUPPOSITORIES

Base	Percent	Base	Percent
PEG 1450	30%	PEG 3350	60%
PEG 8000	70%	PEG 1000	30%
PEG 300	60%	PEG 400	10%
PEG 8000	40%	PEG 8000	30%
PEG 300	48%	PEG 1540	70%
PEG 6000	52%	PEG 8000	40%
PEG 1000	95%	PEG 400	60%
PEG 3350	5%	PEG 8000	20%
PEG 1000	75%	PEG 400	80%
PEG 3350	25%	PEG 8000	60%
PEG 300	10%	PEG 1540	25%
PEG 1540	65%	Cetyl Alcohol	5%
PEG 3350	25%	Water	10%
PEG 8000	50%		
PEG 1540	30%		
PEG 400	20%		

Glycerinated gelatin and PEG bases have many similarities:

- They both dissolve in about 30 to 50 minutes, providing a more prolonged release of drug than cocoa butter.
- Both should be moistened with water before insertion.
- They do not melt in the fingers while being inserted.
- They do not "leak" from body orifices. Thus, they are the preferred bases for vaginal and urethral suppositories because these two organs do not have sphincter muscles to prevent leakage from the orifices.

A disadvantage of PEG bases is that they can produce a stinging or burning sensation in the sensitive tissues of the rectum, vagina, and urethra. When used rectally, they also can cause a defecating reflex. This effect can be minimized by adding 10% water to the PEG base and by the patient's moistening the suppository with water before insertion.

The major disadvantage of the PEG bases, however, is their incompatibility with a large number of drugs. They have been found to be incompatible with silver salts, tannic acid, aminopyrine, quinine, ichthammol, aspirin, benzocaine, iodochlorhydroxyquin, indomethacin, and some sulfonamides. Sodium barbital, salicylic acid, and camphor will crystallize out of PEG suppositories. Also, PEG suppositories should not be stored in polystyrene prescription vials because PEG reacts with the polystyrene.

Drug Release Rate and Absorption

The rate of drug release from suppositories is a complicated process, often resulting in erratic and unpredictable absorption. The rate limiting step in drug release is not the speed at which oleaginous bases melt or PEG bases dissolve. The rate limiting step is the drug partitioning and diffusing out of the base material in the rectal lumen. Therefore, the hydrophilic and hydrophobic characteristics of both the drug and the suppository base must be considered. For drugs that are undissolved in a suppository, the size of the drug particle influences its rate of dissolution and ultimate release. Therefore, drugs present in smaller particle sizes would be expected to have more rapid release.

Notwithstanding the variables, some generalities are possible. The release of a drug from an oleaginous base generally depends on the water:base partition coefficient of the drug in the given suppository base. Most drugs are hydrophobic when present in their unionized form, so if an unionized drug is present in a hydrophobic base, there is little tendency for the drug to leave the base. But if a salt form of the drug is used, a higher water:base partition coefficient would result and the drug release rate should be greater. Emulsifying agents also will increase the release of drugs from oleaginous bases because they create a higher water:oil interfacial area. For this reason, many of the newer suppository bases contain emulsifiers.

Water soluble bases that dissolve in the rectal fluids release both hydrophilic and hydrophobic drugs. Everything being equal, PEG bases should provide more reliable absorption of hydrophobic drugs than oleaginous bases. Table 17.3 summarizes general trends for the release of drugs from suppository bases.

TABLE 17.3: GENERAL TRENDS FOR RELEASE OF DRUGS FROM SUPPOSITORY BASES

Drug Type	Oleaginous Base	Water Soluble/ Miscible Base
Hydrophobic drug	slow release	moderate release
Hydrophilic drug	more rapid release than hydrophobic drug	moderate to rapid release

The actual absorption of the drug can be quite variable once it reaches the rectal mucosa. Because the suppository material may move to various sections of the rectum, the drug may enter different parts of the circulatory system. If the drug is absorbed from the upper part of the rectum into the superior hemorrhoidal vein, it will be transported through the liver first, on its way to the systemic circulation. If the drug can be metabolized in the liver, first-pass metabolism will occur and decrease the drug's bioavailability. If the drug is absorbed from the lower part of the rectum, it will enter the inferior veins and bypass the liver's first-pass metabolism altogether, increasing the bioavailability of the drug.

Methods of Preparation of Suppositories

The common methods used to compound suppositories include hand rolling, compression, and fusion. Of these three, the fusion method is utilized most often.

Hand Rolling

Hand rolling, the simplest method of suppository preparation, may be used when only a few suppositories are to be prepared in a cocoa butter base. This method has the advantage of not having to heat the cocoa butter. A plastic-like mass is prepared by triturating grated cocoa butter and active ingredients in a mortar. The mass is formed into a ball in the palm of the hands, then rolled into a uniform cylinder with a large spatula or a small flat board on a pill tile. The cylinder then is cut into the appropriate number of pieces, which are shaped on one end to produce a conical shape.

Effective hand rolling requires considerable practice and skill. The suppository cylinder, or "pipe," tends to crack or become hollow in the center, especially when the mass is kneaded and softened insufficiently. Even with practice, the suppositories do not have the elegant appearance of suppositories made by fusion.

The steps in hand rolling suppositories are as follows:

1. Weigh the amount of drug and base.
2. Triturate the drug to a fine powder in a glass mortar.
3. Using geometric dilution, mix the drug and the cocoa butter.
4. Put on disposable gloves and collect the mixture in the mortar. Knead the mass into a ball and begin to form a cylindrical pipe.
5. Put the pipe on an ointment slab and, with a broad-bladed spatula, roll the mass into a smooth cylindrical pipe, keeping the ends as square as possible. Use the gauge on the ointment slab or a ruler to determine the proper length of the pipe so equal pieces of appropriate length (appropriate weight) can be cut.
6. Cut the pipe into pieces of equal length and taper one end of each piece into a bullet shape.
7. Weigh each suppository and adjust the weight by slicing thin pieces from the blunt end.

Compression

The compression method is suited for making suppositories that have heat labile components or for suppositories that contain a large proportion of insoluble ingredients. This process provides little opportunity for the insoluble materials to settle. Specialized equipment, however, is required to make suppositories by compression.

The suppository base and other ingredients are blended with kneading mixers inside a warmed mixing vessel. When the mixture is ready, the mass is forced into a mold under pressure. Many different shapes and sizes of molds are available for this operation. When compression is complete, the suppositories are ejected from the mold and the cycle is repeated. Many of the vaginal tablets (inserts) are manufactured using this method. The tablets are formulated to contain lactose as a filler, a disintegrating agent, a dispersing agent, and a lubricant. Vaginal tablets contain the same active drugs as vaginal suppositories—i.e., anti-infectives and hormones.

Fusion

The fusion method involves first melting the suppository base, then dispersing or dissolving the drug in the melted base. The mixture is removed from the heat and poured into a suppository mold. When the mixture has congealed, the suppositories are removed from the mold. The fusion method can be used with all types of suppositories and actually *must* be used with most of them.

Suppository Molds

Industrial molds produce hundreds of suppositories in a single batch. When filling molds, the suppository mixture is placed in the cavities of a closed mold by means of a volumetric pump that meters the melt from a jacketed kettle or mixing tank. An alternative method is to extrude or inject the molten mixture under pressure into molds. Once the suppositories are formed, the molds are opened to retrieve the molded suppositories or the suppositories are ejected from the mold.

Small hand-held molds are made of stainless steel, aluminum, brass, or plastic and come in a variety of

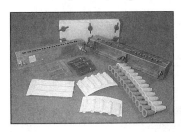

cavity sizes and with different numbers of cavities per mold. Common sizes vary from 1 g to 2.5 g and the number of cavities typically is 6 cavities, but can go up to 100 cavities per mold.

Aluminum metal molds are separated into two halves that typically are held together with several screws and wing nuts, but some molds have only one center screw.

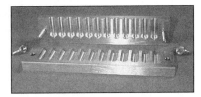

Compounding Suppositories by the Fusion Method

Aluminum molds usually require lubrication before making suppositories. One way is to use a vegetable oil spray. Other lubricants include light mineral oil when water soluble bases are being used, and glycerin or propylene glycol when oleaginous bases are being used. Whatever lubricant is used, only a light coating is needed. If too much lubricant is used, the excess will pool in the tip of the suppository cavity. Any excess lubricant should be wiped off with a tissue.

When using these molds, the suppository mixture is poured into the cavities of a closed mold. Molds should be filled only when they are at room temperature. A cold or frozen mold should not be used, because it can cause fractures and fissures throughout the suppository. Each cavity should be filled slowly and carefully to ensure that no air bubbles are entrapped in the cavity. To prevent layering in the suppositories, the pouring process should not be stopped until all the cavities have been filled. Molds should be allowed to set for 30 minutes at room temperature before opening.

To fill a suppository mold, start pouring the melt at one end and pour continuously without stopping. Do not go to the next cavity until the previous cavity is filled and a slight excess has been poured to overfill the cavity.

When suppository mixtures cool, they contract. Some mixtures and bases (e.g., cocoa butter, PEG) have pronounced contractions, and others (e.g, glycerinated gelatin) have much smaller contractions. The contraction will produce a hole in the blunt end of the suppository, which is undesirable. Pouring the suppository mixture immediately before it reaches its congealing temperature will minimize the contraction. Also, it is helpful to pour a small excess of the suppository mixture on the open end of the

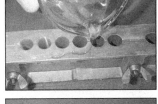

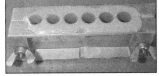

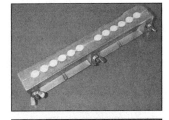

mold. Once the suppositories have hardened, the excess base can be removed by trimming the top of the mold with a warm stainless steel spatula.

The mold then is ready to be separated into its two halves. An efficient way to separate the mold is to remove the wing nuts or to loosen the centered screw and place the mold so the posts rest on the table top. Then apply downward pressure on only the bottom half of the mold. A knife or spatula should not be used to pry apart the two halves, as this will damage the matching mold faces that have been machined to produce a tight seal.

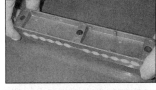

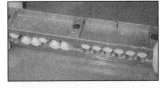

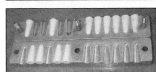

Plastic suppository shells come in long strips that can be torn into any number of cavities. These disposable molds do not require any lubrication

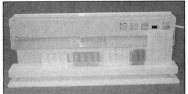

regardless of the suppository mixture. The suppository mixture is poured directly into the shell up to a mark. Using a backfill light helps in visualization of the fill mark on the shell.

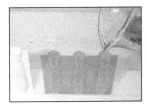

When the mixture has hardened, the plastic mold is heat-sealed.

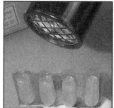 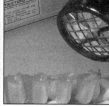 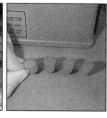

When patients are ready to use a suppository, they select one shell and peel off the sides of the shell to obtain the suppository.

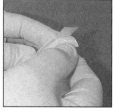 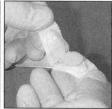 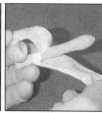

Some suppository molds are made from rubber. When the suppository mixture has congealed in these molds, the finished suppositories are pushed out of each cavity.

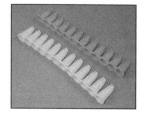

Density Factors

Usually suppositories are made from solid ingredients and drugs that are measured by weight. When they are mixed, melted, and poured into suppository mold cavities, they occupy a volume—the volume of the mold cavity. Because the components are measured by weight but compounded by volume, density factor calculations and mold calibrations are required to provide accurate doses.

When a drug is placed in a suppository base, it will displace an amount of base as a function of its density. If the drug has the same density as the base, it will displace an equivalent weight of the base. If the density of the drug is greater than that of the base, it will displace a proportionally smaller weight of the base. Density factors for common drugs in cocoa butter are available in standard reference texts. The density factor is used to determine how much of a base a drug will displace. The relationship is:

$$\text{Density Factor} = \frac{\text{weight of drug}}{\text{weight of base displaced}}$$

For example, aspirin has a density factor in cocoa butter of 1.3. If a suppository is to contain 0.3 g of aspirin, it will replace 0.3 g ÷ 1.3 or 0.23 g of cocoa butter. If the blank suppository (suppository without the drug) weighs 2 g, then 2 g − 0.23 g or 1.77 g of cocoa butter will be needed for each suppository, and the suppository will weigh 1.77 g + 0.3 g = 2.07 g. So a pharmacist making 12 suppositories would weigh 1.77 g × 12 or 21.24 g of cocoa butter and 0.3 g × 12 or 3.6 g of aspirin.

The weight of the blank suppository is determined easily. A portion of the suppository base is melted, poured into the suppository mold, and allowed to congeal. The suppositories are removed from the mold, and the total weight of the suppositories is determined. The average weight of a blank suppository is determined by dividing the total weight by the number of suppositories.

Table 17.4 gives density factors for common drugs in cocoa butter.

TABLE 17.4: DENSITY FACTORS FOR COMMON DRUGS IN COCOA BUTTER

Drug	Density Factor
Alum	1.7
Aminophylline	1.1
Aspirin	1.3
Barbital	1.2
Benzoic acid	1.5
Bismuth carbonate	4.5
Bismuth salicylate	4.5
Bismuth subgallate	2.7
Bismuth subnitrate	6.0
Boric acid	1.5
Castor oil	1.0
Chloral hydrate	1.3
Cocaine hydrochloride	1.3
Codeine phosphate	1.1
Dimenhydrinate	1.3
Diphenhydramine hydrochloride	1.3
Glycerin	1.6
Ichthammol	1.1
Menthol	0.7
Iodoform	4.0
Morphine hydrochloride	1.6
Phenobarbital	1.2
Phenol	0.9
Potassium bromide	2.2
Potassium iodide	4.5
Procaine	1.2
Quinine hydrochloride	1.2
Resorcinol	1.4
Secobarbital sodium	1.2
Sodium bromide	2.3
Spermaceti	1.0
Sulfathiazole	1.6
Tannic acid	1.6
White wax	1.0
Zinc oxide	4.0
Zinc sulfate	2.8

When the Density Factor is Unknown

When bases other than cocoa butter are used, or when the density factor for a drug in cocoa butter is not known, the density factor can be *estimated by calculation*, or it can be determined experimentally by the *double casting technique*.

Estimation by Calculation: To estimate by calculation, the ratio of the weight of the non-cocoa butter suppository base to the weight of the cocoa butter suppository base must be determined. Each of the bases (i.e., non-cocoa butter and cocoa butter) are fabricated in the same suppository mold, and the ratio then is calculated. As an example of this method, a mold was filled with a PEG base and the average suppository weighed 2.24 grams. The same mold was filled with cocoa butter, and those suppositories weighed 1.87 grams on average. Therefore, the ratio was:

$$\frac{\text{weight of PEG suppositories}}{\text{weight of cocoa butter suppositories}} = \frac{2.24\text{ g}}{1.87\text{ g}} = 1.20$$

If 200 mg of aspirin is to be incorporated into each PEG suppository, it is necessary to determine how much PEG base will be displaced by the aspirin. That displacement amount can be calculated as follows:

density factor of aspirin in cocoa butter = 1.3
(from reference sources)

density of PEG base relative to cocoa butter = 1.20
(the ratio obtained from the calibrations)

$$0.2\text{ g of aspirin will displace } \frac{0.2\text{ g}}{1.3} \times 1.20$$
$$= 0.18\text{ g of PEG base}$$

For each PEG suppository to be formulated, 0.2 g of aspirin and 2.06 g (2.24 g − 0.18 g = 2.06 g) of the PEG base will be needed.

Double Casting Technique In the double casting technique, the total quantity of drug is mixed with an amount of base that is inadequate to fill the number of cavities. The mixture is poured into the mold, filling each cavity only partially.

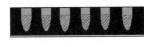

Additional blank base is used to fill the remaining portion of the cavities. When the suppositories have cooled, the excess base is removed from the top of the mold.

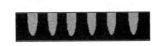

The suppositories then are removed from the mold, remelted, and recast to distribute the active ingredient evenly.

By determining the weights of suppositories at the various steps in the double casting procedure, the density factor can be calculated.

EXAMPLE:

1. Determine a drug's density factor in cocoa butter when the density factor is not known.
2. Using a given mold, the average weight of a blank cocoa butter suppository is 2.0 g. Using the same mold, cocoa butter suppositories each containing 300 mg of drug A averaged 2.1 g. Therefore,

weight of suppository of cocoa butter = 2.0 g

weight of drug in each suppository = 0.3 g

weight of suppository with drug and cocoa butter = 2.1 g

weight of base in medicated suppository = 2.1 g - 0.3 g = 1.8 g

weight of base displaced = 2.0 g − 1.8 g = 0.2 g

Density factor of drug A in cocoa butter = 0.3 g ÷ 0.2 g = 1.5

Obviously, if the density factor of the drug in cocoa butter was known already, there would be no reason to carry out this double casting procedure. The pharmacist would use just the reference source value in any subsequent calculations. But if the pharmacist experimentally determines the density factor, it should be recorded so in the future the value can be used without having to repeat the double casting procedure. Once the density factor is known, it is used to determine the amount of base that the drug will displace.

EXAMPLE: Using the density factor determined above, how much cocoa butter and drug A are needed to make 10 cocoa butter suppositories each containing 0.3 g of drug?

weight of drug A needed = 10 suppositories × 300 mg/suppository = 3,000 mg = 3.0 g

weight of base needed for blank suppositories = 2.0 g/suppositories × 10 suppositories = 20.0 g

weight of base displaced by 3.0 g drug A = 3.0 g ÷ 1.5 = 2.0 g

weight of base needed for medicated suppositories = 20.0 g − 2.0 g = 18.0 g

So 18.0 g of cocoa butter and 3.0 g of drug A are needed to compound this prescription.

The double casting technique can be used to determine the density factor of any drug in any base. The same procedure described for cocoa butter would be carried out, but using instead the base and drug of interest.

EXAMPLE: Determine the density factor of acetaminophen in PEG base.

A PEG base is used, and each suppository is to contain 0.2 g of acetaminophen. Using the double casting technique, the following information is obtained and used to calculate the density factor for acetaminophen in the PEG base.

weight of suppository of blank PEG base = 1.92 g

weight of acetaminophen in each suppository = 0.2 g

weight of suppository with acetaminophen and PEG base = 2.04 g

weight of PEG base only in suppository = 2.04 g − 0.2 g = 1.84 g

weight of PEG base displaced by acetaminophen = 1.92 g − 1.84 g = 0.08 g

$$\text{density factor} = \frac{\text{weight of acetaminophen}}{\text{weight of PEG base displaced}} =$$

$$\frac{0.2\ \text{g}}{0.08\ \text{g}} = 2.5$$

Additional Considerations About Suppositories

- The maximum amount of solid material that can be incorporated into a suppository is about 30% of the blank weight. Therefore, delivering rectal doses of greater than 500 mg may be difficult, but this amount of drug can be incorporated easily into vaginal suppositories.

- The viscosity in some suppository mixtures is too low to support the amount of solid material being incorporated. As the base solidifies, the solids settle out into the tip of the suppository mold. A suspending agent such as silica gel can be added to retard the settling. Generally, 1% to 10% is used, and the most common are the lower concentrations. With oleaginous bases, another approach can be used to increase the viscosity. Ingredients such as fatty acids with longer chain lengths (e.g., C_{16} and C_{18} mono- and diglycerides) can be added to the base. Cetyl, stearyl, and myristyl alcohols and stearic acid in concentrations of about 5% also can be added.

- Solids should be triturated to reduce their particle size before being incorporated into a suppository base. If possible, use the raw powder as the source of the drug. Although crushed tablets, capsules, or injectables can be used as drug sources, the presence of their excipients must be considered in terms of reactivity and bulk mass.

- If the drug is a liquid, mixing it with an inert solid such as starch before incorporating it into the suppository might be helpful. If a large amount of liquid is to be incorporated into a fatty base, it could be emulsified first with cholesterol (2%) or wool fat (10%) into a w/o emulsion. This technique will allow cocoa butter to incorporate about a 15% aqueous solution.

Packaging

Suppositories made in disposable plastic shells or rubber molds can be dispensed directly in the mold. The plastic

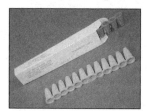

shells can be separated and packaged in a suppository box or other suitable container. The rubber molds can be placed in a sleeve designed for that purpose.

Suppositories that have been made in other molds should be wrapped in aluminum foil before being placed in the dispensing container. The foil can be purchased in 4 inch × 4 inch squares. About 1 inch squares are needed to wrap each suppository.

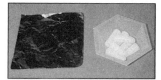

Suppositories and a piece of 4 inch × 4 inch foil.

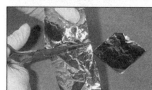

Cut the foil in quarters.

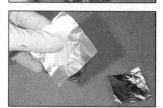

Place the suppository facing two points of the foil.

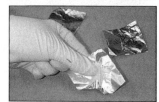

Fold one point of the foil over one end of the suppository.

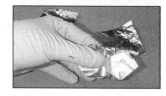

Fold the opposite point over the other end of the suppository.

Fold in one side of the foil over the suppository.

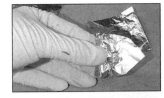

Roll the suppository into the remaining open foil.

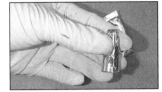

✴ Observing Formulations for Evidence of Instability

Suppositories should be observed for excessive softening. In addition, some suppositories may dry out and harden or shrivel. Either of these changes should be taken as a sign of instability.[2] Suppositories should be examined closely if oil staining is observed on the packaging.

When a manufactured product is used as the source of the active ingredient, USP/NF chapter <795> recommends a beyond use date of "25% of the time remaining until the product's expiration date or 6 months,

whichever is earlier."[3] It is prudent to remember that the formulation manipulations (heating and mixing) can alter the stability of the drugs and excipients. Therefore, the formulation may warrant a shorter beyond use date than the guidelines recommend. As with all compounded formulations, samples of untested formulations should be kept for observation and evaluation.

Suppositories must be stored properly. They should be protected from heat and may be stored under refrigeration but not frozen. Glycerin and PEG base suppositories should be kept in airtight containers because they are hygroscopic.

NOTES

1. Allen, L. V., Jr. Suppositories (chapter 13) in *The Art, Science, and Technology of Pharmaceutical Compounding*, 2nd edition, American Pharmaceutical Association, Washington, D.C, 2002, pp. 189–211.

2. <1191> Stability Considerations in Dispensing Practice: The United States Pharmacopeia 29/National Formulary 24, The United States Pharmacopeial Convention, Inc., Rockville, MD, 2005, pp. 3029–3031.

3. <795> Pharmacy Compounding—Nonsterile Preparations: The United States Pharmacopeia 29/National Formulary 24, The United States Pharmacopeial Convention, Inc., Rockville, MD, 2005, pp. 2731–2735.

CHAPTER EIGHTEEN

Medicated Powder Formulations

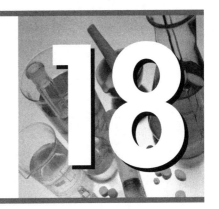

THE VAST MAJORITY OF PHARMACEUTICAL INGREDIENTS occur in the solid state as amorphous powders or as crystals of various morphological structure. The term *powder* has more than one connotation in pharmacy. It can refer to a chemical that is solid in its physical state, or to a dosage formulation that is solid in its physical state. The formulation may be composed of only the active drug, or it may be a mixture of the active drug and other ingredients. Sometimes these are referred to as *medicated powders*, intended for internal or external use.

Although the use of medicated powders per se in therapeutics is limited, the use of powder substances in the preparation of other dosage forms is extensive. For example, powder drugs may be blended with other powder pharmaceutical ingredients to fabricate solid dosage forms such as tablets and capsules, or they may be dissolved or suspended in solvents or liquid vehicles to make various liquid dosage forms. They also may be incorporated into semisolid bases in the preparation of medicated ointments and creams. Granules, which are prepared agglomerates of powder materials, may be used as is for their medicinal value, or they may be prepared for use in various pharmaceutical processes.

Compounded powders offer the following unique advantages:

- Each powder can contain a different dose of active drug.
- Powders can be administered easily to infants and young children who cannot swallow tablets or capsules.
- They will have a rapid onset of drug action because disintegration is not required.
- They can be applied to many body cavities such as ears, nose, tooth socket, and throat.
- The drugs tend to be more stable as a solid than in solution.
- They can be made into many different dosage formulations (capsules, tablets, powders for reconstitution, dusting powders, bulk powders, powders for inhalation, etc.).

Disadvantages of medicated powders are the following:

- They are not suitable for bitter, nauseating, or corrosive drugs.
- Preparation is time-consuming, and therefore more costly.

Properties of Powders

Powders have many characteristics—shape, size, solubility, stability, and so on. These properties are determined early in the development of a pharmaceutical formulation to help make critical decisions about the manufacturing process. Another important use of the information is to guarantee batch-to-batch uniformity of a production procedure. Differences in production batches can come from two sources:

1. The actual manufacturing process, which includes all of the manipulations and machinery involved in creating the product.
2. The powder itself; some drugs require chemical or pharmaceutical modification for therapeutic or formulation reasons before being used in the formulation.

Particle Size

Pharmaceutical powders are formulated to exist as fine particles. Many therapeutic applications and formulation processes are dependent on the particle size of a powder. For example, particle size influences solubility and dissolution rate, both of which in turn influence bioavailability. Powders used for inhalation require that the drug have certain particle sizes to be able to reach the alveoli of the lungs. Some formulations have to be non-gritty (e.g., ophthalmic suspensions and ointments, dermal ointments and creams), which requires smaller particle sizes. From a manufacturing standpoint, particle size influences powder compression, disintegration, wettability, and the ability of a powder to flow in machines.

Powders do not consist of only one-sized particles, and the particles are not perfectly shaped as spheres or

143

cubes. Powders are made up of a distribution of particles of different sizes and shapes. Therefore, the size cannot be described completely with just one parameter such as the length of one side or the diameter. For a powder that is used pharmaceutically, however, a narrow particle size distribution is an advantage. If the particle size distribution is not narrow, the powder can segregate according to the different particle sizes, which may result in inaccurate dosing or inconsistent performance. A narrow particle size distribution ensures a uniform dissolution rate if the powder is to dissolve and a uniform sedimentation rate if the powder is used in a suspension, and it minimizes stratification when powders are stored or transported.

Any mathematical description of particle size will involve a distribution component to account for the different shapes and sizes in the powder. The discipline of *Micrometics* deals with the principles used to describe particle size distributions. The USP/NF provides a qualitative grouping of particle sizes into five categories, as shown in Table 18.1.

TABLE 18.1: USP/NF PARTICLE SIZE CATEGORIES

Description Term	Mesh Opening Size (microns)	Sieve Number
Very coarse	> 1,000	10–2
Coarse	355–1,000	40–20
Moderately coarse	180–355	80–40
Fine	125–180	120–80
Very fine	90–125	200–120

<811> Powder Fineness. The United States Pharmacopeia 29/National Formulary 24. The United States Pharmacopeial Convention, Inc., Rockville, MD, 2005, pp. 2754–2755.

The categories are based on the size of particles that will pass through standard sieves calibrated by the National Bureau of Standards. The sieve number indicates the number of openings per inch in the mesh screen. For example, a #40 sieve has 40 openings per inch in the screen mesh. Particles that can sieve through that mesh are said to be "40 mesh size" and will have a particle size of about 420 microns. Table 18.2 gives the size of the mesh opening in millimeters (1/1,000 of a meter) and microns (1/1,000,000 of a meter).

A sieving method that utilizes a set of standard sieves is used to obtain a quantitative description of the particle size distribution of a powder. The sieves are stacked in order of their number, the powder sample is placed in the top sieve, and the stack is shaken mechanically for a specified period of time. Particles fall through the sieves until they reach the sieve

TABLE 18.2: MESH OPENING SIZES IN U.S. STANDARD SIEVES

Sieve Number	Millimeters (mm)	Microns (μm)
2	9.52	9,520
4	4.76	4,760
8	2.38	2,380
10	2.00	2,000
20	0.84	840
30	0.59	590
40	0.42	420
50	0.297	297
60	0.250	250
70	0.210	210
80	0.177	177
100	0.149	149
120	0.125	125
200	0.074	74

Adapted from "Powders and Granules," by L. V. Allen, Jr., N. G. Popovich, and H. C. Ansel, (chapter 6) in Ansel's Pharmaceutical Dosage Forms and Drug Delivery Systems, 8th edition. (Philadelphia, PA: Lippincott Williams & Wilkins, 2005), pp. 186–203.

that has a mesh opening size that retains the particle. Then the quantity of powder resting on each sieve is weighed.

An example of the information obtained using the sieving method is displayed in Table 18.3. This example is based on the weight of particles. At times, particle size distributions are obtained using the number of particles per category as the dataset. Determining the number of particles in a sample requires a direct observation method such as microscopy.

$$d_{av} = \frac{\Sigma \, (\text{percent retained}) \times (\text{average size})}{100} = \frac{29.232}{100}$$

$$= 0.2923 \text{ mm}$$

TABLE 18.3: EXAMPLE INFORMATION OBTAINED FROM SIEVING METHOD

Sieve Number	Mean of Mesh Opening Size (mm)	Weight Retained (g)	Percent Retained (%)	Percent Retained × Mean Opening Size
20/40	0.630	15.5	14.3	9.009
40/60	0.335	25.8	23.7	7.939
60/80	0.214	48.3	44.4	9.502
80/100	0.163	15.6	14.3	2.330
100/120	0.137	3.5	3.3	0.452
Totals		108.7	100.0	29.232

Adapted from "Powders and Granules," by L. V. Allen, Jr., N. G. Popovich, and H. C. Ansel, chapter 6 in Ansel's Pharmaceutical Dosage Forms and Drug Delivery Systems, 8th edition (Philadelphia, PA: Lippincott Williams & Wilkins, 2005), pp. 186–203.

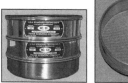

As with any distribution, a statistical descriptor often is used to summarize the data. The mean particle diameter (d_{av}) in the example was calculated by taking the product of the average mesh opening size and the percent of the sample that was retained by those mesh sizes. This sample had a mean particle diameter of 292.3 microns. Thus, this batch of powder can be compared to another batch using only this parameter value. Further comparisons between batches often employ histograms of weight retained or percent retained versus some measure of the particle size. Parameters such as the mode or skewness from the different batches could be used to evaluate batch-to-batch variation.

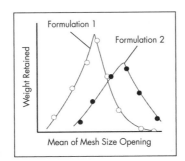

Data often are mathematically transformed into other graphical representations such as cumulative plots, normal-log plots, or probability-log plots to help linearize the data.

WAYS TO DETERMINE PARTICLE SIZES

- Microscopic method
- Sieving method
- Sedimentation method
- Elutriation method
- Centrifugal method
- Coulter counter
- Permeation method
- Adsorption method
- Laser holography

Particle size can be determined in many ways. Sometimes the method used is determined by the anticipated particle size of the sample to be measured. For example, sieving often is used when the particles are about 40 to 9,500 microns in size.[1] Methods such as microscopy, sedimentation rate, laser holography, and cascade impaction are used when particle sizes are smaller than 500 microns. Some methods are selected so the measured particle sizes can be related to the ultimate use of the product. For example, if a powder is to be used in a suspension, more useful information can be obtained by measuring the particle size by sedimentation. Or if the particle surface area is critical in the final formulation, a method that measures surface areas (e.g., gas adsorption, permeability) would be more appropriate.

Microscopy is used to measure particle diameters. The optical measurement involves a calibrated scale that usually is incorporated into the microscope. Gas adsorption methods generally measure the adsorption of nitrogen or krypton as a monolayer on the particles. The particle surface area is calculated as a function of the volume of gas adsorbed, the amount of material occupied by the gas, and the molecular weight and density of the gas. Other determination methods include the electrolyte displace method (the Coulter counter) for particle volumes, and the sedimentation method for particle diameters based on the velocity of sedimentation.[2]

Regardless of the method used to measure the particle size, the measurements will result in a particle size distribution. Various statistical descriptors that measure the central size tendency have been applied to the methods that measure the number, diameter, surface area, or volume of the particles in a powder. Mean particle diameters are the most commonly used parameters because the diameter can be related to the surface area and volume of a particle. The mean particle diameters most commonly used are given in Table 18.4.

TABLE 18.4: DEFINITION OF STATISTICAL DIAMETERS

Type of Statistical Descriptor	Statistical Definition	Particle Property Measured
Arithmetic	$\dfrac{\Sigma nd}{\Sigma n}$	Number of particles
Diameter moment	$\dfrac{\Sigma nd^2}{\Sigma nd}$	Particle diameter
Surface moment	$\dfrac{\Sigma nd^3}{\Sigma nd^2}$	Particle surface area
Volume moment	$\dfrac{\Sigma nd^4}{\Sigma nd^3}$	Particle volume

Adapted from "Micrometics," by A. Martin, (chapter 16) in Physical Pharmacy, 4th edition (Philadelphia, PA: Lea & Febiger, 1993), pp. 423–452.

Particle Shape

The surface characteristics of a powder greatly influence its intrinsic properties. The powder molecules can exist in a crystal system or as amorphous (i.e., without shape) aggregates. Crystal systems are defined by the length of the three sides of the aggregate and the angle that exists at the different apexes. The different structures may be dictated by the morphology of the powder or may be the result of a particular crystallization or precipitation process. Table 18.5 shows the matrix parameters of different crystal systems.

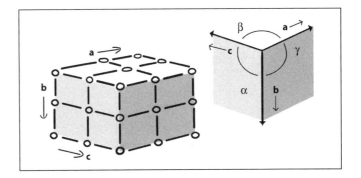

TABLE 18.5: MATRIX PARAMETERS OF DIFFERENT CRYSTAL SYSTEMS

Crystal System	Matrix Parameters
Cubic	$a = b = c, \alpha = \beta = \gamma = 90°$
Monoclinic	$a \neq b \neq c, \alpha = \gamma = 90° \neq \beta$
Triclinic	$a \neq b \neq c, \alpha \neq \beta \neq \gamma$
Orthorhombic	$a \neq b \neq c, \alpha = \beta = \gamma = 90°$
Trigonal	$a = b = c, \alpha = \beta = \gamma \neq 90°$ but $<120°$
Tetragonal	$a = b \neq c, \alpha = \beta = \gamma = 90°$
Hexagonal	$a = b \neq c, \alpha = \beta = 90°$ and $\gamma = 120°$

Crystal habits exist as plates, needles, or cubes and result from the crystallization or precipitation of a compound from solution. If crystal growth occurs equally on the three sides of the aggregate, the original shape will be retained but a larger crystal will result. Therefore, if the shape of the original aggregate was a cube, the crystallized particle also will be a cube. If the crystal growth is inhibited along one or two of the aggregate sides, a plate or a needle crystal is expected to result.

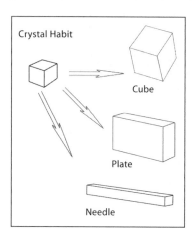

Crystal Habit
Cube
Plate
Needle

Particle Form

A compound can exist in more than one crystalline form. This property is called *polymorphism*. Only one of the polymorphic forms is stable at a given temperature and pressure. The other forms, called *metastable forms*, will convert to the stable form over time. Metastable forms generally have higher solubility and dissolution rates compared to the stable form, but once the crystals have dissolved in solution, the different forms are indistinguishable from one another.

The different shapes (i.e., crystal, amorphous, polymorphs) impart different physicochemical properties to the powders. The pharmaceutical literature contains numerous examples detailing the differences in stability, solubility, dissolution rate, bioavailability, and so on, that result from using different crystalline forms of powders. Thus, knowing the properties of powders that are being used in a formulation process is critical.

Flow

A number of factors, including shape and size, determine how well powders flow. Spherical particles flow better than needle-shaped particles. Very fine particles do not flow as freely as large particles. In general, particles in the size range of 250–2,000 microns flow freely if the shape is suitable. Particles in the size range of 75–250 microns may flow freely or cause problems, depending on shape and other factors. With particles smaller than 100 microns in size, flow rate is a problem with most substances. Flow becomes a critical parameter when powders are used in large scale mixers or machine-fed hoppers. The powder has to flow easily and uniformly to aid in good production results. Good flow properties also are important when packaging powders, filling capsules, and the like.

The *angle of repose* gives an indication of a powder's ability to flow. To determine the angle, the powder flows through a funnel and falls freely onto a surface. As the powder is added to the pile, it slides down the sides until the mutual friction of the particles is in equilibrium with the gravitational force. The height and diameter of the resulting cone are measured and the angle is calculated:

$$\tan \Phi = h/r$$

where

h = the height of the cone
r = the radius

The rougher and more irregular the surface of the particles, the higher will be the angle of repose and the more difficult it will be for the powder to flow easily. Powders with low angles of repose will flow freely.

To improve flow properties, *glidants* frequently are added. Commonly used glidants are magnesium stearate, starch, and talc. The optimum concentration of glidants used in pharmaceutical products seems to be about 1%. Above this concentration a decrease in flow rate often is observed.

Porosity, Volumes, and Densities

Additional considerations in powders are porosity, bulk volumes, true volumes, bulk densities, and true densities. These properties together determine the efficiency of filling equipment used in the manufacturing process and the size of the container to use for the finished product.

Powders of uniform-sized spheres can assume either one of two ideal packing arrangements: (1) a rhombohedral packing (the tightest packing); or (2) a cubic packing (the most open or loosest packing). *Porosity* is the empty space between the particles (i.e., the void space). The theoretical porosity for the rhombohedral packing is 26%, and 48% for the cubic packing.[3]

Powders used as pharmaceutical ingredients are neither spherical in shape nor uniform in size, so most powders will have packing arrangements somewhere between these two ideal extremes. If a large number of fine particles (or "fines") are present in the mixture, they may slip into and fill some of the void space, which will reduce the porosity below 26%.

Porosity (ϵ) and *void space* are related in the following relationship:

$$\epsilon = \text{void space} \times 100$$

Void space can be determined when the *bulk volume* (V_{bulk}) and the *true volume* (V) are known. The bulk volume is the volume that a sample of powder will occupy, which includes the volume of the particles and the void space. For example, if 1 g of powder is poured into a cylindrical graduated vessel and occupies 15 ml, the bulk volume is 15 ml. The true volume of the powder is the volume occupied by the particles alone (exclusive of the voids between the particles).

$$\text{void space} = \frac{V_{bulk} - V}{V_{bulk}}$$

and

$$\epsilon = \frac{V_{bulk} - V}{V_{bulk}} \times 100$$

An equivalent density relationship for the bulk volume is called the *apparent density* (ρ_a). Powders with a low apparent density and a large bulk volume are "light" powders, and those with a high apparent density and a small bulk volume are "heavy" powders.

$$\rho_a = \frac{\text{weight of the sample}}{V_{bulk}}$$

A corresponding density relationship for the true volume is called the *true density* (ρ).

$$\rho = \frac{\text{weight of the sample}}{V}$$

By determining the true density, the true volume can be calculated.

If the powder is nonporous and insoluble in a liquid, its true volume can be determined using a *pycnometer* and measuring the liquid volume displaced when the powder is added. Then, knowing the weight of the sample and the volume it occupied, the true density can be determined.

If the powder is porous, the true density may be determined using a *helium densitometer*. The volume of the empty apparatus is first determined by introducing a known quantity of helium. A weighed amount of powder then is introduced into the apparatus, adsorbed gases are removed from the powder, and helium is introduced again. The pressure is determined, and the volume of helium surrounding the particles and penetrating into the porous areas is calculated. Again, the true density

can be calculated by knowing the weight of the powder sample and the volume it occupied.

The relationship between porosity (ϵ), apparent density (ρ_a), and true density (ρ) can be derived as:

$$V_{bulk} = \frac{\text{weight of the sample}}{\rho_a}$$

$$V = \frac{\text{weight of the sample}}{\rho}$$

$$\epsilon = \frac{V_{bulk} - V}{V_{bulk}} \times 100$$

$$\epsilon = \frac{\dfrac{\text{weight of the sample}}{\rho_a} - \dfrac{\text{weight of the sample}}{\rho}}{\dfrac{\text{weight of the sample}}{\rho_a}} \times 100$$

$$\epsilon = \frac{\dfrac{1}{\rho_a} - \dfrac{1}{\rho}}{\dfrac{1}{\rho_a}} \times 100$$

$$\epsilon = \left(1 - \frac{\rho_a}{\rho}\right) \times 100$$

Comminution (Reduction in Particle Size)

Comminution is the process of reducing the size of particles or aggregates. Reducing the particle size may be a requirement for a formulation being compounded, or a narrower distribution of particle sizes within a powder sample may be desired. Smaller particle sizes are useful to:

- facilitate crude drug extraction
- increase the dissolution rates of drugs
- aid in the formulation process
- enhance absorption
- increase dissolution rate
- increase the suspendability of suspension particles
- create uniformity of liquid mixtures
- increase penetrability of particles for inhalation
- create nongrittiness in ointments, creams, gels.

Large Scale Reduction

Reduction in particle size can be accomplished using a variety of methods. In manufacturing, a variety of mills can be employed. The choice of the appropriate mill is based upon the desired particle shape, the degree of particle size reduction desired, and the chemical properties of the powder. Large scale comminution mills are classified as:

1. course crushers (e.g., jaw, roll, impact crushers)
2. intermediate grinders (e.g., hammer, roller, rotary cutters)
3. fine grinding mills (e.g., ball, hammer, colloid, fluid energy mills).

Course crushers are used when the size of the material is very large (1.5 to 60 inches in diameter). Because most powders are not in that size range, these are not often used in the pharmaceutical setting. Intermediate grinders, however, provide powders that are between 20 and 200 mesh. Fine grinding mills result in particles smaller than 200 mesh, and these are measured in microns.

Mills (or grinders) reduce particle size by attrition, rolling, or impact. Attrition involves rubbing the particles between two surfaces. Most mills use two stone or steel grinding plates that revolve to provide the grinding action. Air jet attrition mills use opposing air jets at 100 psig, which causes particles to colloid with one another. Impact grinders hit the particles with hammers or bars and split them into smaller pieces.

Small Scale Reduction

When particle size reduction is desired on a small scale (e.g., extemporaneous compounding), the three methods of comminution are:

- trituration
- pulverization by intervention
- levigation

Trituration involves the continuous rubbing or grinding of the powder in a mortar with a pestle. This method is used when working with hard, fracturable powders.

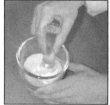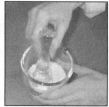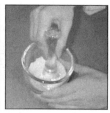

Pulverization by intervention is used with hard crystalline powders that do not crush or triturate easily, or gummy-type substances. The first step is to use an "intervening" solvent (such as alcohol or acetone) that will dissolve the compound. The dissolved powder then is mixed in a mortar or is spread on an ointment slab to enhance evaporation of the solvent. As the solvent evaporates, the powder will recrystallize out of solution as fine particles.

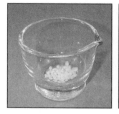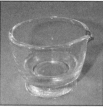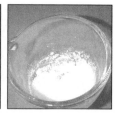

Levigation reduces the particle size by triturating it in a mortar or spatulating it on an ointment slab with a small amount of a liquid in which the solid is not soluble. The solvent should be somewhat viscous, such as mineral oil or glycerin. This method also is used to reduce the particle size of insoluble materials when compounding ointments and suspensions.

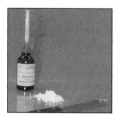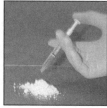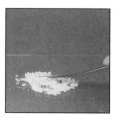

Blending

In the blending process, two or more powders are combined into a homogenous mixture. A homogeneous mixture is needed to ensure that the powder formulation will yield consistent doses. Just as with comminution, there are large scale (manufacturing) and small scale (compounding) blending methods.

Large Scale Blending

Large scale methods involve equipment designed to mix large portions of the powder sample and at the same time reduce particle size segregation. Some types of industrial blenders are double cone *or twin shell blenders*, which rotate about an off-centered axis. Another type of blender is a *vertical impeller mixer*, which is cone-shaped with a screw-type impeller along the interior wall.

Other types include paddle blenders, *fluidized air mixer*, and motionless mixers, which rely on a series of flow-twisting or flow-splitting components. Each blender must be monitored to prove that it produces a powder bed that is mixed uniformly. This is done by analyzing various parts of the mixed powder bed and assuring that the mix composition is similar.

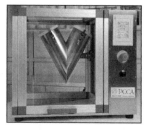

Small Scale Blending

As the name suggests, *spatulation* mixes powders using a spatula. The mixing can be done in a mortar, on an

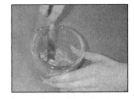

ointment slab, or in a plastic bag. This method produces no reduction in particle size, so the powders must be of fine particle size and of uniform size before the blending begins. Also, no pressure is applied to the mixture as it is blended, so the resulting blend is light and "fluffy."

This is the method to use when mixing *eutectic compounds*, which liquefy when they are brought together. First the compounds should be adsorbed on a "carrier" powder (e.g., magnesium oxide, calcium carbonate, starch, lactose), and then blended by spatulation. Some eutectic compounds are aspirin, benzocaine, camphor, lidocaine, menthol, phenol, resorcinol, salicylic acid, and thymol.

Spatulation using a plastic bag is shown in the following photos.

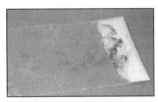

The powders to be blended are placed inside the bag.

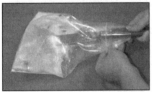

A large stainless steel spatula is placed inside the bag, and the bag is collected around the spatula.

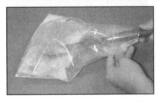

The powders are spatulated inside the bag.

The following photos illustrate the steps in mortar spatulation.

Add the powders to be blended into a mortar.

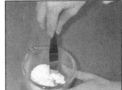

Use a hard rubber spatula and slowly mix the powders together.

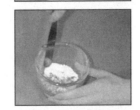

Ensure that all of the powder is incorporated into the mix.

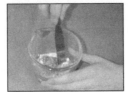

Continue mixing until a uniform mixture is created.

Triturating the powder together in a mortar using a pestle blends powders more intimately than spatulation does. When mixing two powders of unequal quantity, a technique called *geometric dilution* is used. The smaller quantity of powder will be "diluted" by adding it to the larger quantity of powder. To begin, the smaller quantity of powder is triturated with an approximately equal portion of the larger quantity of powder. This first "dilution" then is mixed with an approximately equal portion of the larger quantity of powder and the powders are triturated again. This sequential dilution scheme is continued until all of the two powders have been mixed. The following photos depict the sequence of geometric dilution.

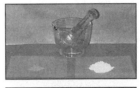

The powders are accurately weighed.

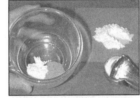

A portion of the larger quantity of powder is mixed with an equal portion of the smaller quantity of powder.

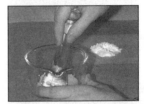

The powders are triturated together.

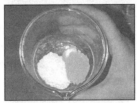

Another portion of the larger quantity of powder equal to the mixture in the mortar is added.

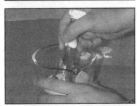

The powders are triturated together.

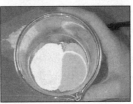

Another portion of the larger quantity of powder equal to the mixture in the mortar is added.

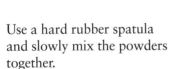
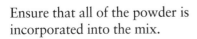

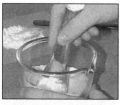

The powders are triturated together.

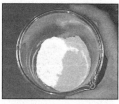

The sequential dilution is continued.

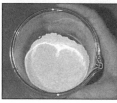

A homogenous powder mixture will result from this technique of mixing.

Types of Compounded Powders

Compounded powders can be prepared as bulk powders or as divided powders (charts).

Bulk Powders

Bulk powders are those that can be reasonably dosed using inaccurate measuring devices such as a teaspoon, the cap, or an insufflator. Bulk powders have a large surface area, which exposes them to potential degradation. For example, some powders are hygroscopic and will absorb moisture from the air. Other powders absorb so much moisture that they liquefy, called *deliquescent powders*. Other powders are volatile and can evaporate if exposed to the air. Therefore, bulk powders should be dispensed in a screw-capped glass container with a wide mouth, large enough to admit a teaspoon. For hygroscopic or deliquescent powders, a desiccant packet can be added to the container.

Oral Bulk Powders

Orally administered bulk powders are basically limited to antacids, dietary supplements, laxatives, and a few analgesics. Most oral powders are fine powder mixtures that the patient empties into a glass of water or juice before ingestion.

Effervescent Granulations

Granules are agglomerations of particles about 4 to 10 mesh (2,000 – 5,000 micrometer) in size. Granules always are made intentionally and consist of an agglomeration of smaller particles of powders. They generally are made by first blending the powders together, then moistening the mixture to form a pasty mass. The mass is passed through a sieve and then dried in air or in an oven.

Granules have less surface area because they are bigger particles, so they hydrate and dissolve more slowly than fine powders do. Granules generally are used as intermediates in the manufacturing of capsules and tablets because they flow more smoothly and predictably than do smaller particles.

The most popular compounded granulation is the effervescent powder, sometimes called effervescent salts. These mixtures of powders dissolve rapidly in water, liberating carbon dioxide. The release of carbon dioxide causes the solution to "fizz." The effervescent granulation is popular because of its taste and psychological impression.

The size of the effervescent granulation must be considered carefully. If the powder has particles that are too small, the powder may effervesce too much when water is added, and overflow the container. If this happens, the mixture should be passed through a sieve with a smaller mesh number.

Usually the formulation contains sodium bicarbonate, citric acid monohydrate, and tartaric acid with citric acid monohydrate and tartaric acid used in the ratio of 1:2, respectively. If citric acid monohydrate is used alone, a sticky mixture that is not easily granulated will result. Tartaric acid is not used alone because the granules are too friable and will crumble. The amount of sodium bicarbonate to be used may be calculated from the reaction that occurs when the granules come in contact with water.

EXAMPLE: How much sodium bicarbonate should be mixed with 1 g of citric acid monohydrate and 2 g of tartaric acid to produce effervescent granules? (sodium bicarbonate mol. wt. = 84; citric acid monohydrate mol. wt. = 210; tartaric acid mol. wt. = 150)

The reaction equation between citric acid monohydrate and sodium bicarbonate is:

$$3\ NaHCO_3 + \underset{\underset{CH_2-COOH}{|}}{\overset{\overset{CH_2-COOH}{|}}{HO-C-COOH}} \cdot H_2O + 4\ H_2O \rightarrow$$

$$\underset{\underset{CH_2-COONa}{|}}{\overset{\overset{CH_2-COONa}{|}}{HO-C-COONa}} + 3\ CO_2 \uparrow + 8\ H_2O$$

Three moles of sodium bicarbonate (3×84 g) will react with one mole of citric acid monohydrate (1×210 g).

Setting up a proportion to determine the amount of sodium bicarbonate that will react with 1 g of citric acid:

$$\frac{1 \times 210 \text{ g citric acid monohydrate}}{3 \times 84 \text{ g NaHCO}_3} = \frac{1.0 \text{ g citric acid monohydrate}}{X \text{ g NaHCO}_3}$$

X = 1.2 g sodium bicarbonate to react with 1.0 g of citric acid monohydrate

Similar calculations show that 2.24 g of sodium bicarbonate react with 2 g of tartaric acid.

$$2 \text{ NaHCO}_3 + \begin{array}{c} \text{COOH} \\ | \\ \text{CHOH} \\ | \\ \text{CHOH} \\ | \\ \text{COOH} \end{array} + 4 \text{ H}_2\text{O} \rightarrow$$

$$(2 \times 84 \text{ g}) \qquad (1 \times 150 \text{ g})$$

$$\begin{array}{c} \text{COONa} \\ | \\ \text{COOH} \\ | \\ \text{CHOH} \\ | \\ \text{COONa} \end{array} + 2 \text{ CO}_2 \uparrow + 6 \text{ H}_2\text{O}$$

$$\frac{1 \times 150 \text{ g tartaric acid}}{2 \times 84 \text{ g NaHCO}_3} = \frac{2.0 \text{ g tartaric acid}}{X \text{ g NaHCO}_3}$$

X = 2.24 g sodium bicarbonate to react with 2.0 g tartaric acid

It has been calculated that 3.44 g (1.2 g + 2.24 g) of sodium bicarbonate is necessary to react stoichiometrically with the 3.0 g of combined acids. To enhance the flavor, the amount of sodium bicarbonate may be reduced to 3.4 gm to allow for a small amount of unreacted citric and tartaric acid to provide a tart taste.

Dusting Powders

Dusting powders are fine powders intended to be dusted on the skin by means of sifter top containers. Although a single medicinal agent may be used as a dusting powder, a base frequently is used to apply a medicinal agent and to protect the skin from irritation and friction. Bentonite, kaolin, magnesium carbonate, starch, and talc are used as inert bases for dusting powders. Powder bases

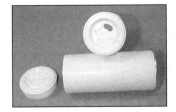

absorb secretions and have a drying effect, and some ingredients can impart a cooling sensation. All extemporaneous dusting powders should be passed through a 100–200 mesh sieve to ensure that they are grit-free and will not mechanically irritate traumatized areas.

Douche Powders

Douche powders are used to prepare aqueous solutions to cleanse the vagina. Most douche powders are used for their hygienic effects but may contain antibiotics.

Because powder is more portable than a bulky solution, douche powders are a matter of convenience for the user. The formula is developed so a teaspoonful or capful of powder dissolved in a specific volume of water provides the desired concentration of active drug. The pH usually ranges between 3.5 and 5. Feminine bulb syringes or fountain syringes are used for vaginal irrigation.

Because many of the ingredients (e.g., menthol, thymol, volatile oils) are volatile, douche powders should be packaged in glass jars with a wide mouth. Some commercial douche powders are available in metal foil packets that contain the proper amount of powder for a single douche. Many douche powders also are available in a single use solution in disposable applicators.

Insufflators

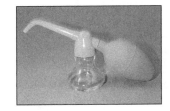

Insufflations are extremely fine powders to be introduced into body cavities. The powder usually is administered using a device called an *insufflator*. Squeezing the rubber bowl causes turbulence within the powder reservoir, forcing some of the powder into the air stream and out of the device.

Divided Powders / Charts

Divided powders or charts—sometimes called *powder papers*—are single doses of a powder formulation individually wrapped in plastic, metallic foil, parchment paper, or white bond paper. The divided powder is a more accurate dosage form than bulk powder because those who use divided powder are not involved in measuring a dose. Powders enclosed in plastic and foil packages are better protected from the environment than are powders enclosed in paper. The user places the package contents in a glass of water or juice, and most of the drug and ingredients dissolve in the liquid before the person drinks it.

When powder papers are compounded extemporaneously, they are packaged in powder papers and dispensed in a telescoping box. A chart (i.e., the paper holding the powder) should fold readily, hold its form, remain clean with handling, protect contents from the atmosphere, be water repellent, and present an elegant appearance. Instructions for folding powder papers are given at the end of the chapter. Methods used to portion the powder blend into the individual unit (or divided) doses are:

- weighing each individual dose
- blocking and dividing the powder blend
- using a powder measure that delivers the appropriate dose
- using a volumetric template that delivers the appropriate dose.

Trituration Aliquot

When compounding a divided chart formulation, the least weighable quantity (L.W.Q.) of the prescription balance may become an important consideration. Many times, the total amount of the active drug in a divided chart formulation is less than the L.W.Q. In these cases, a *trituration aliquot* must be made first to ensure that an accurate amount of active drug is present in the formulation. A trituration aliquot implies that at least two powders are to be *triturated* together, and then an *aliquot* (a portion) of that trituration is to be used in the formulation.

The trituration is made by taking a weighable amount of the active drug and triturating it with an inert powder in such a proportion that a weighable aliquot of the triturate will contain the amount of drug needed. Lactose is the most commonly used diluent (inert powder) because of its low incidence of side effects, its ready availability, and its low cost.

There is a practical reason for making a trituration aliquot even if the amount of drug needed is greater than the L.W.Q. If the amount of drug needed is about 200–400 mg per unit, that is a small amount of material to handle conveniently. Making a trituration aliquot will provide more material per unit, which will aid in handling and administration.

EXAMPLE: Make 10 powders, each containing 0.6 mg atropine sulfate and each weighing a total of 200 mg.

Assume that a Class A balance is being used and that the LWQ is 120 mg. Therefore, any substance weighed on the balance must be at least 120 mg.

Using ratio and proportion, the weight of drug and lactose required to make the trituration, as well as the weight of the aliquot to be used to finish compounding the formulation, can be determined from the following relationship:

$$\frac{\text{(A) Weight of drug in trituration}}{\text{(B) Weight of trituration}} = \frac{\text{(C) Weight of drug in aliquot}}{\text{(D) Weight of aliquot}}$$

To make the trituration:

1. Total weight atropine sulfate required in the formulation (this is C in the proportion)

    0.6 mg/powder × 10 powders = 6 mg

2. Select the *size of the aliquot* to contain the 6 mg of drug (this is D in the proportion)

    Select 120 mg (any amount ≥120 mg will be suitable)

3. Select the amount of drug to weigh for the trituration (this is A in the proportion)

    Select 120 mg (any amount ≥120 mg will be suitable)

4. A, C, and D are now determined. Solve for B (trituration weight)

$$\frac{120 \text{ mg atropine sulfate}}{X \text{ mg trituration}} = \frac{6 \text{ mg atropine sulfate}}{120 \text{ mg aliquot}}$$

    X = 2,400 mg trituration (drug + diluent)

5. Determine the weight of diluent (lactose) required to prepare the trituration by subtracting the weight of atropine sulfate from the trituration weight.

    2,400 mg trituration − 120 mg atropine sulfate = 2,280 mg lactose

To finish compounding the formulation:

Determine the weight of lactose that must be added to the trituration aliquot so each powder will weigh 200 mg.

200 mg/powder × 10 powders = 2,000 mg (drug and lactose)

2,000 mg − 120 mg aliquot = 1,880 mg lactose

This formulation is prepared using the following steps:

1. Weigh 120 mg atropine sulfate and triturate to a fine powder.
2. Weigh 2,280 mg lactose.
3. Mix atropine sulfate and lactose by geometric dilution.
4. Remove 120 mg of the trituration (this aliquot contains 6 mg atropine sulfate).
5. Weigh 1,880 mg lactose and mix with the 120 mg aliquot by geometric dilution.
6. Prepare individual powders each weighing 200 mg.

Suggested Sieve Sizes for Intended Applications

Once powder formulations are made, they should be sieved to obtain an optimum particle size distribution for their intended application. Table 18.6 gives suggested sieve sizes for various types of powders. This should serve only as a guide, as not all sources agree about the optimum particle size.

TABLE 18.6: SUGGESTED SIEVE SIZES FOR VARIOUS POWDERS

Intended Application	Suggested Sieve Size
Granules	2–10
Douche	40–60
Effervescent powders, divided powders	40–100
Dusting	80–120
Insufflations	100–200

Place the sieve on glassine paper. This photo shows a 5" sieve.

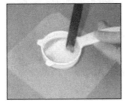

Place the powder inside the sieve. This photo shows a smaller, hand-held sieve.

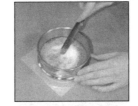

Use a hard rubber spatula to work the powder through the wire mesh.

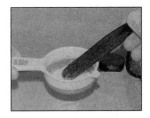

Observing Formulations for Evidence of Instability

The USP Chapter <1191> points out the possibility that dry powders can "cake into hard masses or change color, which may render them unacceptable."[4] And effervescent formulations are particularly sensitive to moisture. If the mass swells or develops a gas pressure, this is a sign of instability indicating that some of the effervescent action has occurred already. Powders and effervescent granules must be protected from "environmental water," so powders should be packaged in a tight, screw-capped glass container to prevent premature wetting of the formulation. Divided powders can be packaged in reclosable zip-lock bags or heat-sealed polyethylene or cellophane bags instead of metallic foil or parchment paper. For hygroscopic or deliquescent powders, a desiccant packet can be added to the container.

Powders can have beyond use dates of 25% of the remaining expiration date if a manufactured product is used as the drug source, or 6 months, whichever is earlier. Manufactured products typically are not used as the drug source. Most often, the pure ingredient is obtained in powder form. If the ingredient is a USP/NF substance, a 6-month beyond use date can be given. It would be prudent to prepare a duplicate formulation for

---

HOW TO FOLD POWDER PAPERS

1. Place the paper on the counter away from wind or drafts.

2. Fold down the top long edge of the paper one-half inch.

3. Place the weighted dose of the drug in the center of the paper.

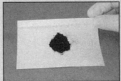

4. Bring the lower edge of the paper up and insert it completely into the top fold of the powder paper. Make a second fold in the top edge of the paper.

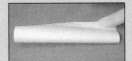

5. Center the folded paper lengthwise over an open powder box of the size intended to be used. Then fold the equal overhanging ends down while pressing in the sides of the box. Be careful not to press too hard, as it may bend the box.

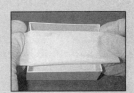

6. Fold the ends of the powder paper completely back, and sharply crease the end folds. Place the filled powder paper into the box, with the folds away from you.

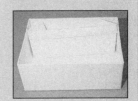

7. Prepare a folded powder paper for each dose. One way to work efficiently is to take one powder paper as a template. Once the correct length of the folds has been determined, the other powder papers can be folded quickly to match the template.

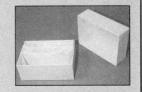

observation if the product is new to the pharmacist, as the beyond use date is long. The appearance of fog or liquid inside the container could signify improper storage conditions. Changes in color and odor might be other indicators of instability.

NOTES

1. Martin, A. Micrometics (chapter 16) in *Physical Pharmacy*, 4th edition. Lea & Febiger, Philadelphia, PA, 1993, pp. 423–452.

2. O'Connor, R. E., Schwartz, J. B., Felton, L. A. Powders (chapter 37) in *Remington: The Science and Practice of Pharmacy*, 21st edition. Lippincott Williams & Wilkins, Baltimore, MD, 2006, pp. 702–719.

3. Martin, Note 1.

4. <1191> Stability Considerations in Dispensing Practice: The United States Pharmacopeia 29/National Formulary 24, The United States Pharmacopeial Convention, Inc., Rockville, MD, 2005, pp. 3029–3031.

ADDITIONAL READING

Vu, N. Quality-Control Analytical Methods: Considerations in Compounding Peroral Solid Dosage Forms. *International Journal of Pharmaceutical Compounding* 11:143–146, 2007.

SELF-CONTAINED FOLDED POWDER PAPER

1. Use a square piece of powder paper. *Note: if the powder is to be double-wrapped, both papers must be folded together.* Fold the paper diagonally from Points "a" to "c" and again from "b" to "d." When you unfold the paper, the two diagonal lines will meet at "e." Fold in "d" to "e" to give "f." Unfold the paper to the open position (Figure A).

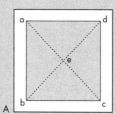

2. Bring "b" to "f" and crease, using a spatula. The fold intersects the "ac" diagonal line at "g" (Figure B).

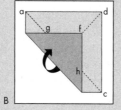

3. Bring "c" to "g" and crease, using a spatula. The fold intersects the "ac" diagonal line at "h" (Figure C).

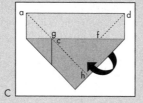

4. Bring "a" to "h" and crease, using a spatula. This fold forms an elongated envelope (Figure D).

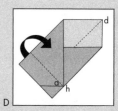

5. Bring the bottom of the envelope up so it divides into thirds and leaves the flap to be tucked into the envelope after filling (Figure E).

6. Place the weighted powder dose into the envelope.

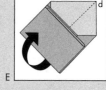

7. Tuck "d" into the opening at the bottom, which previously has been brought up to form the envelope. This secures the powder packet, which then can be placed into a sealable bag and labeled appropriately with the physician's directions (Figure F).

CHAPTER NINETEEN

Capsules

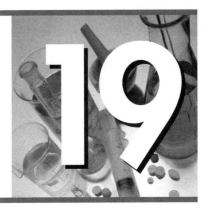

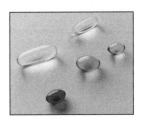

CAPSULES ARE SOLID DOSAGE FORMS THAT CONTAIN the active drug and other excipients in an enclosed shell of gelatin. Administering medicinal ingredients in capsule form is popular with consumers. In market surveys, 44.2% prefer soft gelatin capsules, 39.6% tablets, and 19.4% hard gelatin capsules.[1] The pharmaceutical industry currently does not follow these consumer preferences because it prepares 75% of its solid dosage forms as compressed tablets, 23% as hard gelatin capsules, and 2% as soft gelatin capsules.

Capsules can be either clear or opaque and can be manufactured in a variety of colors that aid in identifying the product. Opaque capsules can hide unattractive ingredients and thereby increase their aesthetic appearance. Another reason for the wide acceptance of capsules is that they are tasteless and odorless.

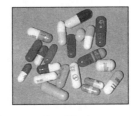

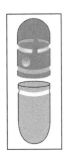

Commercial capsules are classified as either hard or soft, depending on the nature of the gelatin shell. Hard gelatin capsules have little elasticity and are composed of two parts—a longer body and a shorter cap. The cap is designed to fit snugly over the body. Some hard gelatin capsules have a locking cap that keeps the body and cap joined during shipping and handling but can be separated easily for filling.

Soft gelatin capsules are made from a more flexible plasticized gelatin film that forms a one-piece shell. The soft shell is made by adding plasticizers such as glycerin, sorbitol, or propylene glycol to the gelatin. The capsule is completely sealed and cannot be opened without destroying the dosage form. A variety of sizes (0.1 ml to 30 ml) and shapes (spherical, oval, oblong, tube, suppository-type) are available. Soft gelatin capsules most commonly contain liquids, but suspensions, pastes, dry powders, preformed tablets, and semisolids that do not affect gelatin also can be encapsulated.

Powders incorporated into capsules can come from many sources. They may be the raw ingredient or from a tablet. If tablets are the source, the tablet should be crushed and triturated before being encapsulated, and only conventional tablets (not modified release) should be used. Powders can be taken from other capsules. Liquids can be evaporated to dryness on an adsorbent carrier before being placed in the capsule.

Capsules usually are administered orally. Swallowing capsules is easier than swallowing tablets because the gelatin shell hydrates in the mouth and passes easily into the esophagus. Although gelatin is insoluble in cold water, it does soften when hydrated because it can absorb up to 10 times its weight in water. Gelatin is soluble in both hot water and warm gastric fluid, so when capsules are swallowed and enter the gastrointestinal tract, the capsules rapidly dissolve and release their contents, making them available for dissolution and/or absorption.

Soft gelatin capsules are administered orally, but they also can be administered rectally or vaginally. When administered via these routes, the capsule generally is pierced with a pin or needle so the aqueous body fluids can penetrate the capsule shell readily and dissolve its contents more easily.

Hard Gelatin Shells
Manufacturing Hard Gelatin Shells

Hard gelatin capsule shells are made from a mixture of gelatin and water. To this basic mixture, colorants, opacifying agents, and preservatives may be added. Gelatin is obtained by the hydrolysis of collagen obtained from the skin, white connective tissue, and bones of animals. The chemical and physical properties of gelatin can vary depending on the source of the collagen and the manner of hydrolytic reaction. The two basic types are

- type A gelatin derived mainly from pork skins and produced by acid hydrolysis.
- type B gelatin, obtained from bones and animal skins by alkaline hydrolysis.

The two types can be differentiated by their isoelectric points (4.8–5.0 for type B and 7.0–9.0 for type A). They also exhibit different viscosities and film-forming characteristics. Blends of the two types often are used to make gelatin solutions with the desired viscosity and strength. Bone gelatin (type B) contributes firmness, and pork skin gelatin (type A) contributes plasticity and clarity.

The physicochemical properties of gelatin that manufacturers evaluate most often are the bloom strength and viscosity. *Bloom strength* is an empirical measure of gel strength that gives some measure of firmness of the gel. It is measured in a Bloom Gelometer, which determines the weight in grams required to depress a standard plunger a fixed distance into the surface of a 6.67% w/w gel under standard conditions. Desirable bloom strengths for capsules vary between 150 g and 280 g.

The thickness of a gelatin film is determined primarily by the *viscosity* of a gelatin solution. Viscosity is measured in a standard 6.67% w/w gelatin solution at 60°C in a capillary pipette. Viscosities in the range of 30–60 millipoise are used in manufacturing capsules.

Colorants are commonly soluble synthetic dyes or insoluble pigments. Most synthetic coloring agents are made from aniline, a colorless derivative of benzene. Because benzene is a distillation product of coal tar, these synthetic aniline derived dyes sometimes are called "coal tar" dyes. They usually are dissolved in the gelatin solution to provide their coloring property.

Lake dyes are insoluble materials and are dispersed in gelatin solutions to impart color. A FD&C lake dye is made by absorbing or precipitating a dye onto a substratum of alumina hydrate. Opacifying agents such as titanium dioxide are included in the gelatin film to make the capsule opaque. Opaque capsules can be used to hide unattractive ingredients and also protect the contents of the capsule from light.

Capsules are manufactured by dipping plates containing pegs of the desired shape and diameter into a temperature controlled reservoir of a melted gelatin mixture. The pegs on which the caps are formed are slightly larger in diameter than the pegs on which the bodies are formed. This allows the cap to telescope over the body.

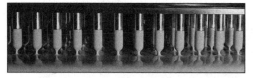

Each plate is lowered to the depth and maintained for the desired time to achieve the proper length and thickness of gelatin coating.

At the appropriate time, the plates are removed from the bath and inverted, and the gelatin shells are dried by a gentle flow of air. After the gelatin dries, the two parts of the capsule are removed from the pegs, trimmed to the proper length, and the body and caps are joined together.

The manufactured capsules then are visually inspected and defective capsules are removed. Some defects are serious (e.g., imperfect cut, dented, long bodies,

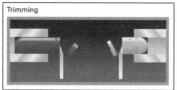
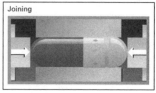

contains holes) and cause the filling machine to stop. Smaller defects that are of aesthetic concern include small bubbles in the shell, specks in the film, or marks at the cut edge.

Filling Hard Gelatin Shells

Hard gelatin capsules are manufactured in one operation and filled in a completely separate operation. Modern capsule filling equipment allows hard gelatin capsules to be filled with a variety of formulations such as beads, tablets, powders, or semisolids. Modified release granules or pellets also can be used because the fill is not crushed or compacted, so the formulation technology used to produce the extended release property will not be affected.

The following four steps involved in filling capsules are common to all capsule filling equipment:

1. All the capsules must be oriented to face in the same direction (rectification).
2. The caps are removed from the capsule bodies.
3. The empty capsule bodies are filled with the desired formulation.
4. The caps are returned to the bodies.

The first two steps are accomplished by the mechanical design of the filling machine. Capsules are to be oriented (rectified) in the same direction (e.g., body down position). The capsules enter a channel that is wide enough for one capsule at a time to enter, and a specially designed apparatus rotates the capsule into the body down position regardless of which end entered the channel. The caps are separated from the bodies by passing the rectified capsules into a split bushing or ring. A vacuum is applied to the capsule bodies, pulling them away from the caps, which are held in place by the ring. The split ring separates, with the caps held by one part of the ring and the capsule bodies held by another part. The bodies now are ready for filling.

The formulation that is used to fill the capsule body must have good flow properties so the body can be filled easily and an accurate dose can be filled each time. In dry powder formulations, the active drug and inactive excipients are blended thoroughly to ensure a uniform mixture. This is critical especially for low dose drugs in which the lack of homogeneity could result in unacceptable content uniformity.

A more uniform filling can be achieved if the density and particle size of all of the components in the fill are similar. To accomplish this, powders sometimes are milled to produce particles of about 50 to 1,000 microns prior to being placed in the capsules. If particles smaller than 50 microns are needed, micronization is employed, which will produce particles ranging from about 1 to 20 microns in size.

The powder must be free flowing to allow a constant and steady flow of the formulation through the various parts of the capsule filling equipment and into the capsule bodies. Adding a lubricant or glidant such as fumed silicon dioxide, magnesium stearate, calcium stearate, stearic acid, or talc will enhance flow properties. Magnesium stearate is a water insoluble material that can retard the penetration of biological fluids into a capsule because of its "waterproofing" characteristics. To overcome this problem, sodium lauryl sulfate, a surface active agent, often is added to the formulation.

When bulking agents are required, diluents or bulk filling materials are added to the formulation to produce the proper capsule fill volume. Lactose, microcrystalline cellulose, and starch are commonly used for this purpose. These materials impart a cohesive property to the powder blend, which is beneficial when transferring the powder blend into the capsule bodies. Disintegrants frequently are included in a formulation to help the powder blend break up once the capsule shell has dissolved. Commonly used disintegrants are pregelatinized starch, croscarmelose, and sodium starch glycolate.

Capsule filling machines are either semi-automatic or fully automatic. Semi-automatic machines require that an operator be present. Depending on the operator's skill, the formulation, and the capsule size being filled, these machines are capable of filling about 15,000–20,000 capsules per hour. The fully automatic machines can fill 120,000–180,000 capsules per hour. These fully automatic machines are classified as either intermittent or continuous motion machines. Intermittent machines must be stopped during the filling sequence because turntables and other parts of the machinery must be changed or moved during the filling process. The continuous motion machines do not have to be stopped during the filling process.

Although capsule filling machines vary widely in their engineering design, the main differences between them is how the formulation is put into the capsules. Some of the filling methods available are described below.

Auger Fill Method

In the augur fill method, the empty capsule bodies are held in a metal ring that rotates on a turntable under the powder hopper. The auger in the powder hopper rotates at a constant speed, and this causes the powder fill to be delivered to the empty capsules at a constant rate. Thus, the primary factor influencing the capsule fill weight is the rotation speed of the metal ring under the hopper. Faster rotation rates produce lighter fill weights because the capsule bodies have a shorter dwell time under the hopper.

Vibratory Fill Method

Here, the capsule bodies first pass under a powder feed frame. The feed frame has a perforated resin plate that is connected to a vibrator. The vibration of the plate helps the powder pass through the holes of the plate into the capsule bodies. Also, powders tend to become fluidized because of the vibration, which further assists in filling the capsules. Each capsule body is overfilled, and then the excess is scraped off. The fill weight is controlled by the speed of the vibrator and the dwell time the capsule body is under the feed frame.

Piston-Tamp Method

Piston-tamp filling machines tamp individual doses of powders into plugs that resemble soft tablets. These plugs then are ejected into a empty capsule body. The two types of piston-tamp fillers are dosing-disk machines and dosator machines.[2]

A dosing-disk has a number of cavities that act as filling chambers for the powder. The powder is placed on the dosing-disk and maintained at a relatively constant level. The dosing-disk rotates under a set of pistons (either three or five), and each piston sequentially compresses the powder in the cavities to form a plug. Because the dosing-disk passes under each of the pistons, the plug is compressed or tamped several times. The plug then is ejected into a empty capsule body. The amount of powder in each plug is controlled by the cavity thickness of the dosing-disk, the powder depth in each chamber, and the tamping pressure of each piston.

Dosator machines have a series of cylindrical tubes fitted with movable pistons. One end of the tube is open, and through the other end the piston is preset to a specified height to define the volume of powder that will be contained in the tube. The series of tubes (called the dosator) is plunged down into the powder bed, which is maintained at a constant level. The powder bed is higher than the piston, so powder enters the open end of the tubes and is compressed slightly against the piston. The piston then gives a tamping stroke, which causes the powder to form into a plug. The dosator then is withdrawn from the powder bed and moved over empty capsule bodies, where the pistons push downward and eject the powder plugs into the capsule bodies. The fill weight is controlled primarily by the initial piston height and secondarily by the height of the powder bed.

Finishing the Process

Finishing the process requires sealing, cleaning and polishing, and packaging.

Sealing

Capsules that have some type of positive or locking closure will not separate during shipping and handling. Hard gelatin capsules are made self-locking by forming indentations or grooves on the inside of the cap and body portions. When the cap is completely placed on the body, the positive interlock is created between the cap and body portions. Some capsules have indentations farther down on the cap. These "pre-lock" indentations keep the capsules joined, yet the capsule can be easily separated for filling. Examples of self-locking capsules are Loxit®, Snap-Fit®, and Coni-Snap®.

Another feature of some capsules is a tapered rim on the body of the capsule, which will help guide the cap onto the body. In high-speed automatic capsule filling machines, this feature can reduce or eliminate the snagging or splitting of capsules.

Hard gelatin capsules may be hermetically sealed by banding. This involves putting an additional layer of gelatin film around the seam of the cap and body or by some form of thermal welding process.

Cleaning and Polishing

Small amounts of powder may adhere to the outside of the capsule after filling. The powder may be bitter or otherwise unpalatable and should be removed before the capsules are packaged. On an industrial scale, many capsule filling machines have attached cleaning vacuums that remove the extraneous material before the capsules leave the equipment.

Packaging

While dry gelatin is stable in air, it can undergo microbial decomposition when it becomes moist. Normally, hard gelatin capsules contain between 13% and 16% moisture.[3] Gelatin can absorb up to 10 times its weight in water, so if the capsules are stored in high humidity, they will absorb additional moisture and may become distorted and lose their rigid shape. This re-shaping can occur with a moisture content of >18%.[4] In extreme dryness (moisture contents <12%) some of the moisture normally present in the gelatin capsules is lost and the capsules may become brittle and crumble when handled.

Prolonged exposure to high humidity also can affect *in vitro* capsule dissolution. These changes have been observed in capsules containing tetracycline, chloramphenicol, and nitrofurantoin.[5] The effect is thought to result from the decrease in the solubility of gelatin in water. During dissolution the capsules develop a "skin" or *pellicle*, which retards water penetration into the gelatin shell. Although the exact mechanism is not known, gelatin cross-linking has been suggested.

Soft Gelatin Capsules

Aqueous liquids cannot be encapsulated in gelatin capsules because the water softens the gelatin, distorts the capsule, and causes the contents to leak. Some liquids that do not affect gelatin, however, may be placed in soft gelatin capsules. The liquids may be the active drug itself or a solvent that has been used to solubilize the active drug. In addition to liquids, soft gelatin capsules may be formulated as suspensions, pastes, dry powders, and pre-formed tablets.

A soft gelatin capsule is a completely sealed dosage form that cannot be opened without destroying the capsule. A wide variety of sizes and shapes is possible, including spherical, oval, oblong, tube, and suppository-type. Sizes may range from about 0.1 ml to 30 ml.

Suitable liquids for soft gelatin capsules are limited to those that do not have an adverse effect on the gelatin shell. The pH of the liquid should be between 2.5 and 7.5. Liquids with a pH that is too acidic tend to hydrolyze the gelatin and cause the contents to leak. Liquids having a pH higher than 7.5 decrease gelatin solubility, which adversely affects the dissolution of the capsule shell. The liquids must flow freely below 35°C because the sealing temperature of the gelatin film during manufacturing is around 37°C–40°C. Examples of suitable liquids are vegetable oils (cottonseed oil, olive oil, soy oil, castor oil, and coconut oil), aromatic and aliphatic hydrocarbons (mineral oil), medium chain triglycerides, and low molecular weight polyethylene glycols (PEG 400, PEG 600).

A potential problem with soft gelatin capsules is that the liquid and the capsule shell have more intimate contact than with dry filled capsules. This greater contact can increase the likelihood of interactions between the gelatin and the liquid contained in the capsule. Another potential interaction could involve the active drug migrating into the shell, which might result in the drug in the shell acting as an "initial dose" of drug before the shell dissolves. Also, the drug might be lost to the environment if it can pass into and through the gelatin shell. Low molecule weight alcohols and ketones can pass through gelatin shells easily.

The soft capsule shell is made by adding plasticizers such as glycerin, sorbitol, or propylene glycol to the gelatin. The ratio of dry plasticizer to dry gelatin determines the "hardness" of the shell and varies from 0.3–1.0 parts plasticizer for a very hard shell to 1.0–1.8 for a very soft shell. Moisture in the finished capsules usually is in the range of 6%–10%. Comparable to hard gelatin capsules, soft gelatin capsules may have a single- or two-tone color and may be imprinted with identifying marks.

They also may contain dyes, opacifying agents, preservatives, and flavors.

Manufacturing Processes

Manufacturing these capsules requires that all of the filling and sealing processes are done in one continuous operation. The oldest commercial process is the *plate process*, in which a set of plates or molds is used to form the capsules. A warm sheet of gelatin is first poured on the bottom plate mold, and then the liquid formulation is poured onto the sheet of gelatin. Another sheet of gelatin is added on top of the liquid, and when the top plate is pressed into the bottom plate, the capsules are formed and sealed simultaneously.

In the *rotary die process*, the machine forms the liquid gelatin, which flows from an overhead tank, into two continuous ribbons and brings them together between twin rotating dies that have cavities machined into them. An injection wedge brings material to the point where the two gelatin ribbons come together as they pass over

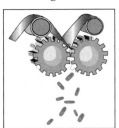

the rotary dies. As the gelatin ribbons pass over the rotary dies, metered fill material is injected forcefully between the ribbons, causing pockets to form in the gelatin ribbon that conform to the shape of the cavities in the dies. These pockets then are sealed by pressure and heat, which also simultaneously release the capsule from the ribbon.

In a variation of the rotary die process, reciprocating filling machines have dies that move together from opposite directions as the gelatin ribbon passes between the dies.

The *Accogel process* is another rotary process, but this is the only process used to fill soft gelatin capsules with powders or granules. The process involves a measuring roll, a die roll, and a sealing roll. The measuring roll rotates directly over the die roll, and the cavities of the two rolls are aligned with each other. The powder or granular fill material is held in the cavities of the measuring roll by vacuum. A plasticized sheet is drawn into the cavities of the die roll under vacuum. As the measuring roll and die rolls rotate, the measured doses are transferred to the gelatin-lined cavities of the die roll. The continued rotation of the filled die converges with the rotating sealing roll, where a second gelatin sheet is applied to form the other half of the capsule. The pressure developed between the die roll and sealing roll seals the capsules and cuts them from the sheets.

A truly seamless, one-piece soft gelatin capsule can be produced by the *bubble method*. A concentric tube dispenser simultaneously discharges the molten gelatin from the outer rim of the tube and the liquid content from the inner part of the tube. By means of a pulsating

pump mechanism, the liquids are discharged from the tube orifices into a chilled oil column. As they are cooled, droplets form, with a liquid core and a molten gelatin envelope. The droplets assume a spherical shape because of surface tension forces.

Extemporaneously Compounded Capsules

Extemporaneously compounded capsules offer several advantages:

- They mask the unpleasant taste, aroma, or appearance of a drug.
- They allow powders to be dispensed in an uncompressed form, allowing for quicker dissolution and absorption of the drug following oral dosing (compared to tablets).
- Almost any dose desired for a variety of administration routes (oral, rectal, vaginal) can be made quickly and cheaply.
- The number of products a person has to take can be reduced by combining several products into one capsule.
- Some people find them easier to swallow than tablets.
- They can be used to alter the release rate of the drug.

Disadvantages or limitations include the following:

- They are easily tampered with (although techniques are available to prevent this).
- They are subject to the effects of relative humidity and microbial contamination.
- They are difficult for some people to swallow.

Selecting a Capsule Size

Eight capsule sizes are available for human use. Size 5 is the smallest, and size 000 is the largest. Typically, the smallest size capable of holding the formulation in the capsule body is selected. The cap is included only to complete the capsule. But some factors may be important in selecting the capsule size. Some people have difficulty handling very small capsule sizes (e.g., 4 and 5), so some formulations must have additional bulk filling materials to allow a larger capsule size. At the other extreme, some patients have difficulty swallowing the larger capsule sizes (e.g., 00 and 000), so some formulations will need smaller doses per capsule, but that requires the person to take more capsules to maintain the same dose.

Capsule sizes can be selected by three methods, described next. In general, the smallest capsule size capable of holding the formulation should be used to reduce the difficulty of swallowing larger capsule sizes (00 and 000). The capsule size, however, should be large enough to

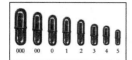

hold the formulation in the *body* of the capsule so the cap will only complete the capsule. Once the capsule is finished, it can be tapped so the contents will distribute throughout the entire capsule.

Powder Similarities

The range of hard gelatin capsule sizes can hold approximately 40 mg to 1.5 g of powdered material. One method of selecting the appropriate capsule size for a given formulation is to compare the capsule size used to encapsulate an equivalent amount of known material with similar characteristics. The chart shown in Table 19.1 can be used for this comparison. If the formulation has a bulk density similar to one of the drugs in the table, the capsule size could be selected based on the amount of formulation needed for one dose.

For example, if the formulation had a bulk density similar to aspirin and 400 mg of formulation is needed for one dose, a size 0 capsule would be selected. When 400 mg is placed in the size 0 capsule, it still will allow room for additional material (i.e., an additional 90 mg). If the capsule appears to be "partially full," the compounder would add more bulk filling material to the formulation so the capsule would be properly filled by the one dose.

If the powder density is known, the approximate amount of material the capsule will hold can be estimated from a chart similar to the one in Table 19.2.

Liquids that do not dissolve gelatin (e.g., absolute alcohol and fixed oils) may be dispensed in capsules. The liquids may be the drug themselves or a solvent that has been used to solubilize the drug into a liquid. Liquids that have been used in gelatin capsules include cottonseed oil, olive oil, soya oil, castor oil, and coconut oil. The approximate volumes that can be placed in different sized capsules are given in Table 19.3. The size of the capsule

TABLE 19.2: CAPSULE CAPACITY BASED ON SELECT POWDER DENSITIES

Powder Density (g/ml)	Fill Amount (mg) By Capsule Size						
	00	0	1	2	3	4	5
0.3	285	204	150	111	90	63	39
0.4	380	272	200	148	120	84	52
0.5	475	340	250	185	150	105	65
0.7	665	476	350	259	210	147	91
1.0	950	680	500	370	300	210	130
1.3	1,235	884	650	481	390	273	169
1.5	1,425	1,020	750	555	450	315	195

Adapted from "Oral Solid Dosage Forms," by E. M. Rudnic and J. B. Schwartz , (chapter 45) in Remington: The Science and Practice of Pharmacy, 21st edition (Baltimore, MD: Lippincott Williams & Wilkins, 2006), pp. 889–928.

TABLE 19.3: APPROXIMATE VOLUME CAPACITY OF CAPSULE SIZES

Capsule Size	Volume (ml)
000	1.36
00	0.95
0	0.67
1	0.48
2	0.37
3	0.27
4	0.20
5	0.13

should be chosen so the liquid does not completely fill the body.

Rules of Sixes

The *Rule of Sixes* is based on the experimental observation that the bulk densities of many powders average about 0.6 g/ml. The steps for using this rule are as follows:[6]

Step 1:	Put in six "6"s	6	6	6	6	6	6
Step 2:	List the capsule sizes	0	1	2	3	4	5
Step 3:	Determine the fill-weight difference (in grains)	6	5	4	3	2	1
Step 4:	Convert grains to milligrams	390	325	260	195	130	65

This method gives the weight of powder that can be placed in capsules sizes 0 to 5 if the apparent bulk density

TABLE 19.1: CAPSULE CAPACITY BASED ON POWDER SIMILARITIES

Capsule Size	Lactose (mg)	Aspirin (mg)	Sodium Bicarbonate (mg)	Quinine Sulfate (mg)
000	1,250	975	1,430	650
00	850	650	975	390
0	600	490	715	325
1	460	335	510	227
2	350	260	390	195
3	280	195	325	130
4	210	130	260	97
5	140	65	130	65

of the formulation is about 0.6 mg/ml. The apparent bulk density of a powder formulation can be determined by adding a known amount of powder to a 100 ml graduated cylinder. For example, if 60 grams of powder fills a 100 ml graduated cylinder, the apparent bulk density is 60 grams/100 ml or 0.6 g/ml. Many literature references give the bulk density of individual ingredients, but in a compounded formulation that contains many ingredients, the apparent bulk density can be determined experimentally as above.

Rule of Sevens

Another method to determine the appropriate capsule size is to use the *Rule of Sevens*. This method will work only if the calculated values are less than –3 or more than 5.[7] To use the method:

1. Convert the weight of the formulation to be in each capsule to grains.
2. Subtract the number of grains from 7.
3. Match the result with the chart below.

If the resulting number is . . .	choose this capsule size
–3	000
–2	00
–1 or 0	0
1	1
2	2
3	3
4	4
5	5

Preparing the Capsule Formulation

If the amount of active drug required per dose is large enough, a capsule can be filled with just the drug. But many times the dose is too small to be placed alone in a capsule. In these cases a formulation is created that will contain a bulk agent. Lactose, microcrystalline cellulose, and starch are commonly used for this purpose. These materials also impart a cohesive property to a powder blend that aids in filling the capsule bodies. Filling operations also are improved if a powder blend has a uniform particle size. For extemporaneous compounding, triturating a powder blend in a mortar with a pestle will increase the uniformity of particle size.

If powders that are being mixed before encapsulation are light and fluffy and "difficult to manage," add a few drops of alcohol, water, or mineral oil. As an alternative, mix these powders in a plastic bag. If the powders seem to have a "static charge," use about 1% sodium lauryl sulfate.[8]

Magnesium stearate (less than 1%) can be added to powders to increase their "flowability," which makes filling capsules easier. Magnesium stearate, however, is a hydrophobic compound and may interfere with dissolution of the powders.

Liquids that do not dissolve gelatin may be dispensed in capsules. When filling such capsules, measure the liquid with a pipet or calibrated dropper and put the liquid in the capsule body without touching the opening of the body. Locking capsules are best for these formulations. The capsules should be placed on a paper and inspected for leakage before dispensing.[9]

Drugs also can be incorporated into a semisolid substance and then encapsulated. Examples of some of the semisolid materials that could be used are carnauba wax, cocoa butter, beeswax, lanolin, cetyl or stearyl alcohol, palmitic or stearic acid, Plastibase™, and Fattibase®.

Semisolid formulations can be encapsulated into a capsule using one of the following techniques.

- If the material has adhesion properties, roll the formulation into the shape of a pipe with a diameter slightly less than the capsule opening. Cut the pipe to the correct length that will contain the desired weight of formulation. Then place the pieces of pipe into individual capsule bodies. If the formulation is difficult to insert into the capsule, dust it with corn starch prior to insertion.

- If the semisolid formulation is too firm to be formed into a pipe but has a suitable melting temperature, melt it and pour it into the capsule bodies. After the melt has cooled and solidified, place the caps on the body. It is a good idea to use a holding device (either homemade or a capsule machine) that can keep the bodies in an upright position.

Methods for Extemporaneously Filling Hard Gelatin Capsules

Two methods of filling hard gelatin capsules shells are given here. In both methods some powder will be lost in the process; therefore, using extra powder is recommended. Some references suggest using 10% extra, and others suggest using enough extra powder to fill two extra capsules. If a powder blend is to be used, triturate the ingredients in a mortar with a pestle and pass the powder blend through a 60–100 mesh sieve before beginning either filling process.

Punch Method

When filling a small number of capsules, the punch method is used. The steps are as follows.

1. Place the powder on an ointment slab. Smooth and block the powder with a spatula to a height approximately one-third to one-half the length of the capsule body.

2. Wear gloves or finger cots to prevent hand contact with the powder and the capsule body and cap. Alternatively, use the cap from a capsule as a holder slipped over the body of the capsule to be filled.

3. Place the exact number of empty capsules on the powder paper or ointment slab. This will prevent the pharmacist from preparing the wrong number of capsules and will avoid contaminating the empty capsules in the original manufacturer's package with drug powder that cling to the hands. Separate the capsule bodies and caps.

4. Hold the body of the capsule vertically, and repeatedly push or "punch" the open end into the powder until the capsule is filled. When punching the capsule, rotate the capsule slightly as it enters the powder and passes through the powder. This will aid in packing the powder in the capsule. Some powders will not pack inside the capsule body even with repeated punching. In these cases, place the body on its side and use a spatula to guide the powder into the body. Take care not to scrape or scratch the capsule body. Some granular powders also are difficult to punch into a capsule because they are not cohesive. Many times, reducing the particle size makes the particles more cohesive.

5. When the body is filled with powder, place the cap on the body to close the capsule.

6. Weigh each filled capsule, using an empty capsule as a counterweight. Add or remove powder until the correct weight of powder is contained in the capsule.

practice site. The brands of machines differ slightly in their operation, but the steps are the same.

1. Load empty hard capsules into the machine. Most machines come with a capsule loader, which correctly aligns all of the capsules body down in the machine base.

2. The machine has plates on its base that can be moved by turning adjustment screws. Tighten the screws so the plates bind the capsule bodies in place, and remove the caps all at one time in a top plate.

3. Loosen the adjusting screws, allowing the capsule bodies to drop so their tops are flush with the working surface of the plate.

4. Pour the formulation powder onto the plate and use special spreaders and combs to fill the individual capsules. Some manufacturers have special shakers that will help spread the powder and fill the capsules. Spread the powder evenly over the plate, and use the comb to tamp and pack the powder into the capsules. Repeat these two processes until the capsule bodies are filled with the powder.

5. Release the caps on the capsule bodies, and remove the closed capsules from the machine.

These machines have the advantage of filling many capsules in a timely manner, but there is a tendency to pack the capsules in the middle of the plate with more powder than the capsules along the periphery. Practice is required to ensure that each capsule contains the same amount of drug. A quality control procedure should be executed with each batch of capsules produced with the machine. One such procedure has been published.[10]

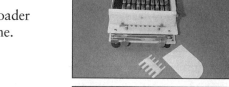

The capsule loader on the machine.

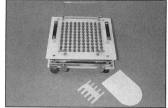

Capsules loaded in the machine.

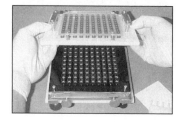

Capsule tops removed from capsule bodies.

Hand Operated Machines

Small capsule machines are available for filling 50, 100, or 300 capsules and often are used at a pharmacy

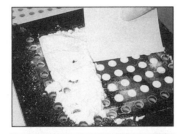

The spreader is used to distribute the powder.

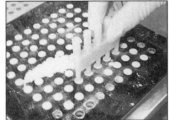

The comb is used to pack the capsule bodies.

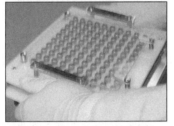

The powder is packed in the capsule bodies.

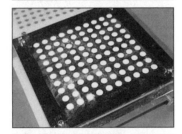

The capsule tops are reattached to the capsule bodies.

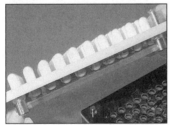

The capsules are removed from the machine.

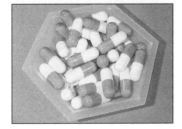

The capsules are removed from the top.

Finishing Procedures

Once a capsule is filled, the pharmacist may want to "seal" the capsule. The best way to produce a sealed capsule is to use locking capsules in the compounding process. If these are used, the cap is not locked (i.e., completely closed) onto the body until after the correct weight of the powder is in the capsule. If locking capsules are not used, a seal can be made by touching the outer edge of the body with a moist towel to soften the gelatin. Alternatively, a cotton swab dipped in warm water can be rubbed around the inner edge of the cap. When the cap is closed on the body, slightly twist it to form the seal.

When compounding and sealing are complete, the capsules may require cleaning to remove fingerprints, traces of body oils, or loose powder. Fingerprints and oils cannot be cleaned effectively from capsules, so the best way to prevent these problems is to wear gloves or finger cots during the compounding process. Any clinging powder can be removed by rolling the capsules between the folds of a towel.

Another proposed cleaning method is to put the capsules in a container filled with sodium bicarbonate, sugar, or sodium chloride, and gently roll the container. Then the container contents can be poured into a 10 mesh sieve so the "cleaning salt" will pass through the sieve.[11]

Physical Appearance Tests

Capsules should be visually inspected and checked for the following:

- *Product color check*: Check the description on the Formulation Record. It may be advisable to use a color chart for determining the actual color of the formulation.
- *Uniformity*: Check capsules for uniformity in appearance and color.
- *Extent of fill*: Check capsules for uniformity in extent of fill to ensure that all capsules have been filled.
- *Locked*: Check capsules to ensure that they all have been tightly closed and locked.

Physical Stability Test

- Prepare an additional quantity of capsules; package and label (for physical stability observations).
- Weekly, observe the capsules for signs of discoloration or change.
- At each observation interval, record a description on the form.

Packaging

Capsules are dispensed most often in capsule vials. These vials are available in various sizes to accommodate different numbers and sizes of capsules, and they have both child-resistant and non-child-resistant closures. Cotton can be placed in the top of the vial to keep the capsules from rattling in the container.

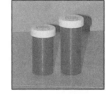

Observing Formulations for Evidence of Instability

The USP/NF chapter <1191> has comments for the stability of solid dosage forms in general:

> Many solid dosage forms are designed for storage under low moisture conditions. They require protection from environmental water, and therefore should be stored in tight containers or in the container supplied by the manufacturer. The appearance of fog or liquid droplets, or clumping of the product, inside the container signifies improper conditions. The presence of a desiccant inside the manufacturer's container indicates that special care should be taken in dispensing.[12]

Specifically for capsules, the pharmacist should observe the gross physical appearance or consistency of any compounded capsules. A change in the softness or hardness of the capsule shell is a primary indicator of instability. Another sign of instability is the release of gas from the capsule. This most likely is seen as a distended seal on the capsule.

NOTES

1. Rudnic, M., and Schwartz, J. Oral Dosage Forms (chapter 45) in *Remington: The Science and Practice of Pharmacy*, 21st edition. Lippincott Williams & Wilkins, Philadelphia, PA, 2006, pp 889–928.

2. Augsburger L. Hard and Soft Shell Capsules (chapter 11) in *Modern Pharmaceutics*, 4th edition, edited by G. S. Banker and C. T. Rhodes. Vol. 121: *Drugs and the Pharmaceutical Sciences*. Marcel Dekker, New York, NY, 2002, pp. 335–380.

3. Jones B. E. Hard Gelatin Capsules and the Pharmaceutical Formulator. *Pharmaceutical Technology* 9:106–112, 1985.

4. Scott, D. C, Shah, R. D, and Augsburger, L. L. A Comparative Evaluation of the Mechanical Strength of Sealed and Unsealed Hard Gelatin Capsules. *International Journal of Pharmaceutics* 84:49–58, 1992.

5. Murthy, K. S., and Ghebre-Sellassie, I. Current Perspectives on the Dissolution Stability of Solid Oral Dosage Forms. *Journal of Pharmaceutical Sciences* 82:113–126, 1993.

6. Nash, R. A. The "Rule of Sixes" for Filling Hard-Shell Gelatin Capsules. *International Journal of Pharmaceutical Compounding* 1:40–41, 1997.

7. Al-Achi, A., and Greenwood, R. B. The "Rule of Seven" for Determining Capsule Size. *International Journal of Pharmaceutical Compounding* 1:191, 1997.

8. Allen, L. V., Jr .Featured Excipient: Capsule and Tablet Lubricants. *International Journal of Pharmaceutical Compounding* 4:390–392, 2000.

9. Allen, L. V., Jr. Preventing Leakage in Oil-Filled Capsules. *International Journal of Pharmaceutical Compounding* 3:364, 1999.

10. Allen, L. V., Jr. Standard Operating Procedure for Quality Assessment of Powder-Filled, Hard-Gelatin Capsules. *International Journal of Pharmaceutical Compounding* 3:232–233, 1999.

11. Allen, L. V., Jr. Capsules (chapter 10) in *The Art, Science, and Technology of Pharmaceutical Compounding*, 2nd edition. American Pharmaceutical Association, Washington, DC, 2002, 133–159.

12. <1191> Stability Considerations in Dispensing Practice: The United States Pharmacopeia 29/National Formulary 24, The United States Pharmacopeial Convention, Inc., Rockville, MD, 2005, pp. 3029–3031.

ADDITIONAL READING

Allen, L. V., Jr. Featured Excipient: Capsule and Tablet Diluents. *International Journal of Pharmaceutical Compounding* 4:306–310, 2000.

Newton, D. W. Capsule-Weighing and Trituration Calculations. *International Journal of Pharmaceutical Compounding* 5:192–194, 2001.

CHAPTER TWENTY

Introduction to Tablets

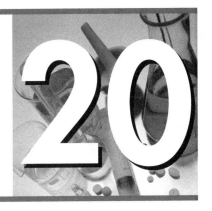

THE COMMERCIALLY MANUFACTURED TABLET IS THE most popular dosage formulation today. A tablet is a solid dosage form containing an active drug and several pharmaceutical excipients. Usually tablets are administered orally, but tablets are administered by other routes such as the sublingual tablet (under the tongue), the buccal tablet (cheek pouch), the pellet (subcutaneous implant), and the vaginal insert. Tablets vary in size, shape, color, weight, hardness, thickness, disintegration speed, and dissolution rate.

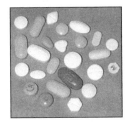

Types of Tablets

Types of tables include compressed, multiple compression, chewable, sugar coated, film coated, gelatin coated, enteric coated, buccal or sublingual, and effervescent.

Compressed Tablets

Compressed tablets are made by taking powdered materials and compressing the mixture into the desired tablet size and shape. The molding and compression usually are done in a tableting machine. Powdered

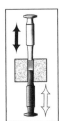

material flows into die cavities that have both an upper and a lower punch. The upper punch exerts great pressure when it compacts the powdered material. The lower punch then pushes the tablets out of the die, the die is refilled, and the process is repeated. After compression, the tablets may be coated with various materials.

The powdered material contains many ingredients in addition to the active drug. These include:

1. diluents or fillers, which add the necessary bulk to prepare a tablet of the desired size,

2. binders or adhesives, which promote cohesion of the various ingredients,

3. disintegrants or disintegrating agents, which help the tablet break up into smaller particles after being administered, and

4. glidants or lubricants, which enhance the flow of the powdered material into the tablet dies during manufacturing; the use of lubricants also minimizes the wear on punches and dies.

Other adjuvants that might be used include colorants and flavors.

Multiple Compressed Tablets

Multiple compressed tablets, sometimes called layered tablets, are prepared by subjecting the powdered material to more than a single compression. Layered tablets are prepared by initially compacting a portion of the powdered material and then adding material to the dies and compressing it again. This results in a two- or three-layered tablet depending on the number of separate fills. Each layer may contain a different active drug, separated from one another for reasons of chemical or physical incompatibility. Or each layer may have

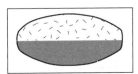

a different drug release characteristic. Or the reason for layering tablets may be simply to lend a unique appearance to the tablet.

Multiple compression tablets also can result in a tablet within a tablet—the inner tablet being the core and the outer portion being the shell. These "press-coated" tablets are prepared by feeding a previously compressed tablet into a special tableting machine and compressing another granulation layer around the pre-formed tablet. Press-coated tablets can be used to separate incompatible drugs, mask the taste of the drug in the core tablet, or provide a means to impart an enteric coating to the core tablets.

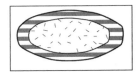

Chewable Tablets

Chewable tablets are chewed or allowed to dissolve in the mouth before swallowing. Chewable tablets are especially useful when administering large tablets to children or when adults have difficulty swallowing solid dosage forms. Chewable tablet products include antacids, antibiotics, anti-infective agents, anticonvulsants, and various cold/allergy combination formulations.

These tablets are prepared using minimal compression to produce a soft tablet. Because the tablet will be in the mouth for an extended time, it generally has a creamy base of specially flavored and colored mannitol. Mannitol is about 70% as sweet as sucrose and produces a cool feel in the mouth because of its negative heat of solution. In many chewable tablet formulations, mannitol accounts for 50% or more of the weight. Sometimes other sweetening agents (e.g., sorbitol, lactose, dextrose, and glucose) are substituted for part or all of the mannitol.

In the preparation of sugar-free chewable tablets, xylitol may be used. Xylitol is sweeter than mannitol and also has the negative heat of solution that produces the cooling sensation in the mouth. To enhance the appeal of the tablets, colorants and tart or fruity flavors frequently are incorporated.

Sugar Coated Tablets

Compressed tablets may have a sugar coating that provides a color, protects the enclosed material from the environment, and masks objectionable tasting or smelling materials. The coatings also enhance the appearance of the compressed tablet and permit the manufacturer to imprint identifying information. The major disadvantage of sugar coated tablets is the time and expertise required to perform the coating process. In addition, coated tablets cause an increase in the size, weight, and shipping cost of the tablets. Sugar coated tablets may be 50% larger and heavier than comparable uncoated tablets.

Film Coated Tablets

Film coated tablets are compressed tablets coated with a thin layer of a polymer. Film coated tablets have an advantage over sugar coated tablets in that film coated tablets are more durable and less bulky, and less time is required to apply the coating.

Gelatin Coated Tablets

Gelatin coated tablets are often called GelCaps and are capsule shaped compressed tablets coated with gelatin, which allows the product to be about one-third smaller than a capsule containing an equivalent amount of powder. The gelatin coating also facilitates swallowing.

Enteric Coated Tablets

Enteric coated tablets are designed to delay the release of active drug. They pass unchanged through the stomach into the intestines, where the tablets disintegrate and dissolve. Enteric coatings are used when the active drug is destroyed by gastric acid or is particularly irritating to the gastric mucosa, or when absorption can be enhanced by making the drug available in the intestines.

Buccal or Sublingual Tablets

Buccal or sublingual tablets are flat, oval tablets intended to dissolve in the buccal pouch (buccal tablets) or beneath the tongue (sublingual tablets) for absorption through the oral mucosa. They enable the absorption of drugs that are destroyed by gastric acid and/or are poorly absorbed from the gastrointestinal tract. Buccal tablets are designed to erode slowly, whereas sublingual tablets dissolve promptly and provide rapid pharmacological effects.

Lozenges (or troches) are disc-shaped semisolid dosage forms in which the drug is contained in a hard candy or sugar base formulation. They dissolve slowly in the oral cavity and usually produce a localized effect, although some are formulated for systemic absorption.

A newer approach is to make tablets that melt at body temperatures. When the tablet melts, the drug is already in solution and available for the absorption, eliminating the dissolution rate limiting step for poorly soluble compounds.

Effervescent Tablets

Effervescent tablets are prepared by compressing granulations that contain sodium bicarbonate and organic acids, usually tartaric and citric acids. In the presence of water, these additives react, liberating carbon dioxide that acts as a disintegrator and produces the effervescence (i.e., fizzing). The effervescent granulation is popular because of its taste and psychological impression.

Tablet Ingredients

In addition to the active drug, tablets contain a number of inert materials called *excipients*, which may be classified according to their role in the finished product. One group of excipients imparts processing and compression characteristics to the formulation—diluents, binders, glidants, and lubricants. Another group of excipients provides additional desired physical characteristics to the finished tablet; in this group are disintegrants, colors, flavors and sweetening agents and, in the case of modified release tablets, polymers or waxes that retard diffusion or dissolution. The same excipient commonly is used for several different purposes within the same formulation.

Although the term *inert* has been applied to excipients, abundant evidence shows that excipients play an important role in the performance of the various dosage forms. Studies have demonstrated repeatedly their influence on disintegration, dissolution, and bioavailability.

Diluents

In a single tablet, the dose of active drug is usually small, and ingredients are added to increase the bulk of the tablet to make it a practical size for compression. For example, dexamethasone tablets contain 0.75 milligrams of steroid per tablet; hence, other materials obviously must be added to make tableting possible. These added ingredients are called diluents. Common diluents include dicalcium phosphate, calcium sulfate, lactose, microcrystalline cellulose (Avicel®), kaolin, mannitol, sodium chloride, dry starch, and powdered sugar. Certain diluents (e.g., mannitol, lactose, sorbitol, sucrose, and inositol) are used in chewable tablets. Among the most preferred fillers are lactose because of its solubility and compatibility, and microcrystalline cellulose because of its compactibility, compatibility, and the consistent uniformity of supply.

Manufacturers use one or two diluents in their tablet formulations based on their experience and the associated cost. Most important, the compatibility of diluents with the active drug must be considered. For example, calcium salts used as diluents in a tablet containing tetracycline have been shown to interfere with the drug's absorption from the gastrointestinal tract. Highly adsorbent substances such as bentonite and kaolin should not be used in tablets in which the active drug is present in a small dosage, as the small amount of drug may be adsorbed onto the adsorbents after administration, which decreases the drug's bioavailability.

Binders

Agents that give a cohesive quality to the powdered material are called binders or granulators. Binders ensure that the tablets will remain intact after compression. In addition, they improve the free-flowing qualities of the powdered material by forming granules of desired hardness and size. Materials commonly used as binders include starch, gelatin, and sugars such as sucrose, glucose, dextrose, and lactose. Natural and synthetic excipients include acacia, sodium alginate, carboxymethylcellulose, methylcellulose, and polyvinylpyrrolidone.

Alcohol and water are not binders, but because of their solvent action on some ingredients such as lactose, starch, and the celluloses, they enhance the formation of granules, and the residual moisture in the granules enables the materials to adhere to each other when compressed.

The quantity of binder used has a marked influence on the characteristics of the compressed tablets. If too much binder or too strong a binder is used, this will result in hard tablets that will not disintegrate easily. Also, this condition causes excessive wear of the punches and dies in the tableting machine. If an insufficient amount or too weak a binder is used, powdered materials will not have adequate free-flowing properties and the tablets will not remain intact after compression. Obviously, materials that have no cohesive qualities of their own

will require a larger amount or stronger binder than those with some cohesiveness.

Binders are used both as a solution and in the dry form, depending on the other ingredients in the formulation and the method of preparation. The same amount of binder in solution will be more effective in reaching and wetting each particle within the powdered mass than if it were dispensed in a dry form and moistened with the solvent. This is because each particle in a powder blend has a coat of adsorbed air on its surface and the dry form is not as efficient in penetrating this film as a solution is. Also, with the dry binder, a period of time is necessary for the binder to dissolve in the moistening agent and become completely available for use. These dry form binder variables make it preferable to use binding agents that are solutions. And, because of the increased effectiveness of solution binders, lower concentrations often are possible.

Lubricants

Lubricants have a number of functions in the tablet manufacturing process. They prevent the powdered material from adhering to the surfaces of the dies and punches, reduce inter-particle friction, facilitate ejection of the tablets from the die cavity, and improve flowability of the tablet granulation. Commonly used lubricants are talc, magnesium stearate, calcium stearate, stearic acid, and polyethylene glycol. Most lubricants, with the exception of talc, are used in concentrations below 1%. When used alone, talc may require concentrations as high as 5%.

In most cases, lubricants are hydrophobic materials. If an inappropriate lubricant is used, or if the concentration is too high, the tablets may become "waterproofed"; i.e., water cannot come in contact with the tablet surface. When this happens, the tablets will have a delayed disintegration or dissolution time or rate. In some cases, sodium lauryl sulfate is added to overcome this limitation. Lubricants have to be used to decrease adherence to the punch and dies because most tablet formulations expand after they are compressed and have a tendency to bind or stick to the side of the die.

Lubricants are added to a granulation formulation as a powder, as a suspension, or as an emulsion. If added as a powder, the lubricant is finely divided and passed through a 60–100 mesh sieve onto the granulation. After adding the lubricant, the granulation is tumbled or mixed gently to distribute the lubricant without coating the particles too much or breaking them down into finer particles. If the granulation is blended too much, the tablet hardness, disintegration time, and dissolution performance can be changed. When lubricants are added as suspensions or emulsions, the amount of time for many operational procedures is reduced, shortening the overall production time.

Glidants

A glidant is a substance that improves the free-flowing property of a powder mixture. These materials always are added in the dry form just prior to compression. The most commonly used glidant, colloidal silicone dioxide, is generally used in low concentrations of 2% or less. Talc also is used and may serve the dual purpose of lubricant/glidant. It is important to optimize the order of addition and the mixing process for these materials, to maximize the glidant effectiveness and minimize their lubricant properties in the formulation.

Disintegrants

A disintegrant is an excipient or mixture of excipients added to a tablet formulation to facilitate the breakup or disintegration of a tablet after administration. By this disintegration action, the disintegrated tablet particles can start to dissolve and the active drug will begin to be released from the formulation. Factors other than the presence of disinte-grant can affect the disin-tegration time of tablets significantly. For example, binders, tablet hardness, and lubricants have been shown to influence the disintegration time.

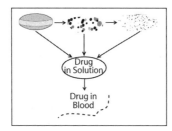

Commonly used disintegrants are starches, clays, celluloses, gums, and cross-linked polymers. The oldest and most often used disintegrants are corn and potato starch powders. Starch has a large affinity for water, and it swells once moistened, facilitating rupture of the tablet. Starch 5% is generally used, but if a more rapid disintegration is desired, 10% or 15% may be needed. Other specific excipients include Veegum®, methylcellulose, carboxymethylcellulose, agar, bentonite, alginic acid, and guar gum.

A subgroup of materials is known as the *super disintegrants*. With these ingredients, lower concentrations (2% to 4%) can be used. Croscarmelose, crospovidone, and sodium starch glycolate represent examples of a cross-linked cellulose, a cross-linked polymer, and a cross-linked starch, respectively. Sodium starch glycolate and croscarmelose disintegrate tablets because of their ability to swell when wetted. Sodium starch glycolate swells sevenfold to twelvefold in less than 30 seconds, and croscarmelose swells fourfold to 28-fold in less than 10 seconds. Crospovidone swells very little, so the mechanism of disintegration is thought to result from wicking or capillary action.

The evolution of carbon dioxide is another effective way to cause the disintegration of compressed tablets. Tablets containing a mixture of sodium bicarbonate and an acidulant such as tartaric acid or citric acid

monohydrate will effervesce when added to water. One drawback to this type of disintegration is that the tablets must be protected from moisture during manufacture, storage, and packaging. The reaction equation between citric acid monohydrate and sodium bicarbonate is given below to illustrate the evolution of this gas.

$$
3\, NaHCO_3 +
\begin{array}{c}
CH_2\text{-}COOH \\
| \\
HO\text{-}C\text{-}COOH \cdot H_2O \\
| \\
CH_2\text{-}COOH
\end{array}
+ 4\, H_2O \rightarrow
$$

$$
\begin{array}{c}
CH_2\text{-}COONa \\
| \\
HO\text{-}C\text{-}COONa + 3\, CO_2 \uparrow + 8\, H_2O \\
| \\
CH_2\text{-}COONa
\end{array}
$$

The disintegrant usually is mixed with the powdered materials prior to granulation. Sometimes the disintegrant is added to the powder blend in two different portions. The first part is added to the powder blend prior to the granulation step, and the second portion is added prior to compression. In this manner, the disintegrant serves a dual purpose: (1) the proportion added prior to compression breaks down the tablet to granules, and (2) the part mixed with the active drug and other excipients prior to granulation disintegrates the granules into smaller particles.

Coloring Agents

Coloring agents are used in pharmaceutical preparations for aesthetic reasons. Colors also serve as a means of identification to the user. A distinction should be made between chemicals that have inherent color and the excipients employed as colorants. Certain chemicals—sulfur (yellow), cupric sulfate (blue), ferrous sulfate (bluish green), and red mercuric iodide (vivid red)—have inherent color and are not thought of as pharmaceutical colorants in the usual sense of the term.

Most of the colorants used today are of synthetic origin. These agents were first prepared in the middle of the 19th century from coal tar. Coal tar, a byproduct in the destructive distillation of coal, contains anthracene, benzene, naphtha, creosote, and phenol. About 90% of the pharmaceutical dyes are synthesized from aniline, a derivative of benzene. Aniline dyes today usually are made from petroleum.

The use of color additives in foods, drugs, and cosmetics is regulated by the Food and Drug Administration through provisions of the federal Food, Drug, and Cosmetic Act of 1938, as amended in 1960 by the Color Additives Amendments. The approval and certification status of colorants is reviewed continuously in light of current toxicological findings, and changes in certification, classification, or approval are made as needed.

Within each certification category are various basic colors and shades (reds, yellows, oranges, greens, blues, and violets). By selecting combinations of the different colors and shades, distinctive colors can be created. In some instances, multiple dyes are used to give a purpose-fully heterogeneous coloring and form the speckling on compressed tablets.

Colorants are used in pharmaceutical formulations in very low concentrations, ranging between 0.0005% and 0.001% depending on the colorants and the depth of color desired. The exact amount must be reproduced accurately each time the formulation is prepared or each production batch would have a different appearance. Because of their color potency, dyes generally are added to pharmaceutical preparations as diluted solutions rather than concentrated dry powders. This permits greater accuracy in measurement and more consistent color production.

The most common method of adding color to a tablet formulation is to dissolve the dye in the binding solution prior to the granulation process. Another approach is to adsorb an aqueous solution of the dye on starch or calcium sulfate and blend the dried powder with the other excipients. These methods can be used because most dyes are water soluble. Water soluble dyes, however, can be made into insoluble pigments called *color lakes*. A lake dye is a water soluble dye adsorbed onto aluminum hydroxide. The resulting product is not water soluble but does exist in a powdered form.

If the color lake is to be used as the colorant, it can be blended with the other dry ingredients. FD&C lakes are subject to a certification process and must be made from water soluble dyes that have been certified previously. Lakes do not have a specific dye content but range from 10% to 40% pure dye. Blends of various lakes may be used to achieve a variety of colors.

When coloring pharmaceuticals, lakes can also be used in the form of fine dispersions or suspensions. Different vehicles might be used to disperse the lakes, such as glycerin, propylene glycol, or a sucrose syrup, and these result in particle sizes ranging from 1 to 30 microns. The finer the particle, the less is the chance of color speckling in the finished product.

Both dyes and lakes are used to color many of the sugar coated and film coated tablets. Traditionally, sugar coated tablets are colored with syrup solutions containing varying amounts of the water soluble dyes. The initial coats start with very dilute dye solutions, but the concentration is increased as additional coats are applied. As many as 30 to 60 coats may be applied. With the color lakes, fewer coats are needed. Appealing tablets have been made with as few as 8 to 12 coats, using lakes dispersed in syrup. Water soluble dyes in aqueous

vehicles or lakes dispersed in organic solvents also may be sprayed on tablets to achieve attractive film coatings.

Colors in wet granulations have a tendency to migrate during the drying process. This migration results in an uneven distribution of the color in the granulation. Tablets will have a mottled appearance if such granulations are used, because of the uneven color distribution. Color migration may be reduced by slowly drying the granulation at low temperatures and stirring the granulation while it is drying. The affinity of several dyes for natural starches has been used to prevent color migration. Other additives that have been shown to act as dye migration inhibitors include tragacanth (1%), acacia (3%), attapulgite (5%), and talc (7%). Lake dyes do not have the problem of color migration because they are insoluble. Another way to prevent mottling is to use lubricants and other excipients that have been colored similarly to the granulation prior to their use. Table 20.1 lists colors that have been approved for use in pharmaceutical dosage forms.

Sweetening Agents

Most tablet formulations do not have sweetening excipients. The one exception is the chewable tablet

TABLE 20.1: COLORS APPROVED FOR USE IN PHARMACEUTICAL DOSAGE FORMS

Color	Other Names
FD&C Red 40	Allura Red AC
D&C Red 33	Acid Fuchsin D
D&C Red 36	Naphthalene Red B
Canthaxanthin	Food Orange 8
D&C Red 22	Eosin Y
D&C Red 28	Phloxine B
D&C Red 3	Erythosin B; Acid Red 51; Food Red 14
Cochineal extract	Natural Red 4; Carmine
Iron Oxide—Red	
FD&C Yellow 6	Sunset Yellow FCF
FD&C Yellow 5	Tartrazine; Acid Yellow 23
FD&C Yellow 10	Quinoline Yellow WS
Beta carotene	
Iron Oxide—Yellow	
FD&C Blue 1	Brilliant Blue FCF; Erioglaucine; Acid Blue 9
FD&C Blue 2	Indigotine; Indigo Carmine; Carmine Blue
FD&C Green 3	Fast Green FCF
Iron Oxide—Black	
Caramel	
Titanium dioxide	

Adapted from "Oral Solid Dosage Forms," by E. M. Rudnic and J. B. Schwartz, (chapter 45) in Remington: The Science and Practice of Pharmacy, 21st edition (Philadelphia, PA: Lippincott Williams & Wilkins, 2006), pp. 889–928.

because it will remain in the mouth long enough to sense the sweetness of the formulation. The diluents used in chewable tablets (e.g., mannitol, lactose) impart a sweetness on their own, but in some cases additional sweetening agents may be included. Formally, the cyclamates with or without saccharin were widely used as these additional sweetening agents. Because cyclamates have been banned and saccharin has an indefinite ban status, however, new natural sweeteners are being sought. Most of these newer sweeteners have the advantage of being used in less quantity, so the bulk volume of the tablet is reduced. Also, because they are present in smaller quantities, the newer sweeteners do not affect the physical characteristics of granulations.

Some desired properties of sweeteners include: colorless, odorless, completely soluble in water at the concentrations needed for sweetening, and pleasant tasting with no aftertaste. Syrup USP, 70% sorbitol solution, sodium saccharin (0.05%), aspartame (0.1%), and dextrose have many of these properties. Table 20.2 compares the sweetening property of some agents compared to sucrose.

TABLE 20.2: SWEETENING AGENTS AND THEIR SWEETENING CAPACITY

Sweetener	Approximate Sweetness Compared to Sucrose
Sucrose	1.0
Sorbitol	0.5–0.6
Mannitol	0.7
Saccharin	60 mg equivalent to 30 g
Sodium saccharin	500
Aspartame	200
Stevia	250–300

Methods of Manufacturing Tablets

Tablets contain the active drug and a number of excipients that are mixed or blended and brought together in tableting equipment designed to produce thousands of tablets per minute. To facilitate such high speed production, the ingredient mixture or blend must possess a number of physical characteristics such as the ability to flow freely, form a cohesive mass, and provide lubrication. The basic mechanical unit in all tablet compression equipment includes a die and a set of punches. The lower punch fits into the die from the bottom, and an upper punch (with the same shape and dimension as the tablet) enters the die from the top. The upper punch enters the die cavity after the die cavity has been filled with material.

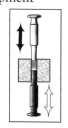

The tablet is formed when pressure is applied on the punches. Once the tablet is formed inside the die, it is ejected from the die by the lower punch, new material enters the die, and the process is repeated. The weight of the tablet is determined by the volume of the material that fills the die cavity. Therefore, the ability of the material to flow freely into the die is important to ensure a complete and uniform fill. If the material does not possess good cohesive properties, the tablet will crumble and fall apart after compression. The material must provide lubrication to assist the punches to move freely in and out of the die, and to minimize friction as the compressed tablet is ejected from the die.

After tableting, the tablets must have a number of additional attributes such as appearance, hardness, appropriate disintegration and dissolution, and so on. These attributes are influenced both by the method of tableting and by the materials making up the tablet formulation.

Wet Granulation Method

Of the several methods used to commercially produce tablets, the most widely used is the wet granulation method. This method has more operational manipulations and is more time consuming than the other methods and is not suitable for drugs that are thermolabile or hydrolyzable by the presence of water.

The general steps involved in a wet granulation process are to:

1. weigh and blend the ingredients,
2. prepare a damp mass,
3. screen the damp mass into granules,
4. dry the granulation,
5. size the granulation by dry screening,
6. add lubricant, and
7. tablet the granulation by compression.

Weighing and Blending

Specified quantities of active ingredient, diluent, and other required formulation ingredients are mixed by mechanical blenders or mixers until a uniform powder blend is obtained. Several different types of blenders might be used. For larger quantities of powder, the twin shell blender can effect precision blending in a short time. Planetary mixers (e.g., the Glen mixer and the Hobart mixer) have been used in the pharmaceutical industry for many years. Other types of blenders include ribbon blenders, sigma blade type mixers, high speed high shear mixers, and fluid bed granulators.

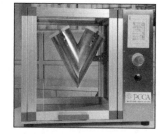

Preparing the Damp Mass

The liquid binder is added to the blended mixture to facilitate adhesion of the powdered particles. A damp mass resembling dough or brown sugar is formed and is used to prepare the granulation. A good binder results in appropriate tablet hardness and does not alter the drug release from the tablet. If the granulation is too wet, the granules would require more pressure to form the tablets and the resulting tablets would be hard. In addition, the resulting tablets may have a mottled appearance. If the powder mixture is too dry, the resulting granules may be too soft and will tend to break down during compression.

Screening the Damp Mass into Granules

The wet mass is pressed through a screen (usually No. 6 or 8 mesh) to prepare the granules. This may be done by hand, using a manual screen with small batches. For larger batches, comminuting mills can be used. Some of these mills include the Stokes oscillator, the Colton rotary granulator, and the Fitzpatrick comminuting mill. For continuous production, extruders such as the Reitz extructor have been adopted for the wet granulation process. The extruder mixes the powder in a chamber and then gradually forces the wet mass through a perforated screen.

Drying the Granulation

Granules may be dried on racks in thermostatically controlled drying cabinets or in fluid bed dryers. When tablets are dried by fluidization, the material is suspended and agitated in a warm air stream while the granulation is maintained in motion. Fluidization drying is much faster than tray drying. In addition to the decreased drying times, the fluidization method has better control of drying temperatures, lower handling cost, and the opportunity to blend lubricants and other materials into the dry granulation directly in the fluidized bed.

For continuous granulation operations, radio frequency drying and infrared drying have been used successfully. Some of this equipment allows oxygen to be excluded and lower temperatures to be used. This minimizes the degradation of the ingredients during the drying cycle.

During the drying process, a residual amount of moisture has to be maintained in the granulation to keep the various granulation ingredients in a hydrated state. The residual moisture also reduces the static electric charges on the particles. Water soluble drugs and colorants can migrate toward the surface of the granulation during the drying process. If the colorant migrates, the tablets have a mottled appearance. If the drug migrates, the content uniformity of the tablets may be compromised. Migrations can be reduced by drying the granulation slowly at low temperatures or using a granulation in which the major diluent is present in large size granules.

Sizing the Granulation by Dry Screening

After drying, the granules are passed through a smaller mesh than was used to make the original granulation. The degree to which the granules are reduced depends upon the size of the desired tablet. In general, the smaller the tablet, the smaller the granules. Finer granules are needed in small dies to provide rapid and complete filling of the die cavity. Table 20.3 gives recommended mesh sizes for the various tablet diameters.

TABLE 20.3: RECOMMENDED MESH SIZES FOR VARIOUS TABLET DIAMETERS

Tablet Diameter (inch)	Recommended Mesh Size
Up to 3/16	20 mesh
7/32 to 5/16	16 mesh
11/32 to 13/32	14 mesh
7/16 inch and larger	12 mesh

Adding Lubricant

A finely screened (60 to 100 mesh) lubricant is dusted over the dried granules. After a final blending operation, the granules are ready to be tableted. If too much fine powder is added to the blend, the granules may not feed into the die evenly. Also, too many "fines" make it necessary to clean the machine frequently because the fine powder blows out around the upper punch and down past the lower punch. Every blend will have some fines, and most problems likely can be avoided if the percentage of fines is kept to about 10%–15%.

Wet Granulation with Fluid Bed Granulators

Fluid bed drying technology has allowed the wet granulation process to be completed as a continuous process in a single piece of equipment. The powder blend is suspended in a vertical column of a rising air stream, and while the particles are suspended, a granulating solution or solvent is sprayed onto the particles. Typical liquid binders include aqueous solutions of acacia, hydroxypropyl cellulose, or povidone. There is a gradual particle buildup as the process continues, resulting in a granulation that is ready to be compressed after a lubricant is added.

The properties of the granulation will influence the ultimate tablet performance. Characteristics such as the rate of addition of the granulating solution, temperature in the bed of particles, and air properties including temperature, volume, and moisture content all have been shown to influence tablet performance. Fluid bed granulation generally produces less dense particles than conventional methods do, and this will affect the subsequent compression behavior and the final tablet performance.

Some commercial technologies can produce "micropellets," which are granules in the range of 10–600 microns with active drug loads approaching 90%.

Other Methods of Making Wet Granulations

Spheronization refers to the formation of spherical particles from wet granules. A wet granulation containing the active drug and additional excipients is passed through an extruding machine to form rod-shaped cylindrical segments ranging in diameter from 0.5 to 12 mm. After extrusion, the segments are placed into specialized equipment, where they are shaped into spheres by centrifugal and frictional forces. The spheres then are dried, mixed with suitable lubricants, and compressed into tablets. The advantage of this process is that granules are produced with uniform shape, size, and surface characteristics. Also, fewer fines are produced.

The *microwave vacuum processing* method allows the powder blend to be mixed, wetted, granulated, and dried in a single piece of equipment. Batch processing time is generally in the range of 90 minutes—about a one-fourth time savings compared to other methods. The granules then are removed, mixed with lubricants, and compressed into tablets.

Dry Granulation Method

In the dry granulation method, the powder mixture is compacted into large pieces and subsequently broken down or sized into granules. When using this method, either the active drug or the diluent must have the necessary cohesive properties. Dry granulation is especially applicable to materials that cannot be prepared by a wet granulation method because of their degradation by moisture or by the elevated temperatures required for drying the granules. The powder blend can be compacted in two ways: slugging and roller compaction.

1. *Slugging:* The powder mixture is compressed into large flat tablets or pellets (called slugs) about one inch in diameter. The slugs are broken up by hand (in small batches) or by mills (in larger batches), and the granules are sized by passing the pieces through a mesh screen. Lubricant then is added and the granules are ready for tableting. Aspirin is a good material (active drug) for making granules via the slugging method. Other suitable materials include thiamine hydrochloride, ascorbic acid, and magnesium hydroxide.

2. *Roller compaction*: The powder blend is compacted between high-pressure rollers that increase the density of the powder. The material then is broken up, sized, and lubricated, and the resulting granulation is tableted. A potential disadvantage of the roller compaction method is that the excessive pressures used to compact the powder blend may result in a prolonged disintegration or dissolution rate.

Direct Compression Method

Direct compression means that the tablets are made directly from the powder blend without any modification of the blend itself—i.e., no granulation is made. Clearly, this method is limited to just a few formulations that have the required physical properties (i.e., cohesiveness, flowability) to make a good tablet. Active drugs that have these properties include potassium salts (chloride, bromide, iodide, permanganate), ammonium chloride, and methenamine. If the active drug alone constitutes a major portion of the total tablet weight, additional excipients are not necessary. If the tablet will contain 25% or less of the active drug that has the necessary properties, however, excipients generally are added to impart the necessary properties to the powder blend.

Some common diluents used in direct compression tablets are spray dried lactose, microcrystalline cellulose (Avicel®), granulated mannitol, compressible sugar, hydrolyzed starch, and dicalcium phosphate. Disintegrating agents include direct compression starch, sodium carboxymethyl starch, cross-linked carboxymethylcellulose fibers, and cross-linked polyvinylpyrrolidone. Common lubricants include magnesium stearate, talc, and fumed silicone dioxide.

Tablets made by direct compression may exhibit *capping*, *splitting*, or *laminating* if air is entrapped during the compression step. If excess fines are present at the compression step (generally greater than 10% to 20%), air entrapment can be a significant problem. When air is entrapped, the resulting tablets expand when the compression pressure is released, and this expansion causes splits or layers in the tablets. Mechanical devices such as forced feeders and induced feeders on the tableting equipment can reduce air entrapment. These devices make the powder blend more dense and amenable to compaction. Other factors that may cause tablets to cap or split may be worn or imperfect punches, identifying designs or emboss marks that are too deep and heavy, and tablets that are stored improperly.

Tablet Machines

The numerous types of tableting machines all have the same basic function and operation. They all compress the tablet formulation within a steel die cavity with the pressure being exerted by the movement of two steel punches—a lower punch and an upper punch. As the lower punch drops inside the die, the feeding mechanism of the tablet machine (e.g., hopper, shoe) fills the die with the material to be compressed. The feeding mechanism retracts and scrapes away any excess material from the previous compression cycle and also levels the fill material in the die cavity. The upper punch lowers into the die and compresses the fill material. This compression stroke results in the formation of a tablet that assumes the size and shape of the punches and dies used. The upper punch retracts as the lower punch rises and ejects the tablet from the die. The feeding mechanism again moves over the die cavity, which also moves the tablet aside that was made in the compression stroke. The die is filled with material again, and the cycle continues. The tablets that are pushed aside are gathered in a collection container.

Tablets can have many shapes—round, oval, capsule-shaped, square, triangular, or other irregular shapes. The tablet shape is created by the curvature on the punch faces. Punch faces with ridges are used to produce "scores," or breaking lines in tablets. Punch faces also have the designs necessary to create engraved or embossed symbols or initials on the tablets.

Single Punch Machines

The simplest tableting machines are those having a single punch design. Some of the available machines are hand-operated, but most are power driven. The compression stroke for a single punch machine was described above. Single punch machines produce up to 100 tablets per minute. The weight of the tablet is determined by the volume of the die cavity. The lower punch is adjustable to increase or decrease the volume of the die cavity so the weight of the tablet can be increased or decreased as needed.

Rotary Tablet Machines

Rotary tablet machines were developed to increase production output. In these machines, revolving heads carry a number of sets of punches and dies. The heads revolve continuously, and compression takes place as the upper and lower punches passed between a pair of rollers. This action compresses the material in the die cavity from the top and bottom and provides a chance for entrapped air to escape. The lower punch lifts up and ejects the tablet. Adjustments in tablet weight and hardness can be made while the machine is in operation.

A single rotary press with 16 stations (16 sets of punches and dies) may produce up to 1,100 tablets per minute. Rotary machines with up to about 70 stations are available. Some machines have dual compression points and are referred to as double rotary tablet machines. These machines are capable of producing two tablets in each die and may exceed a production rate of 10,000 tablets per minute.

The main concern with such high speed tableting machines is to ensure that the dies are filled accurately before each compression stroke. Various forced feeding methods or induced feeding methods have been developed to overcome this difficulty. The high speed production also increases the occurrence of lamination (horizontal striations) and tablet capping (top of the tablet separating from the whole). Generally, these undesired attributes can be reduced by decreasing the tableting speed.

Multiple Compression Tablet Machines

Multiple layered tablets (one to three layers) are produced by the multiple feeding and multiple compression of material in a single die. Originally, layered tablets were prepared by a series of single compression strokes. The first component of the table was prepared in a single compression method. The dies then were filled with a different granulation and the compression stroke was repeated, forming a layered tablet. The problem with this method was that the lines of the various layers tended to be irregular. Rotary tablet machines have been developed in which the granulation receives a precompression stroke after the first and second fill, which lightly compacts the granulation and maintains a well defined separation between each layer.

Tablets having an inner core tablet are prepared by machines that take a previously compressed tablet and compress another granulation around the core tablet. These machines have a special feeding apparatus that strategically places the core tablet in the die so the addi-tional fill material can be compressed around the core.

Contamination Control

There usually is a fine powder or dust on tablets collected from a tableting machine. Also, uncompressed granulation material has to be removed from the tablets and the tableting machines. Vibrating screens or vacuum devices are used to accomplish this post-tableting clean-up. Critical problems include possible cross-contamination between different drug formulations that use the same tableting machine and the potential exposure of personnel to airborne dust or residual quantities of drugs that might cause hypersensitive reactions. Some tableting machines have been designed so the compressing compartment is completely sealed off from the outside environment. These have a designated air supply and vacuum equipment that maintain a dust free compartment.

Tablet Coating

After a tablet is made by one of the methods described above, it is a functionally complete dosage form, but many tablet formulations subsequently are coated for a number of reasons:

- to protect the drug from the environment (particularly air, moisture, and light) with a view to improving stability
- to mask an unpleasant taste or odor
- to increase the ease at which the patient can ingest the product
- to provide a product identity
- to facilitate post manufacturing handling in automated packaging machines or counters in pharmacies
- to improve product appearance and aesthetics
- to reduce the risk of interaction between incompatible ingredients
- to improve product mechanical integrity
- to modify drug release such as an enteric coat, repeat action, or extended release
- to protect nonpatients from inadvertent contact (e.g., Proscar® tablets).

The three major techniques for applying coatings to tablets are:

1. sugar coating
2. film coating
3. compression coating

Sugar Coating

Sugar coating is the oldest method of tablet coating. In this method, aqueous solutions of sucrose are deposited repeatedly on the tablets until a smooth, aesthetic pleasing coat is formed. Of all the sugars available, sucrose is almost always used because it produces coats that are essentially dry and tack-free at the end of the process. Originally, sugar coatings were applied manually, so the finished product was highly dependent on the skill of the technical personnel doing the work. Also, those original techniques were not automated, so the sugar coating process often was protracted and tedious, sometimes requiring several days. Using newer techniques and automation, however, processing times have been reduced to about one day.

Tablets intended to be coated are thin-edged and highly convex to allow the coatings to form rounded rather than angular edges. The entire coating process is conducted in acorn-shaped coating pans made of galvanized iron, stainless steel, or copper. The pans are partially opened in the front and have diameters ranging from 1 to 4 feet. The pans operate at a 40° angle to keep the tablets inside the pan while allowing the operator access to the tablets.

During the coating process, the pan is rotated at moderate speeds. The tablets tumble over each other

while the coating solutions are poured or sprayed onto the tablets. Because the coating process builds up multiple layers on the tablets, the coating solutions are added in portions and the tablets are dried between each addition. During the process, warm air is blown into the pan to speed up drying and to prevent the tablets from sticking together. In many cases a dusting powder is added between the individual coating solutions.

The sugar coating process is tedious, time consuming, pan-specific, and requires the expertise of skilled technicians, and it also results in coated tablets that may be twice the size and weight of the original uncoated tablets. Also, sugar coated tablets may vary slightly in size from batch to batch and within a batch.

Tablet friability is also a concern because in the sugar coating process, the tablets are constantly tumbling over other tablets. If the tablets are too soft or have a tendency to laminate, they may break up and the fragments may adhere to the surface of otherwise good tablets. The entire coating process (i.e., rotating pans, tumbling tablets, putting coating solutions on the tablets) potentially can create nonuniform distribution of coating materials on the tablet surfaces, which in turn can lead to unacceptable characteristics such as uneven coloring of tablets and tablets of poor aesthetic quality.

Overuse of dusting powders can result in a soft coating. If too much dusting powder is used, particularly during the subcoating stage, the quantity of powder will exceed the binding capacity of the coating solution applied to the tablet core. Thus, the coats will not be bonded as strongly to the core and will have an increased tendency to crack.

Sugar coating is a multistep process that can be subdivided into the following main coating steps:

1. waterproofing and sealing
2. subcoating
3. smoothing and final rounding
4. coloring and finishing
5. polishing

Waterproofing and Sealing Coats

Coats are applied directly to the tablet core to waterproof the core from the aqueous coatings that will be applied in the subsequent steps. These sealing or waterproofing coatings protect the core from moisture and enhance the stability of the final product. The coatings also strengthen the tablet core. Sealing coats usually consist of alcoholic solutions (approximately 10% to 30% solids) of pharmaceutical shellac, zein, cellulose acetate phthalate, or polyvinyl acetate phthalate. If an enteric coated product is being produced, additional sealing coats are applied and polyvinyl acetate phthalate or cellulose acetate phthalate is used.

The quantities of material applied as a sealing coat depend primarily on the tablet and batch size. The porosity of the tablet also is important. Highly porous tablets absorb more of the first coating solution, which prevents it from spreading evenly across the surface of the tablet. Additional coats will be necessary to ensure that the tablet cores are sealed effectively.

Because most sealing coats have some tackiness during the drying process, a dusting powder (commonly asbestos-free talc) is added to keep the tablets from sticking together in the pan. If too much powder is applied, the tablets "slip" over each other instead of "tumbling" over each other, and this creates difficulty in getting a uniform coating. Too much powder also makes the core difficult to wet, which causes an inadequate subcoat buildup on the edges.

Subcoating

After the tablets are waterproofed, multiple subcoats are applied to build up the coating on the tablet. These coats help bond the sugar coating to the tablet core, give the tablet rounded edges, and also significantly increase the tablet weight. The process of sugar coating increases the tablet weight by 50% to 100%, and most of that increase is a result of the number of subcoats applied.

Subcoats typically consist of sucrose syrup that also contains gelatin, acacia, or polyvinylpyrrolidone. After the subcoat solution is applied and while the tablets are partially dried, the tablets are sprinkled with a dusting powder to reduce tack and facilitate the coating buildup. The dusting powder usually is a mixture of powdered sugar and starch, but talc, acacia, or precipitated chalk may be added to the mixture. Warm air is applied to the rolling tablets, and when they have dried, another application of the subcoat solution is applied and the procedure is repeated until the tablets are of the desired shape and size.

Smoothing and Final Rounding

After the tablets have been subcoated, a few additional coatings of a thick syrup are applied to complete the rounding and smoothing of the tablets before the color coating is applied. The syrup is approximately 60% to 70% sucrose, sometimes containing additional ingredients such as starch and calcium carbonate. Often the smoothing syrup contains titanium dioxide (1% to 5%) as an opacifier. This will make the subsequent color coating more reflective, which will result in a brighter, cleaner final color.

Coloring and Finishing

When coats are applied in this process, two outcomes are obtained: (1) the final shape and smoothness of the tablet coat is achieved, and (2) the tablets get the appropriate color. Again, many coats of a syrup solution (60% to 70% sugar solids) are used, but this syrup solution contains the requisite coloring agents. Up to 50 or 60 individual applications of the colored syrup solution may be required to attain the final desired product. Because the tablets must be dried thoroughly and slowly after each application, the processing time in this step can be quite protracted.

The two types of coloring materials are *water soluble dyes* and *water insoluble pigments* (i.e., *lake dyes*). Water soluble dyes produce a more elegant coated tablet with cleaner and brighter final colors. Water soluble dyes, however, can migrate as the coat is dried and moisture is lost. Irregularities in appearance also can be caused by "washing back" the color from a previous coat. If too much color syrup solution is used, it may redissolve some of a previously applied coating. To minimize these problems, small quantities of coloring syrups are added (just enough to wet the surface of tablets) and the tablets are slowly dried. The coats must be dried thoroughly before subsequent coats are applied. Otherwise moisture may become trapped in the coating and may cause the tablets to "sweat" upon standing.

Tablet color coating with pigments offers some significant advantages. Because the pigments are water insoluble, they will not migrate as moisture is removed from the tablets during drying. Therefore, the color remains where it was deposited by the syrup solution. In addition, if the pigment is opaque or is combined with an opacifier such as titanium dioxide, the desired color can be developed much more rapidly using fewer, thinner coats. Because thinner coats can be dried much more rapidly, processing times between coats can be reduced significantly. And because fewer coats are needed, the processing time can be reduced further.

Pharmaceutical pigments can be classified either as *inorganic pigments* (e.g., titanium dioxide, iron oxide) or as *certified lakes*. Certified lakes are produced by adsorbing water soluble dyes on an insoluble substrate such as aluminum hydroxide. Therefore, incorporating pigments into the syrup solution is not as easy as with water soluble dyes because the pigments must be wetted completely and dispersed uniformly.

Polishing

Sugar coated tablets have to be polished to achieve a final elegance. Polishing can be accomplished in several ways:

1. Special drum-shaped pans or ordinary coating pans lined with fabric or canvas cloth impregnated with agents such as carnauba wax, beeswax, or hard paraffin wax may be used to polish tablets as they tumble in the pan.

2. Pieces of wax may be placed in the polishing pan and the tablets allowed to tumble over the wax until the desired sheen is attained.

3. The tablets may be sprayed with a organic wax solution; two or three coats of wax may be applied, depending upon the desired gloss.

Tablets must have a smooth surface before proceeding to the polishing step. If the surface is rough, polishing will result in a marbled appearance because the wax will build up in the small depressions on the tablet surface.

Imprinting

All solid dosage forms for human consumption, including both prescription only and over-the-counter drug products must be imprinted with product specific identification codes or distinctive symbols. Some exemptions to this requirement are allowed, but most commercially manufactured tablets are imprinted. The imprinting is done either before or after the polishing step.

Technically, the imprinting may be debossed, embossed, engraved, or printed on the tablet surface with pharmaceutical branding inks.

- *Debossed* means imprinted with a mark below the surface.
- *Embossed* means imprinted with a mark raised above the surface.
- *Engraved* means imprinted with the code that is cut into the surface during production.

Film Coating

Film coating deposits a thin polymer film onto the tablet surface. Unlike sugar coating, film coating is applied to formulations other than tablet cores. For example, powders, granules, nonpareil particles, and capsules can be film coated. Film coating was introduced in the 1950s to combat the shortcomings of the sugar coating process. The coatings were applied with volatile organic solvents to enable the film to adhere quickly to the surfaces and have short drying times, but some of these solvents were flammable or toxic, causing environmental concerns.

Significant advances have been made in process technology and equipment design, so the emphasis has shifted from using volatile organic solvents in traditional pans to using aqueous solvents in side-vented pans or in fluid bed equipment.

Film coating has many advantages including

- minimum weight increase (typically 2% to 3% of tablet core weight)
- significant reduction in processing time
- increased flexibility in coating different formulations
- improved resistance to chipping of the coating
- skin-tight coating so embossed identifying codes can be seen.

The major components used in film coating are a polymer, a plasticizer, a colorant, and a solvent. A typical film coating formulation may contain 5% to 20% solids in the solvent, in which 60% to 70% of the solid is the polymer, 6% to 7% is the plasticizer, and 20% to 30% is the pigment.

Ideal properties for the polymer include solubility in a wide range of solvent systems, an ability to produce coatings that have suitable mechanical strength, and solubility in gastrointestinal fluids so as to not compromise the bioavailability of the active drug. Cellulose ethers are the preferred polymers in film coating. Hydroxypropylmethyl cellulose often is used, but hydroxypropyl cellulose and methylcellulose also may be used. Hydroxypropyl cellulose may produce slightly tackier coatings, and methylcellulose may retard drug dissolution. Other polymers that have been used are methacrylate and methyl methacrylate copolymers, polyvinyl alcohol, ethylcellulose pseudolatex, or cellulose acetate phthalate. Many of the polymers are available in a range of molecular weight grades, and the different grades have significant influences on the properties of the coating, such as solution viscosity and mechanical strength and flexibility.

Incorporating a *plasticizer* into the coating solution improves the flexibility of the coating, reduces the risk of the film packing, and improves adhesion of the film to the tablet surface. The plasticizer must be compatible with the polymer and be retained permanently in the film. If the plasticizer is used in conventional tablets, it must have sufficient solubility in or permeability to biological fluids such that the bioavailability of the active drug is not affected. Examples of typical plasticizers are glycerin, propylene glycol, polyethylene glycols, triacetin, castor oil, and phthalate esters (e.g., diethyl phthalate).

Colorants are used in film coating processes in a manner similar to those in the sugar coating processes. Colorants improve the appearance of the product and facilitate product identification. In addition, the color coating may act as a moisture barrier for the product. Water soluble dyes cannot be used with organic solvents because of their lack of solubility in the solvent system. Therefore, water insoluble dyes are used for their solubility, but they also protect the tablet from moisture and tend to be more light stable than water soluble dyes are. Because the pigments are solids, they also can be used to add bulk to the overall solid content of the coating dispersion.

Mottling can occur when using pigments and organic solvents, similar to the situation of using soluble dyes with aqueous film coatings. The color pigment can migrate as the organic solvent evaporates, or it can migrate if it is soluble in the plasticizer. Uneven color distribution also can occur from inadequate dispersion of the pigments in the coating solution.

Solvents are used as vehicles for the materials. The solvent is applied to the surface of the tablet, and when it dries, the film coating is left behind. A solvent system is selected that will ensure a controlled deposition of the polymer onto the surface so a uniform and adherent film is applied. The solvent also should enable the polymer to reach its maximum chain extension. This will produce films with the greatest cohesive strength. The most common solvents used are alcohols, ketones, esters, chlorinated hydrocarbons, and water.

As a result of both the expense and the environmental concerns of organic solvents, manufacturers have begun moving to aqueous based film coating solutions. One of the problems, however, is the slow evaporation of the aqueous solution compared to the volatile organic solvent. Commercially available aqueous based solutions tend to have low viscosity, so less water can be used, which allows for shorter drying times.

Certainly other ingredients may be included in a film coating solution. These might include surfactants to enhance spreadability of the film over the surface, an opacifier for rapid color development, and sweetening agents. The film coated tablets also may be polished in a manner similar to that of sugar coated tablets.

Softer tablets have a tendency to *laminate* while being coated. When the tablets are sugar coated, this is not a significant problem because sugar coatings are very thick and can easily hide the laminations. When using much thinner film coats, however, such imperfections cannot be easily hidden. Thus, laminated tablets should be identified prior to the coating process, as subsequent recovery of the tablets may be extremely difficult after the coating has been applied.

The actual process of film coating can cause a *picking* or *orange peel appearance* in the tablets. When the delivery of the film coating solution exceeds the drying capacity of the process, some tablets stick together and subsequently break apart. A portion of the coat will be missing where it was pulled off the surface (i.e., picked off the surface). An orange peel (or rough) appearance results from premature drying of small droplets of the coating solution on the surface.

When the film is drying, the coating can crack if the internal drying stress is greater than the tensile strength of the film. Cracking also can occur if the tablet formulation has a tendency to expand after it has been compressed. Another problem can arise if the drying stress of the coat is greater than the adhesive bonds between the coating and the tablet surface. Here, the coat pulls away from the surface of the tablet and can cause engraved or embossed identifying codes in the tablet surface to disappear.

Modified Release Film Coatings

Film coatings can be applied to pharmaceutical products to modify the release of active drug from the product. The two types of modified release dosage forms are *delayed release* and *extended release*. Delayed release products prevent the drug from being released in the upper part of the gastrointestinal tract. Film coatings used to prepare this type of dosage form are called *enteric coatings*.

Enteric Coatings

Enteric coated tablets remain intact as they pass through the stomach but then disintegrate and dissolve in the intestines. Their purpose is to protect the drug from degradation in the gastric contents or to protect the user from nausea or gastric bleeding caused by a drug-induced irritation of the gastric mucosa. These coatings also can be used to produce a simple repeat action effect. An inner core of the drug formulation can be enteric coated, and additional drug formulation can be applied over the enteric coat. The outer portion of the product will be released in the stomach, and the enteric coated portion will be released further down the gastrointestinal tract.

Enteric coating also can be applied to granules, which then are fabricated into capsules and tablets. Different coating thicknesses can be applied to the granules, and if a variety of these are in the fabricated product, a more continuous extended drug release can be achieved. The thinly coated granules would be available for absorption in the upper gastrointestinal tract, and the thicker coated granules would be available in the lower part of the tract.

The most commonly used enteric coating materials are synthetic polymers. Polymers are selected that have pH-sensitive solubilities such that they are insoluble at low pHs (i.e., in the gastric contents) but are soluble at the higher pHs found in the gastrointestinal tract. The most effective coating polymers have a pKa of 3 to 5. The most extensively used polymer is cellulose acetate phthalate. The compound becomes soluble at pHs greater than 6. Coatings with cellulose acetate phthalate are more permeable to moisture and gastric fluid as compared to other enteric coating polymers, and are susceptible to hydrolytic decomposition. Polyvinyl acetate phthalate is less permeable to moisture and gastric fluid, more stable to hydrolysis, and able to solubilize at the lower pHs, resulting in earlier release of the drug. Other polymers that have been used in enteric coatings are hydroxypropylmethyl cellulose phthalate, polyvinyl acetate phthalate, cellulose acetate phthalate, ethyl phthalate, carboxymethylethyl cellulose, and hydroxypropylmethyl cellulose acetate succinate.

Modified Release Formulations

Modified release formulations were developed to reduce the dosing frequency in multiple dosing regimens or to provide a more constant drug blood concentration profile over an extended time. Film coating is one method available to achieve modified release and is used to coat granules, nonpareil beads, drug crystals, and drug-ion exchange resins, as well as the intact tablets. Smaller units—granules, crystals, etc.—subsequently can be formulated into tablets or other dosage forms. For example, a small tablet (called a mini tablet) that is film coated can be placed in a capsule with bulk material added to fill the capsule volume.[1] Many materials have been used as modified release coatings, including beeswax, carnauba wax, glyceryl monostearate, stearic acid, cetyl alcohol, ethylcellulose, cellulose acetate (diacetate and triacetate), and silicone elastomers.

Compression Coating

Compression coating compacts a drug coating around a tablet core. This process uses a modified tableting press that centers the core in an enlarged die before the granulated coating material is applied. Compression coating provides a more uniform coating and uses fewer coating materials than sugar coating. The tablets are lighter, smaller, and less expensive to package and ship. Another advantage of compression coating is that solvents (either aqueous or organic) are not required. Therefore, this technique can be used to apply coats to moisture labile drugs. The major disadvantage is that the process is mechanically complex and finds utility primarily in applying special coatings to novel drug delivery systems.

Tablet Coating Equipment

Sugar coating—the first coating process to be used with tablets—was carried out in coating pans. The coating solution was ladled onto a cascade of tumbling tablets, and the tablets were allowed to dry as they tumbled in the pan. Some pans had a drying air supply that directed warm air over the tablets to facilitate drying. In addition, some pans were fitted with an exhaust system to remove moisture and dust from inside the pan.

Film coating techniques were essentially the same as those used for sugar coating techniques, with some exceptions. Liquid coating solutions were applied more commonly by spray techniques in conventional coating pans that were fitted with the spraying hardware. With the advent of aqueous film coating solutions, improved coating pan designs were developed, such as the Pellegrini coating pan, which rotates on a horizontal axis and has an angular-shaped pan.

Fluid bed technology also was introduced as a method of film coating powders, granules, beads, or tablets when organic solvents were the predominant coating solutions. The material to be coated is suspended in a vertical cylinder by a column of air coming from the bottom of the cylinder. The suspended particles rotate both vertically and horizontally in the air stream, which helps to evenly

apply the coating solution. The spray coating can be introduced in one of three places:

1. The top spray directs the spray toward the bottom of the cylinder.
2. The bottom spray directs the spray toward the top of the cylinder so the spray moves in parallel with the suspended particles.
3. The tangential spray has the spraying hardware on the side of the container.

The top spray coating method is recommended when taste masking, enteric release, or barrier films on particles or tablets is a priority and the coatings are aqueous solutions, latexes, or hot melts. The bottom spray coating method is recommended for modified release and enteric release products. The tangential method is good for modified release coatings applied to a wide range of multiparticulates. Production variables include the distance of the spray nozzle from the material bed, size of the spray droplet, spray rate, spray pressure, and volume of fluidized air. Other variables include drying time, air temperature, moisture content, and size of the processing cylinder.

Evaluation of Tablets

Tablets must meet a number of compendial specifications and requirements. Some of the criteria involve the *appearance* of the tablets, and other specifications involve the *performance* of the tablets. The purpose of the evaluations is to ensure that each batch of tablets is equivalent to other batches that have been produced. If the specifications are met, the tablets will be expected to have the same therapeutic efficacy and aesthetic acceptance. Evaluated specifications include

- size
- shape
- appearance
- hardness
- weight variation
- content uniformity
- disintegration time
- dissolution characteristics

Size, Shape, and Appearance

Size, shape, and appearance are the criteria that are used to evaluate the apparent or visible features of the finished tablets. The size and shape of the tablet are determined by the die and punches used in the tableting process, but production variables, such as the amount of fill material permitted to enter the die, the compactibility of the fill material, and the force or pressure applied during compression, can alter the size of the tablets. Other visually obvious defects are capping, splitting, or cracks in the coating. Color appearance, identification codes, and other engraved information must be reproduced uniformly from batch to batch. There should be no mottling of colorants, logo bridging, or obvious picking or roughness in the tablets.

Thickness, Hardness, and Friability

The thickness of a tablet is determined by the same factors that influence the size of the tablet. Tablet thickness should be measured during the tableting process, either manually with a hand gauge or by automated equipment. Variations of ±5% may be allowed, depending on the size of the tablet.

The correct tablet thickness is critical in several steps of the production process. If the thickness varies too much, equipment may malfunction when larger than specified tablets become wedged in channels or *shots* that are adjusted for a particular tablet thickness. In terms of packaging the finished product, tablet thickness determines how many tablets will be placed in the shipping container. If the thickness varies too much, the tablet count may be altered.

Tablets should be sufficiently hard to withstand the mechanical stress encountered during production, shipping, and handling by the consumer, yet soft enough to disintegrate properly after administration. Tablet hardness is a measure of the ability of a batch of tablets to meet these requirements. During production, the determination of tablet hardness is a quality control measurement of the compression force applied to the tablets by the tableting machines. Tablet hardness is measured by either a dedicated piece of equipment or by a multifunctional system that applies a force to the radial axis of the tablet until it breaks.

Orally administered tablets normally have a hardness of 4 to 8 kg. Chewable tablets are much softer (3 kg), and some modified release tablets are much harder (10–20 kg). Different hardness testers use different units of measurement such as pounds or arbitrary units, so care must to taken when comparing units between different testers.

A tablet property related to hardness is *friability*, which is a measure of the tablet's ability to withstand abrasion or crumbling in packaging, handling, and shipping. Friability may be determined with a *friabilator*, which rolls the tablets and causes them to fall inside a rotating wheel. To conduct the test, a number of tablets are weighed and placed in the apparatus. After a specified number of rotations, the tablets are re-weighed and any loss in weight is calculated. A maximum weight loss of not more than 1% is considered acceptable for most products.

Weight Variation and Content Uniformity

Compendial standards exist for tablets which are given in the USP/NF chapter <905> Uniformity of Dosage Units.[2] The standards state, "The uniformity of dosage units can be demonstrated by either of two methods, weight variation or content uniformity." Under the section "Weight Variation," instructions are given to individually weigh a number of tablets, perform an assay of the combined tablets, and then calculate the average of the active drug in each tablet, assuming a homogenous distribution. Content uniformity differs from weight variation in that the tablets are analyzed individually and the average of those individual analyses is calculated. In both cases, additional tests are to be conducted if the tablets fail to meet the requirements.

Tablet Disintegration

For the active drug in a tablet to become fully available for therapeutic activity, the tablet first must disintegrate into smaller particles, and the smaller particles subsequently must dissolve. Therefore, tablet disintegration is a critical variable in product performance.

It is fully recognized that an *in vitro* tablet disintegration test will not accurately predict the *in vivo* therapeutic response of the drug. The disintegration test measures the time required for a group of tablets to break into particles and pass through a 10 mesh screen. As such, it is most useful as a quality assurance tool to ensure equivalency between production batches. It is not meaningful for chewable tablets, for modified release tablets, or for tablets containing an active drug that is not intended to be absorbed from the gastrointestinal tract (e.g., antacids and anti-diarrheals).

All USP-approved tablets must pass a disintegration test in an official *in vitro* testing apparatus. The apparatus consists of a basket rack assembly containing six open-ended transparent tubes of specified dimensions held vertically on a 10 mesh stainless steel wire screen. During testing, one tablet is placed in each of the six tubes of the basket, and through the use of a mechanical device, the basket is raised and lowered in the immersion fluid at a frequency between 29 and 42 cycles per minute. The rise and fall of the basket rack maintains the wire screen below the level of the immersion fluid.

For uncoated tablets, buccal tablets, and sublingual tablets, the immersion fluid consists of water maintained at 37°C unless otherwise specified in the individual monograph. Complete disintegration is defined as "that state in which any residue of the unit, except fragments of insoluble coating or capsule shell, remaining on the screen of the test apparatus is a soft mass having no palpably firm core."[3]

The specific tablet disintegration times are specified in the individual monographs but usually vary between

10 and 30 minutes for uncoated tablets. Coated tablets may have acceptable disintegration times of up to 2 hours. Sublingual tablets have very brief disintegration times— 5 minutes or less. Enteric coated tablets are tested in Simulated Gastric Fluid for 1 hour and meet the requirements if no disintegration, cracking, or softening is observed. Then they are immersed in Simulated Intestinal Fluid and should disintegrate within a specified time.

Tablet Dissolution

As noted above, disintegration time is a useful tool for production control, but it does not imply that the active drug has been released from the formulation. A tablet can have a rapid disintegration time, yet be ineffective therapeutically because it has not released the active drug from the granules or aggregates formed when the tablet disintegrates. Therefore, the dissolution rate of the drug from the disintegrated particles of the tablet is the critical factor in drug absorption and is the rate limiting step in many formulations. For this reason, the dissolution time has been found to better correlate with *in vivo* therapeutic activity than disintegration time.

When analyzing dissolution rate data, four sets of factors must be considered. One set is the influence that differences in the tablet formulation will have on dissolution. A large body of scientific evidence indicates that the dissolution rate of active drugs is influenced markedly by changes in the formulation. As an example, starch, a commonly used diluent, was shown to affect the dissolution rate of salicylic acid tablets. Increasing the starch content from 5% to 20% resulted in an almost threefold increase in the dissolution rate.

The effect of the tableting process also influences the dissolution rate. For example, it is well documented that a higher compression force during tableting will decrease the dissolution rate. The increased pressure will result in a harder tablet and a decrease in solvent penetrability. The decreased penetrability may be a result of fewer surface pores being available, or it may be the result of increased waterproofing created by greater compaction of the lubricant in the formulation. The method of granulation and factors such as size, density, moisture content, and age of the granules all contribute to the dissolution rate characteristics of the final product.

The other set of factors consists of the method of dissolution testing used in the analysis. The USP/NF describes an Apparatus 1 and Apparatus 2 that are used primarily for immediate release solid dosage forms (such as uncoated and coated tablets). Each apparatus has a variable speed stirrer motor, uses about 1–2 liters of dissolution medium in a covered glass vessel, and has a water bath to maintain the temperature of the vessel. Apparatus 1 has a cylindrical stainless steel basket, and Apparatus 2 has a paddle affixed to a shaft. The tablet is

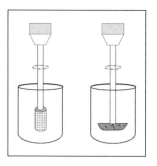

placed inside the basket and the basket is rotated in the medium, or it is placed in the glass vessel and the paddle is rotated in the medium. The shafts of the stirring elements go through the center of the cover on the glass vessels. The cover also has additional ports for the removal of a sample and for the placement of a thermometer. Abundant evidence documents the influence of factors such as agitation speed and composition of the dissolution medium (e.g., pH, viscosity, surface tension, temperature) on observed dissolution performance.

The final set of factors consists of considerations of the tablet itself undergoing dissolution. These variables include the wetting characteristics, the penetration ability of the dissolution medium, and the swelling or disintegration behavior of the tablets. The speed of wetting depends directly on the interfacial tension and the contact angle between the solid tablet surface and the dissolution medium. Incorporating a surfactant in the tablet formulation can improve wettability. After the tablets disintegrate into granules and/or aggregates, predominant factors become the penetration characteristics of the surrounding fluid into the aggregates and the action of the disintegrant to further break up the aggregates.

Dissolution testing also is performed on modified release formulations. Four types of apparatus are used in these tests: Apparatus 1 and 2 are the same as for immediate release tablets, Apparatus 3 is a reciprocating cylinder type, and Apparatus 4 is a flow-through cell type. Apparatus 3 consists of a cylindrical, flat-bottom glass vessel that has a set of glass cylinders in which one end is closed with a polypropylene mesh screen. The product is placed inside the glass cylinder and a motor and drive assembly reciprocate the cylinders vertically inside of the vessel. Apparatus 4 consists of a flow-through cell. The product is placed inside, and dissolution medium is pumped through the cell in a laminar flow pattern. The flow-through cell is mounted vertically with the filter system, preventing the loss of undissolved particles from the top of the cell.

There are many interrelationships between the formulation, production, and performance variables mentioned above. To gain meaningful dissolution rate data, it is generally necessary to hold many of the factors constant and change only one or two variables at a time. In this manner, an understanding of the interplaying relationships can be obtained. As might be assumed correctly, a great deal of time and effort is expended on dissolution testing in a commercial setting. To optimize this process, numerous parts of dissolution testing schemes have been automated.

In Vitro–In Vivo Correlations

As mentioned above, *in vitro* dissolution testing has been shown to be a better predictor than disintegration testing of a conventional tablet's *in vivo* bioavailability. A system has been developed that attempts to predict the likelihood of achieving a successful *in vitro–in vivo* correlation using information about a drug's solubility (high or low) and its intestinal permeability (high or low).[4] Possible combinations and expected outcomes proposed in the system are summarized in Table 20.4.

TABLE 20.4: IN VITRO-IN VIVO CORRELATIONS

Drug Properties	In Vitro–In Vivo Correlation Expectations	Rate Limiting Step
High solubility High intestinal permeability	Yes if dissolution rate < gastric emptying rate	Gastric emptying rate
Low solubility High intestinal permeability	Yes	Drug dissolution
High solubility Low intestinal permeability	Limited expectations	Intestinal permeability
Low solubility Low intestinal permeability	No expectations	Solubility and/or permeability

For modified release tablets, the FDA published a guidance document entitled, "Extended Release Oral Dosage Forms: Development, Evaluation, and Application of In Vitro/In Vivo Correlations."[5] The guidance provides methods for developing *in vitro–in vivo* correlations and evaluating their predictability using dissolution specifications, and how to apply *in vitro–in vivo* correlations to document bioequivalence during the approval process or during the post-approval process of certain manufacturing changes.

The following three categories of *in vitro–in vivo* correlations are included in the document:

1. Level A: a predictive mathematical model for the relationship between the entire *in vitro* dissolution time course and the entire *in vivo* response time course; e.g., the time course of drug blood concentrations or amount of drug absorbed.

2. Level B: a predictive mathematical model of the relationship between summary parameters that characterize the *in vitro* and *in vivo* time courses; e.g., models that relate the mean *in vitro* dissolution time to the mean *in vivo* dissolution time, the mean *in vitro* dissolution time to the mean residence time *in vivo*, or the *in vitro* dissolution rate constant to the absorption rate constant.

3. Level C: a predictive mathematical model of the relationship between the amount dissolved *in vitro* at a particular time or percentage and a summary parameter that characterizes the *in vivo* time course (e.g., C_{max} or AUC).

Level A is the most commonly developed *in vitro–in vivo* correlation model. It generally is developed by using different formulations with different release rates, obtaining *in vitro* dissolution profiles and *in vivo* drug blood concentration profiles for these formulations, then estimating the *in vivo* absorption or dissolution time course for each formulation using appropriate mathematical approaches.

NOTES

1. Porter, S. C., and Ghebre-Sellassie, I. Key Factors in the Development of Modified-Release Pellets (chapter 10) in *Multiparticulate Oral Drug Delivery*, Ghebre-Sellassie, editor. Marcel Dekker, New York, NY, 1994, pp. 217–284.

2. <905> Uniformity of Dosage Units. The United States Pharmacopeia 29/National Formulary 24, The United States Pharmacopeial Convention, Inc., Rockville, MD, 2005, pp. 2778–2785.

3. Guidance Document: Dissolution Testing of Immediate Release Solid Oral Dosage Forms. U. S. Food and Drug Administration, Center for Drug Evaluation and Research, issued 8/1997. Accessed August 10, 2007 from http://www.fda.gov/cder/guidance/

4. Amidon, G. L, Lennermas, H., Shah, V. P., and Crison, J. R. A Theoretical Basis for a Biopharmaceutic Drug Classification: The Correlation of In Vitro Drug Product Dissolution and In Vivo Bioavailability. *Pharmaceutical Research* 12:413–420, 1995.

5. Guidance Document: Extended Release Oral Dosage Forms: Development, Evaluation, and Application of In Vitro/In Vivo Correlations. U. S. Food and Drug Administration, Center for Drug Evaluation and Research, issued 9/1997. Accessed August 10, 2007 from http://www.fda.gov/cder/guidance/

CHAPTER TWENTY-ONE

Compounded Tablets

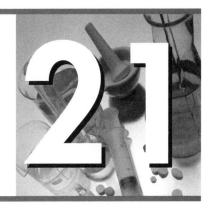

Commercially manufactured tablets offer many advantages, including

- accurate dosage with minimum variability
- elegance of product
- good acceptance by consumers
- convenient to store and carry (light and compact)
- low cost
- ease of administration
- availability of modified release profiles
- suitability for large-scale production
- best overall properties of all oral dosage forms.

The primary limitation of commercially manufactured tablets is that they are available only in fixed dosage strengths and combinations. To provide the flexibility of different dosage strengths, pharmacists can extemporaneously prepare molded and compressed tablets for their patients. Molded tablets are compounded using a tablet mold. Compressed tablets can be made using a pellet press or a single punch tableting machine. The many types of compounded tablets and unique characteristics are summarized in Table 21.1.

Molded Tablets

Tablet triturates and *rapid dissolve tablets* are considered molded tablets. These types of tablets are prepared in a mold of appropriate size for the intended dosage form and use.

One of the advantages of molded tablets is that they disintegrate quickly in the presence of moisture. Also, the pharmacist can easily adjust the composition for a wide range of dosages. Molded tablets generally are prepared by mixing the active drug with lactose, dextrose, sucrose, mannitol, or some other appropriate diluent that can serve as the base. This base must be readily water soluble and should not degrade during preparation of the tablets. Lactose is the preferred base, but mannitol adds a pleasant, cooling sensation and additional sweetness in the mouth.

TABLE 21.1: TYPES OF COMPOUNDED TABLETS

Type of Tablet	Characteristics
Sublingual molded tablets	Tablets are placed under the tongue and dissolve rapidly; the drug substances are readily absorbed, or they can be swallowed.
Buccal molded tablets	Tablets are administered in the cheek pouch and dissolve rather quickly; the medication can be absorbed or swallowed. The excipients can be manipulated between hydrophilicity and hydrophobicity based on the desired release rate.
Sintered tablets	Tablets can be prepared to either dissolve in the mouth, if they are flavored, or to be swallowed; they generally contain the active drug, a diluent, and a meltable binder such as PEG 3350.
Chewable tablets	Tablets must be chewed and swallowed and formulated to be pleasant tasting; they typically contain sugars and flavoring agents.
Soluble effervescent tablets	Tablets contain a mixture of acids and sodium bicarbonate, which in the presence of water releases carbon dioxide, which acts as a disintegrator and produces effervescence.
Implants or pellets	Small, sterile, solid masses containing a drug with or without excipients; generally administered subcutaneously.

Tablet Triturates

Tablet triturates are small, cylindrical tablets containing small amounts of potent drugs. They have the property of dissolving rapidly and completely in water. Therefore, only a minimal amount of pressure is used in making these tablets. Tablet triturates weigh between about 30 and 250 mg. In past times, these tablets served as dispensing tablets (a source of drug in compounding other formulations or solutions) or hypodermic tablets (dissolved in sterile water for injection prior to administration). Today, tablet triturates can be made by hand using a special hand mold or by using a tablet triturate machine.

Most tablet triturate machines use a mold as the basis for forming the tablets, but some others use a punch and die set to form the tablets by compression. These compression machines can produce up to 2,500 tablet triturates per minute. The moistened powder is funneled into a feed plate (the mold), compacted with a pressure foot, and then ejected from the feed plate by a punch. The tablets are dried, usually on a conveyor belt under infrared drying lamps. Obviously, this method of drying can be used only if the drug is chemically stable in these drying conditions. These tablet triturates are compressed with punches that have flat faces.

The base typically used for molded tablet triturates is lactose containing 10%–20% sucrose, the latter added to make a harder tablet. Drugs that react chemically with sugars require special bases such as precipitated calcium carbonate, precipitated calcium phosphate, kaolin, or bentonite. A liquid is added to moisten the powder mixture so it will adhere while being pressed into the mold cavities. Mixtures of alcohol and water in varying proportions (typically about 50%–80% alcohol) are employed; the alcohol will speed drying of the added liquid, and the water will cause the sugars to dissolve slightly and bind the tablet. If the tablet contains ingredients that are highly soluble in water, water can be omitted altogether and alcohol alone can be used.

When using a hand mold, the moistened blend of the active drug and diluents (usually lactose, dextrose, sucrose, mannitol, calcium carbonate, kaolin) is forced into a mold, extruded from the mold, and then allowed to air dry. The mold consists of two plates. One plate (i.e., the cavity plate) has holes or cavities in it; the other plate (i.e., the peg plate) has a corresponding number of projecting pegs that fit into the cavities. Hand molds vary in size from 50 to 500 cavities and are made from polystyrene plastic, hard rubber, nickel or plated brass, or stainless steel.

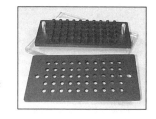

The mold will indicate the capacity of one cavity in the cavity plate, but that indication is only an approximation. Typical plate cavity sizes are 60 mg and 100 mg.

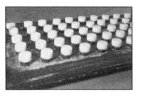

The volume of the cavities always remains constant, but the weight of the tablet made depends on the nature of the material. Different bases and drugs have different densities, so the mold must be calibrated (this is the same reason that all molds must be calibrated).

Preparation of Ingredients

To compound tablet triturates:

1. Prepare the powder mixture using proper techniques, and sieve the mixture through an 80–100 mesh sieve. At this point, you could use either of two methods of preparation: (a) mortar and pestle, or (b) pill tile and hard rubber spatula.

2. Moisten the powder mixture with the wetting solution until the mass adheres to either the pestle or the hard rubber spatula without crumbling. If the powder mixture is too dry, it will appear powdery and crumbly with streaks. If the mixture is too wet, it will appear shiny and mushy.

3. Place the cavity plate on the pill tile and press the wetted mass into the cavities of the plate using a hard rubber spatula. Apply sufficient pressure to pack each cavity tightly. Be sure to fill all cavities equally, especially the marginal cavities. Do not spread the powder mixture over the entire mold at one time, as this will allow the wetting solution to evaporate too quickly. Instead, fill the cavities one or two rows at a time.

4. When the cavity plate is filled, place the plate on the peg plate so the pegs are aligned with the holes. Then press the cavity plate carefully onto the peg plate. As the cavity plate falls, the tablets are pushed out of the cavity plate onto the tops of the pegs.

5. Leave the tablets on the pegs to dry, or place them on a sheet of cheesecloth that is stretched slightly above the table as a drying rack.

Some tablet triturates are made by first making a granulation in the same manner as ordinary compressed tablet granulations, with lactose generally used as the diluent. Tablet triturates made from this type of powder mixture generally are not as satisfactory with respect to solubility and solution characteristics.

The photos below illustrate how to make tablet triturates.

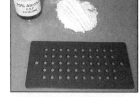

The powder mixture is prepared.

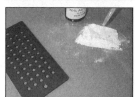

The powder mixture is wetted with a hydroalcoholic solution.

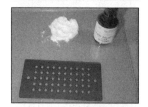

The powder is wetted until it first adheres to the pestle (if using a mortar and pestle) or a hard rubber spatula.

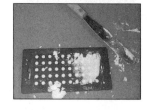

The powder is pressed into the cavity plate, filling one or two rows at a time.

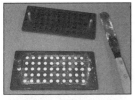

All of the cavities are packed uniformly and filled to capacity.

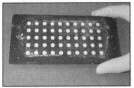

The cavity plate is placed on the peg plate.

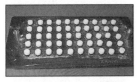

The tablets are removed from the cavity plate.

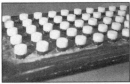

The tablets are allowed to dry on the pegs.

Rapid Dissolve Tablets (RDTs)

RDTs disintegrate or dissolve within minutes of being placed in the mouth. This is an advantage when administering these dosage forms to children, to elderly people, or to anyone who has difficulty swallowing tablets. The tablets liquefy on the tongue, and then the patient swallows the liquid.

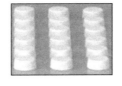

Among the techniques used commercially to manufacture RDTs are lyophilization and soft direct compression. When compounding these tablets, a soft direct compression technique is used.

RDT tablets contain a number of ingredients in a base formulation. These ingredients generally are extremely water soluble and are used to wick water into the RDT to aid in dissolution of the tablet. The base ingredients also provide some friability to the tablet. The RDT will have sweeteners and flavoring agents as well as the active drug. A typical RDT formulation might contain the ingredients shown in Table 21.2.

Preparation of Material

From Table 21.2, the powder base will be sucrose, citric acid, sodium bicarbonate, mannitol, and PEG 3350. The active drug portion of the formulation will include the sweetener, flavor, and bitterness reducing ingredients along with the active drug.

To prepare the RDT:

1. Preheat a convection oven to 110°C.
2. Weigh all of the formula ingredients, and triturate them thoroughly in a mortar with a pestle.

TABLE 21.2: TYPICAL RDT FORMULATION

Ingredient	Use in Formulation
Active drug	
Powdered sucrose	Base
Citric acid, anhydrous	Base
Sodium bicarbonate	Base
Mannitol	Base
Polyethylene glycol 3350	Base
Silica gel	Remove bitterness
Stevioside, acesulfame potassium	Sweeteners
Flavors	Flavors

3. Pour approximately half of the formula powder onto the bottom plate of the RDT mold and fill all of the holes, adding more powder if necessary. Tap the plate on the counter to settle the powder into the holes. Again, add more powder as necessary, and tap again. Continue adding powder and tapping until no more powder formulation can be added.
4. Remove the excess powder between the holes and retain the excess.
5. Put the top plate of the RDT mold onto the bottom plate, and press down with your hands.
6. Remove the top plate and fill the holes again with the remaining formulation powder in the same manner as step 3.
7. Repeat steps 3–5.
8. Repeat the filling procedure one more time (for a total of three times).
9. Remove the top plate and heat only the bottom plate in the oven for 30 minutes.
10. After 30 minutes, remove the bottom plate from the oven, and allow the plate to cool at room temperature for 15 minutes.
11. Remove the tablets from the bottom plate by inverting it onto a pill tile and tapping the inverted plate with a spatula handle. Lift the bottom plate off the RDTs.
12. Allow the RDTs to cool an additional 15 to 30 minutes before packaging.

Compressed Tablets

The pharmaceutical industry uses high speed tableting machines to create millions of tablets in a short time. The compounding pharmacist uses a variation of these machines, which make one tablet at a time, called a single punch tablet press. To make a tablet, the powder material is placed onto the bottom piece of the punch and the handle is depressed and released. The powders are compressed and occupy the size of the gap designed in the punch.

Punches come in many sizes. This allows for the production of tablets of different sizes and compression strengths. Each punch is a matched set, and the top and bottom pieces of different punches cannot be interchanged.

Chewable tablets and effervescent tablets can be made using a single punch tablet press. Chewable tablets generally are made using mannitol because it has a sweet, cooling taste and is easy to manipulate. Other ingredients include binders (e.g., acacia), lubricants (e.g., stearic acid), colors, and flavors. The powder mixture is prepared, then the desired quantity of mixture is weighed and pressed with a single punch tablet machine.

Effervescent tablets generally contain ingredients such as tartaric acid, citric acid, and sodium bicarbonate. These powders are mixed appropriately and pressed into tablets using the same procedure that is used for chewable tablets. The powders do not require a disintegrant because they will effervesce when placed in water.

Using Solid Ingredients in a Mold

When solid ingredients are used in a mold, they will occupy a volume of the cavity. Therefore, the addition of active drug to a base requires that some of the base be removed from the formulation to maintain the fixed volume of the mold. The amount of base that must be removed is termed *amount of base displaced*. The amount of base displaced will be influenced by the density and amount of the active drug in each cavity.

Regarding the *density* of the active drug, if the ingredients have the same density as the base, they will displace an equivalent weight of the base. If the density of the active drug is greater than that of the base, it will displace a proportionally smaller weight of the base. The *amount* of solid ingredients placed in each cavity certainly will influence the amount of base displaced in a direct relationship.

This concept (amount of base displaced) is discussed most often when preparing suppositories. *Density factors* for common drugs in common suppository bases can be obtained readily from standard references or easily determined (see Chapter 17, Suppositories). Density factors are determined from three pieces of information:

1. weight of a dosage form with just the base alone
2. weight of active drug in each dosage form
3. weight of a dosage form with the active drug included in the base.

Density Factor Determinations in Large Volume Molds

The best possible method to determine the density factor of a drug in a tablet formulation is to first fill the mold

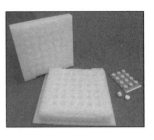

with base alone and determine the average weight of each dosage form.[1] Next, mix the required amount of active drug with about half of the base needed, and pack it in the mold. Then add sufficient base to fill the mold cavities completely, and determine the average weight of these medicated tablets. At this point, the density factor can be determined. If the tablets are to be dispensed, they will have to be reprocessed because the active drug distribution in each tablet is not uniform. These steps can be used to calibrate a RDT mold.

The Paddock method often is used to carry out the necessary calculations.

$$df = \frac{B}{A - C + B}$$

A = weight of dosage form with just base
B = weight of drug alone in each dosage form
C = weight of medicated dosage form
    (base + drug)

EXAMPLE: Using a given mold, the average weight of a blank cocoa butter suppository is 2.0 g. Using the same mold, cocoa butter suppositories each containing 300 mg of drug A averaged 2.1 g. What is the density factor of drug A in cocoa butter suppositories?

weight of suppository of cocoa butter = 2.0 g

weight of drug in each suppository = 0.3 g

weight of suppository with drug and cocoa butter = 2.1 g

$$df = \frac{B}{A - C + B} = \frac{0.3\,g}{2.0\,g - 2.1\,g + 0.3\,g} = 1.5$$

In the above equation, the amount of cocoa butter displaced by drug A is the denominator (i.e., A − C + B). Dividing this number into the amount of drug A contained in each dosage form will give the density factor (df). So 0.3 g of drug A displaces 0.2 g of cocoa butter in each dosage form, giving the density factor of 1.5.

Density Factor Determinations in Small Volume Molds

When dealing with molds used to compound tablet triturates, the individual cavity volumes are quite small. These small volumes make it impractical to carry out the type of density factor determination described above. Therefore, two methods have been used to deal with this limitation: the volume displacement method and the weight displacement method.

Volume Displacement Method[2]

The mold should first be tested by filling with lactose, properly moistened, and the resulting tablets thoroughly dried and weighed. This gives the capacity of the mold in lactose alone. A trial lot of tablets is then made as follows. The medicinal ingredients and also the sugar for fifty (or the desired number of) tablets are weighed. A portion of the sugar equal in bulk (as accurately as can be judged) to the medicinal ingredients is then set aside, and the rest is mixed with the medicinal ingredients, moistened, and filled into the mold. If all the holes are filled and none of the mass is left, the amount used can be ascertained by weighing the sugar which was set aside, and a formula made up for any number of tablets. If there is excess mass it indicates that too much sugar was used, and the excess should be dried, weighed and added to the sugar just set aside, to calculate the quantity which should have been used. If the mold is not completely filled, some of the lactose set aside is moistened and used to complete the filling of the mold. After this has been done the material in the mold may be remassed and again tried. Formulas which have been worked out in this should be recorded for future use.

In this description, an aliquot of sugar is removed from the total amount needed as a base that is "equal in bulk"— i.e., it appears to have the same volume as the medicinal ingredients. So this determination of "equal in bulk" is made by sight. Others have suggested using a small conical graduate to measure the volume of the medicinal ingredients, and then remove an equal volume of base (i.e., determination made by volume).

Weight Displacement Method[3]

The amount of moistened diluent necessary to fill a certain number of holes in the mold should be determined. This is done by molding a certain number of tablets using the moistened diluent and then drying and weighing the resulting tablets. A determination of this kind should be made for each new mold and kept on record for future use. From the figure thus obtained the weight of diluent needed for the required number of triturates is calculated. The weight of medicament to be used is subtracted from the weight of diluent, leaving the amount of diluent to be used.

In this method, the subtraction of the weights implies that the medicaments have the same density as the diluent. Because this may not be the case, it is suggested that a trial batch be formulated to determine if the calculated quantities exactly fill the cavities. Adjustments will be necessary in the weight of diluent needed if the cavities are overfilled or underfilled.

A more direct method to calibrate a tablet triturate mold follows these steps:

1. Tablets that contain only the powder base are made first. The tablets produced are weighed as a batch, and the average weight per tablet of the base is calculated.

2. The average weight per tablet of the active drug is determined. Tablets containing only the active drug are made, and the average weight per tablet for the drug is calculated. Usually, just a few cavities are used in this determination because pure drug is being used.

3. The quantity of drug that will be required in the prescription per tablet is divided by the average weight per tablet of the active drug. This will give a percentage of the cavity volume that the active drug will occupy.

4. Subtracting the percentage in step 3 from 100% will give the percentage of the cavity volume that the tablet base will occupy.

5. The percentage of active drug in the cavity volume and the percentage of base in the cavity volume are used to calculate the appropriate amounts of base and drug to weigh. For example, if the mold contains 50 cavities and each will hold approximately 100 mg, then 5,000 mg of mixture will be needed to fill the mold. The amount of base and drug to weigh can be determined by multiplying 5,000 mg by the two different percentages determined in the preceding steps.

6. Preparing a slight excess of powder mixture (5%–10%) is prudent. This will allow for any variance in the approximate and actual capacity of the mold and also will allow for powder loss during the compounding procedure.

Evaluation of Tablets

Tablets are evaluated using a variety of methods as described in Chapter 20, Introduction to Tablets. Most pharmacies do not have the specialized equipment to carry out analytical drug determinations or tablet hardness tests and dissolution rate determinations, but they can make and use a simple disintegration apparatus as follows:

1. Support a 10 mesh screen about 2 inches above the bottom of a 1,000 ml beaker.

2. Fill the beaker with 1,000 ml of water.

3. Add a stirring bar.

4. Place the beaker on a magnetic stirring plate.

5. Stir at moderate speed.

6. Drop the tablets onto the mesh screen.

7. Record the time needed for the tablets to disintegrate.

A reasonable disintegration time is between 15 and 30 minutes, although the time will depend on the product and the stirring speed.

Observing Formulations for Evidence of Instability

The USP/NF chapter <1191> gives a description of changes in physical appearance for uncoated tablets that could indicate tablet instability.[4] Evidence of physical instability

> …may be shown by excessive powder and/or pieces (i.e., crumbling as distinct from breakage) of tablet at the bottom of the container (from abraded, crushed, or broken tablets); cracks or chips in tablet surfaces; swelling; mottling; discoloration; fusion between tablets; or the appearance of crystals that obviously are not part of the tablet itself on the container walls or on the tablets.

Compounded tablets should be stored under low moisture conditions—which means that they should be packaged in tight containers. The appearance of fog or liquid droplets inside the container likely would indicate that the tablets should not be administered. Sometimes it is advisable to include a desiccant package inside the container to ensure low moisture conditions. One way to determine if this is necessary is to look inside the manufacturer's container. If a desiccant is in the manufacturer's package, it probably should be included in the compounded package. With molded tablets, to put a cotton plug in the package is also advisable because these tablets can be friable.

Effervescent tablets pose a unique problem because they are particularly sensitive to moisture. Swelling of the mass or development of gas pressure is a specific sign of instability, indicating that some of the effervescent action has occurred prematurely.

Chapter <795> sets beyond use dates for solid formulations depending on the source of the active drug. If the active drug comes from a manufactured product, the beyond use date is 25% of the time remaining on the product's expiration date, or 6 months, whichever is shorter. If the active drug is a USP/NF substance, the beyond use date cannot be more than 6 months. These beyond use dates can be extended if additional stability information is applicable to the specific drug and formulation.[5]

NOTES

1. Ohmart, L. M. Dosage Forms (chapter 4) in *Textbook of Pharmaceutical Compounding and Dispensing*, 2nd edition, Lyman, R. A., Sprowls, J. B., editors, J. B. Lippincott Co., Philadelphia, PA, 1955, pp. 51–92.

2. Jenkins, G. L., Francke, D. E., Brecht, E. D., and Sperandio, G. J. Tablets (Chapter 5) in *Scoville's The Art of Compounding*, 9th edition, McGraw-Hill Book Co., New York, NY, 1957, pp. 81–114.

3. Sadik, F. Tablets (chapter 4) in *Dispensing of Medication*, 9th edition, King, R. E., editor, Mack Publishing Co., Easton, PA, 1984, pp. 52–72.

4. <1191> Stability Considerations in Dispensing Practice: The United States Pharmacopeia 29/National Formulary 24. The United States Pharmacopeial Convention, Inc., Rockville, MD, 2005, pp. 3029–3031.

5. <795> Pharmaceutical Compounding—Nonsterile Preparations: The United States Pharmacopeia 29/National Formulary 24, The United States Pharmacopeial Convention, Inc., Rockville, MD, 2005, pp. 2731–2735.

CHAPTER TWENTY-TWO

Modified Release Drug Delivery Systems

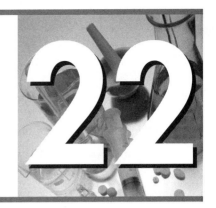

A NY DRUG DELIVERY SYSTEM DELIVERS AN APPROPRIATE amount of active drug to a proper anatomical site and achieves a desired therapeutic drug concentration. A *modified release drug delivery system* adds to that spatial placement concept a temporal component suggesting that the rate of drug activity has been altered in some manner compared to a standard. Research efforts in this area of pharmacy have been ongoing since the 1950s. Initially, strides were made in developing dosage forms that had extended rates of drug release but little spatial direction beyond the systemic circulation.

During the 1970s and 1980s, better understanding about the routes of administration and endogenous barriers to drug distribution led to several novel drug delivery systems that developed a spatial component as well as the temporal component. Research in the 1990s and 2000s has been directed at optimizing and expanding modified release drug delivery systems to better utilize their full potential.

Rationale

The value of modified release drug delivery systems can be appreciated when compared to conventional drug delivery systems. Consider a single dose of a drug whose disposition can be described with a linear one-compartment pharmacokinetic model.

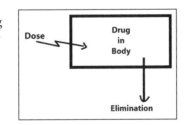

Depending on the route of administration (i.e., enteral or intravenous), the *conventional dosage form* will produce a blood concentration time profile similar to that shown below.

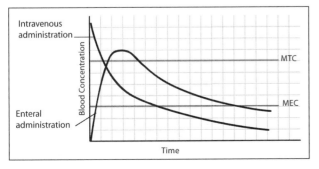

With enteral administration, the blood concentration begins at zero when time is zero (i.e., when the dosage form is administered) because all of the drug is still in the dosage form and none of the drug has been absorbed into the blood. As time goes on, the blood concentrations begin to rise as the drug leaves the dosage form and enters the systemic circulation. Initially, there is no pharmacological effect because most drugs must achieve a *minimum effective concentration* (MEC) before an effect is produced. At the MEC, enough drug is present at the site of action to elicit a therapeutic response. The time at which the MEC is reached initially is called the *onset of action*. The blood concentrations continue to rise to a peak and then start to decline. As the blood concentrations continue to increase, so will the *intensity of the effect*, because the drug in the blood is in equilibrium with the drug at the site of action.

Most drugs have a range of blood concentrations that will produce the desired therapeutic effect without increasing the risk for undesired effects. Concentrations above this range significantly increase the risk of producing an undesired effect. These concentrations are above what is called the *maximum effective concentration*, or the minimum toxic concentration (MTC). The concentration range between the MEC and the MTC is called the *therapeutic window*. The last part of the profile shows that after blood concentrations reach the *peak concentration*, they will decline if no other dose is given. Ultimately these concentrations will fall below the MEC. The time between the onset of action and the time when the MEC is reached by the declining blood concentrations is called the *duration of action*.

When drugs are administered intravenously, the onset of action is instantaneous because all of the drug is placed directly into the blood without an absorption phase. The intensity of effect will be based on the initial blood concentration achieved immediately after administering the dose. The duration of effect will continue as long as the blood concentrations remain above the MEC.

Conventional dosage forms (i.e., those that are *not* formulated specifically to have a modified drug release component) do not maintain blood concentrations within the therapeutic range for extended periods of time. One way to increase the duration of action is to increase the initial dose. The dotted lines on the graph below represent the new blood concentration profiles that would result from this strategy. The blood concentrations will be above the MTC sooner and to a greater extent, and this obviously is undesirable.

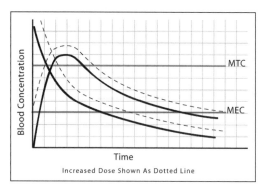

Increased Dose Shown As Dotted Line

An alternative approach is to administer the drug repeatedly using a constant dosing interval. This is a multiple dosing regimen (a fixed dose at a fixed dosing interval). It is shown below for the enteral route of administration and is the mainstay of conventional drug therapy. Multiple daily dosing can be inconvenient for the patient, however, and often results in missed doses, made-up doses, or patient noncompliance, which limits optimum daily therapy.

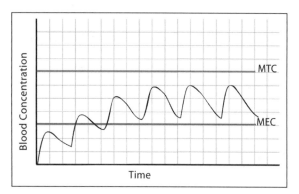

A third alternative is to "modify" the rate of drug release so the drug undergoes a longer absorption phase into the systemic circulation. Using this approach, the duration of action would be extended as illustrated below. In the earliest of these products, modest increases in the duration of action were achieved.

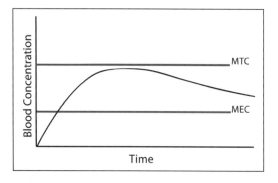

Today, significant extensions of the duration of action have been achieved. Examples are Ocusert®, Prozac Weekly®, Progestasert®, Zoladex®, Estring® Vaginal Ring, and Implanon™. Some of these delivery systems can deliver active drug for years. These results can be achieved because the delivery systems operate independently from their route of administration environment and release the drug at a constant rate of release—a *zero order release*. A constant intravenous infusion of a drug will attain and maintain a nonfluctuating steady-state concentration as long as the infusion continues. These delivery systems mimic the same type of pharmacokinetic behavior.

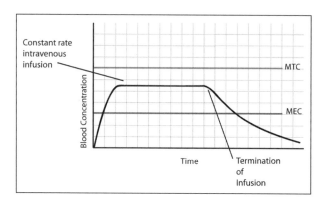

Terminology

Through the years, many terms have been used to identify drug delivery systems that extend the duration of action. Some of these include sustained release (SR), sustained action (SA), extended release (ER), prolonged action (PA), controlled release (CR), time release (TR), and long-acting (LA). Often these terms were used interchangeably even though the product designs and performances were different. For the most part, these terms were used to describe orally administered dosage forms.

In recent years, *modified release* has become the term to describe drug delivery systems that provide time course and/or directed site administration outcomes that are not available in conventional or immediate release dosage forms. The USP/NF categorizes modified release dosage forms as extended release or delayed release in several of its chapters.

> Extended release: a dosage form that allows a reduction in dosing frequency compared to a conventional dosage form (e.g., a solution or an immediate release dosage form).
>
> Delayed release: a dosage form that releases the drug from the dosage form at a time other than promptly after administration. The absorption of the drug into the systemic circulation is not altered, but the time that the drug is freed from the dosage form is altered. The delayed release may be based on time or on the influence of environmental conditions such as gastrointestinal pH. Enteric coated tablets are an example of a delayed release dosage form.

Another type of modified release dosage form is termed *repeat action*. Repeat action tablets might be considered an alternative method of extended release because multiple (generally two) doses of the drug are contained within a single dosage form and each dose is released at a different time. The first dose is released immediately after administration, and the second dose is released a few hours (e.g., 4–6 hours) later. The dosage forms are made with the immediate release dose in the outer coating and the second dose in the inner core. The two are separated by a slowly permeable barrier coating. An example of this type of dosage form is Polaramine® Repetabs. Repeat action dosage forms are best suited for chronic conditions when repeated dosing is necessary.

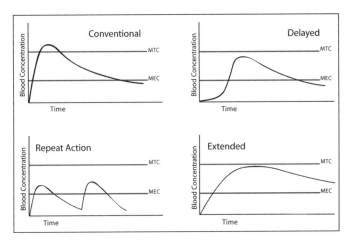

Most practitioners now clearly understand the terminology *extended*, *delayed*, and *repeat action* drug delivery systems, but terminology used to describe delivery systems that provide a longer duration of action independent of the administration site still not is applied uniformly. Some practitioners term these types of temporal systems as *controlled release*, and others use *rate controlled release*. Many of these delivery systems incorporate methods to localize the drug at an active site (i.e., spatial placement). If this is the only feature of the drug delivery system, terms such as *site specific*, *targeted delivery*, and *receptor targeting* have been used. The best terminology to use for systems that provide a longer duration of action, independent drug release, and targeted delivery is still unclear.

Advantages and Limitations

The major rationale for using modified release drug delivery systems is to improve and optimize drug therapy outcomes. Using delivery systems that reduce the steady state fluctuations in drug blood concentrations will minimize the time that patients may be at increased risk for side effects and maximize the time the blood concentrations are within the therapeutic window.

Modified release systems achieve this objective in several ways.

1. Dosing is less frequent because the systems provide a longer duration of action.
2. Many of these systems can protect the active drug from degradation at the site of administration.
3. Some systems allow drugs to be administered at sites different from their conventional counterparts.

The latter two features increase the bioavailability of the drug, which allows for either less frequent dosing or administration of a smaller dose that also will result in fewer side effects.

Advantages

General advantages of drug delivery systems are summarized in Table 22.1. Advantages of the system are compared to an appropriate conventional dosage form such as immediate release tablet, capsule, solution, and so on.

Disadvantages

The primary disadvantage is the cost of some of these drug delivery systems. The costs have to be weighed in

TABLE 22.1: ADVANTAGES OF MODIFIED RELEASE DRUG DELIVERY SYSTEMS

Advantage	Explanation
Reduction in drug blood concentration fluctuations at steady state	By controlling the rate of drug release, peaks and valleys in steady state blood concentrations can be reduced or eliminated.
Improve bioavailability	Delivery systems can protect drugs from degradation in some sites of administration, or can allow the drug to be administered at new sites of administration.
Requires less total drug	Reduced steady state fluctuations and more efficient drug absorption strategies use less total drug.
Reduction in dosing frequency	The system delivers more than one therapeutic dose.
Improved patient compliance	Patient convenience, and therefore compliance, is increased with less frequent dosing, especially from multiple doses per day to once-a-day dosing. Some systems offer much more extended dosing intervals (i.e., weeks, day, years) and also have the ability to be dosed at more convenient times.
Reduction in adverse side effects	Because steady state concentrations remain in the therapeutic window longer, fewer adverse side effects occur and/or occur less frequently.
Reduction in overall health care costs	The increased cost of the drug delivery system is more than offset by enhanced therapeutic benefit, fewer side effects, and reduced professional time to dispense and administer drugs and monitor patients.

"Modified-Release Solid Dosage Forms and Drug Delivery Systems," by L. V. Allen, Jr., N. G. Popovich, and H. C. Ansel, (chapter 9) in Ansel's Pharmaceutical Dosage Forms and Drug Delivery Systems, 8th edition (Philadelphia, PA: Lippincott Williams & Wilkins, 2005), pp. 260–275.

light of the improved therapeutic benefit versus the cost of the system itself and the cost of professional personnel needed to assist the patient if the system is not used. Patients' confidence is another factor. They want to have some control over their medical treatments, and if they can accomplish all or part of the treatment physically and it is a successful treatment, they are more willing to take the necessary responsibility for their care.

Some disadvantages pertain directly to the systems themselves. A good drug delivery system may be available to deliver a drug via a particular route of administration, but the drug being considered cannot be absorbed from that region. Another problem is "dose-dumping" if the system fails. Most systems have more drug than is needed for an equal number of doses from a conventional dosage form, so if the system fails, multiple doses of the drug will be released into the patient all at once. Another disadvantage is that many of these systems are not retrieved readily. If their removal becomes necessary, professional personnel may be required.

Candidates for Modified Release Drug Delivery Systems

The design of effective drug delivery systems must take into consideration many interrelated factors, such as route of administration, materials in the delivery system, length of therapy, and so on. One of the most important variables is the physicochemical properties of the drug. Not all drugs are candidates for a modified release product. Pharmaceutical experience and research have shown that the following characteristics and properties of drugs are necessary for successful modified release drug delivery systems.

Dose

The therapeutic *dose* of the drug has to be small. This is more a physical limitation of the site of administration than a therapeutic necessity. The modified release product will have to be administered at a site in the body and will have to contain all of the dose (and generally more than the dose) for the intended length of therapy. If too much drug is required to meet these requirements, the product will be too large for convenient or even possible administration. For orally administered products, a dose size of 0.5–1.0 g is the upper limit to fit conveniently in a single unit. If injectible parenteral routes of administration (i.e., intramuscular, subcutaneous) are being used, the dosing volume will be limited to a few milliliters.

Half Life

The *half life* of the drug will have an indirect effect on the dose required to be administered. If the drug has a brief half life (i.e., less than 2 hours), too much drug will

be required in the delivery system to maintain any useful extended period of therapy. Some drugs, however, have an inherently long half life but do not have to be in a delivery system because they can be dosed once a day from a conventional dosage form. When looking at orally administered delivery systems, drugs with half lives of 8 hours are considered to be the upper limit for successful delivery systems. This assumes that the drugs will be absorbed uniformly throughout the gastrointestinal tract and have a good residence time.

Aqueous Solubility and pKa

For any drug to be biologically active, it must have the ability to dissolve in aqueous body fluids and in most cases be able to partition through biological membranes. Therefore, the physicochemical properties of *aqueous solubility* and dissociation potential are required in a successful drug. In modified release systems, these properties are of greater concern than in conventional dosage forms.

The aqueous solubility of the drug influences its dissolution rate, which in turn establishes the drug concentration in solution, which is the driving force for diffusion across membranes. Some drugs with very low solubilities might be inherently extended release for a particular route of administration. For example, orally administered drugs with solubilities less than 0.01 mg/ml (e.g., digoxin, griseofulvin, salicylamide) tend to be extended release. But using these drugs in a modified release system whose rate limiting step is diffusion of the drug through a polymer would not be successful. At the other extreme, drugs with very high solubilities and, therefore, rapid dissolution rates often cannot be used in modified release products. The major difficulty here is to decrease their dissolution rate to a useful range. One often used method is to use a less soluble form of the drug, such as one of its salts, another crystalline form, etc.

The ability of a drug to exist in the undissociated form is based on the environment pH and the drug's *pKa*. According to the pH partition hypothesis, the undissociated form of a weak acid (or base) will transport preferentially through biological membranes by passive diffusion. Acids have favored absorption in lower pH environments, and bases are better absorbed at higher pHs. So the dissociation potential of the drug may dictate which delivery system might be used or by which route the drug can be administered.

Partition Coefficient

From the time a drug leaves the site of administration and ultimately is eliminated from the body, it must diffuse through a variety of biological membranes. These membranes are predominately lipid in nature, and the potential of a drug to cross biological membranes often is measured by the partition coefficient. The *partition coefficient* is defined as the ratio of the drug in an oil phase to that of an adjacent aqueous phase. Therefore, drugs with larger partition coefficients are predominantly lipid soluble and should pass through biological membranes. These drugs also persist in the body longer than drugs with lower partition coefficients because they can be localized in lipid membranes of cells.

A drug's partitioning potential also affects its ability to diffuse through polymers, so the choice of diffusion rate limiting membrane material will be made largely on the drug's partitioning characteristics. Partition coefficients are determined by:

$$PC = \frac{C_o}{C_w}$$

where

C_O = equilibrium concentration of all forms of the drug (e.g., ionized and unionized) in an organic phase

C_W = equilibrium concentration of all forms of the drug in an aqueous phase

Stability

Formulators of drug delivery systems must consider two types of *stability* issues. One, in common with their conventional counterparts, is the stability of the drug inside a dosage form outside of the body. But delivery systems may be inside the body for extended times, so the stability of the drug in the system inside the body also must be considered. These stability issues may be either positive or negative. On the positive side, the drug may be protected from enzymatic degradation inside the delivery system so can remain in the body longer. A negative could be that the drug is trapped and concentrated in an area (i.e., inside the system) where penetrating fluids could produce higher rates of degradation.

Mechanisms of Modified Release

Many strategies of modified release have been used over the years. The methods discussed here are the more common and more successful mechanisms, but by no means are the only ones developed for modified release dosage forms.

Membrane Dissolution

The membrane dissolution mechanism has been used a long time because of its low cost and ease of production. The rate limiting factor is the dissolution of a membrane that surrounds the drug. The rate of dissolution depends on membrane properties such as thickness, composition, porosity, tortuosity, and applied compression force. Studies have shown that the result of changing one or many of these properties generally yields the anticipated

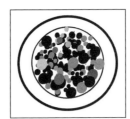

outcomes. For example, thicker membranes tend to take longer to dissolve, which postpones drug release. Membrane materials that are hydrophobic tend to dissolve more slowly than hydrophilic materials. Membranes that are more compressed tend to dissolve more slowly than less compressed membranes.

The drug core of the modified release particle may be made up of just the active drug, or may contain other excipients. In one type of system, groups of particles are made that have different membrane thicknesses, compositions, and so forth, and that will release the drug at different rates or times. These membrane coated particles are combined with uncoated particles (about a two-thirds to one-third ratio) and packaged inside the single dosage form (e.g., a capsule). When the dosage form is administered, the uncoated particles provide an immediate release of drug, which will act as a loading dose. Then a continuous release of drug will ensue, in which particles with very thin coats will release the drug first and particles with thicker coats will release the drug later. Because a spectrum of different membrane thicknesses is employed, a more uniform drug absorption will occur, which will result in a more uniform blood concentration profile. Many times, identifying colors are associated with the different groups of particles.

Some dosage forms are made using one drug core surrounded by one membrane (i.e., the whole tablet is one particle). In these cases there will not be a continuum of drug release, just one modified release rate.

In another type of membrane dissolution controlled delivery system, a layer of drug is coated on a nonpareil seed and then coated with the slowly dissolving membrane material. Another layer of the drug is applied, followed by another coat of the membrane material. The outermost layer typically is a layer of drug that will serve as a loading dose. Using this multiple-layer scheme, a pulsed-type delivery mechanism can be achieved. If just a few coats (two or three) are present and the drug dosage is the same in each layer, a repeat action delivery system can be achieved.

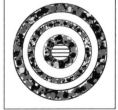

The underlying mechanism in all of the membrane dissolution controlled systems is that the dissolution of the membrane is the rate limiting step. Dissolution of the drug in the core is assumed to be rapid in comparison to the membrane, so once the membrane dissolves, the drug is released.

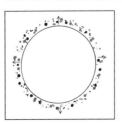

The dissolution process occurs as the membrane dissolves at the interface of the membrane material and the aqueous environment within the site of administration. The dissolved membrane molecules diffuse through an unstirred or static layer of aqueous solution that forms at the interface. The dissolution process is described by the Noyes-Whitney equation:

$$\frac{dc}{dt} = KS(C_s - C)$$

where

$\dfrac{dc}{dt}$ = dissolution rate of the membrane

K = dissolution rate constant of the membrane material in the aqueous medium

S = total membrane surface area

C_s = solubility of the membrane material in the aqueous medium

C = concentration of membrane material in the aqueous medium

The dissolution rate constant is a composite constant of the diffusion coefficient of the membrane material in the unstirred layer and the thickness of the unstirred layer. Using this expression to predict the rate of membrane dissolution, it can be seen that a constant dissolution rate will be maintained if the surface area, diffusion coefficient, unstirred layer thickness, and concentration difference ($C_s - C$) remain constant. As dissolution proceeds, however, the surface area available for dissolution certainly does change and the other variables may change as well. Therefore, these types of delivery systems are expected to produce extended release through a slow first order release rate.

Many coating materials have been used in the various delivery products. The most commonly used coating materials include gelatin, carnauba wax, pharmaceutical shellac, methylcellulose, cellulose acetate phthalate, beeswax, and polyvinyl acetate. The membrane coating can be applied to the surface of the drug cores in a number of ways. Pan coating and fluid bed coating are two that are commonly used.

A useful technique for applying polymeric membranes to small particles is *microencapsulation*. The process first was widely used to make "carbonless" reproduction paper. Dyes in small gelatin microcapsules were released under the pressure of a typewriter key or pen.

Microencapsulation can be accomplished using a variety of techniques including the following:

1. *Coacervation:* utilizes the interaction between two oppositely charged polyelectrolytes to form the membrane around the particles.

2. *Interfacial polymerization:* disperses an organic phase containing the drug particles into an aqueous phase containing polymeric monomers; the monomers react at the organic:aqueous interface to form the membrane.

3. *Hot-melt techniques:* mechanically drop the particles into a melt at an elevated temperature and then cool it.

4. *Solvent evaporation:* disperses the drug and membrane material in an aqueous solution, which subsequently is evaporated.

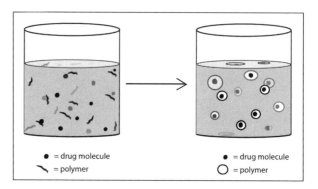

● = drug molecule   ● = drug molecule
↘ = polymer   ○ = polymer

The net outcome of each technique is that the membrane material encapsulates a small amount of drug in a micron-sized particle. The membrane thickness for most materials can be varied from approximately 1–200 microns by changing the amount of membrane material or the microencapsulation technique employed. A typical delivery system would be composed of about 67%–75% microencapsulated particles, and the remaining portion would be uncoated drug particles. This would provide a portion of the dose for immediate release, and then a sustaining reservoir from encapsulated particles.

Table 22.2 gives examples of membrane dissolution drug delivery products.

TABLE 22.2: EXAMPLES OF MEMBRANE DISSOLUTION DRUG DELIVERY PRODUCTS

Delivery System Name	Manufacturer	Examples
Spansules	Glaxo SmithKline	Dexedrine®
Sequels	Lederle	Diamox®

Matrix Dissolution

In the matrix dissolution delivery system, the drug is interspersed in a tablet, disk, or device (called a matrix) that undergoes slow dissolution. As the matrix dissolves and erodes, the drug is released. Layered tablets can be prepared with the inner core containing the drug in matrix material and the outer layer containing a portion of the dose that is not embedded in matrix material. Thus, the outer

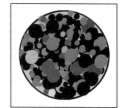

shell releases its portion of the dose immediately and the inner core serves as a reservoir to extend the drug release.

In another variation, the drug is dispersed in a series of different sized granules made of the matrix material. Different size granules will have different dissolution times, so a continuum of extended drug release can be achieved by using a variety of granule sizes in a single dosage form (e.g., a capsule). This spectrum of different sized granules will provide a more sustained drug blood concentration profile. These matrix granules often are combined with granules that have no matrix material, again providing a portion of the dose that is released immediately and a portion that serves as a reservoir.

Two general methods are used to prepare this type of delivery system:

1. *Congealing,* in which the drug (and necessary excipients) is mixed with the matrix material and congealed. The resulting material then is sieved to the desired size.

2. *Aqueous dispersion,* in which the materials are mixed and sprayed in or on water and the resulting particles are collected. Aqueous dispersion delivery systems typically have faster release rates than congealed systems because some water becomes entrapped in the particles, which aids in the dissolution of the matrix.

Matrix tablets are made by direct compression of the mixture of drug, matrix material, and excipients.

The underlying drug release mechanism in all of the matrix dissolution controlled systems can be described in the same manner as the membrane dissolution controlled systems. The dissolving component, however, is the matrix material, so the parameters of the Noyes-Whitney equation are applied to the physiochemical properties of the matrix material. The released drug or drug particle is assumed to dissolve at a faster rate than the matrix material and, therefore, will not be the rate limiting step.

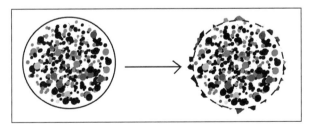

As the matrix material dissolves, the surface area of the matrix system will not remain constant. Therefore, these delivery systems are not expected to provide a constant zero order release rate. Rather, an extended release is expected to occur because of a slow first order release rate.

To overcome the problems of the changing surface area, several geometric shapes for delivery systems have been investigated. The goal has been to find a shape in which the surface area will increase (and thereby stay constant) as the matrix dissolves. Theoretically, such devices would give a more extended release because the release rate would approach a zero order process. Some of the shapes examined with various success are thin wafers, thin-walled cylinders, cylinders with wedge-shaped apertures, inward hemispheres, and matrices with nonuniform drug distribution. Table 22.3 gives examples of matrix dissolution drug delivery products.

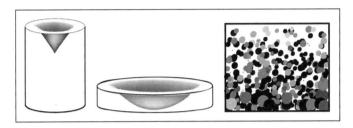

TABLE 22.3: EXAMPLES OF MATRIX DISSOLUTION DRUG DELIVERY PRODUCTS

Delivery System Name	Manufacturer	Examples
Extentab	Robins	Dimetapp®
Timespan	ICN	Mestinon®
Dospan	Aventis	Tenuate®
Chronotab	Schering-Plough	Disophrol®
Repetab	Schering-Plough	Polaramine®

Membrane Diffusion (Reservoir)

One characterization of reservoir devices is to have a core of drug (i.e., the reservoir) in an impervious shell on three sides, and an insoluble polymeric membrane that will allow the drug to diffuse through it. This characterization is termed a "slab" configuration. Because the membrane does not dissolve during the life of the delivery system, drug dissolution into and diffusion through the membrane are important steps. For membrane diffusion to be the rate limiting step, the drug dissolution process must be more rapid than the diffusion process. An additional formulation strategy is to ensure that more drug is in the core than is needed for the intended life of the system. Generally, an amount of drug that is twice the solubility concentration is used when employing this strategy.

Membrane diffusion controlled systems can provide zero order drug release, and the release can be modified by changing the physicochemical properties of the membrane material. The predominant drawback of many of

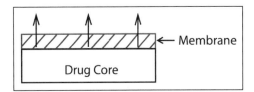

these systems is that they can be difficult to remove from inside the body if this becomes necessary. This is an important considera-tion with implantable systems that are intended to be ef-fective for months or years. With orally administered systems, a naive patient might be alarmed by the appear-ance of a drug depleted reservoir system in the stool.

Release of drug from a slab membrane diffusion controlled system can be described by Fick's first law of diffusion, which states that the amount of drug passing across a unit area is proportional to the concentration difference across the plane. The equation is:

$$J = -D\frac{dc}{dx}$$

where

J = flux or diffusion rate

D = diffusion coefficient of the drug in the membrane material

$\frac{dc}{dx}$ = rate of change in C relative to a distance x in the membrane

If the assumption is made that the drug on either side of the membrane is in equilibrium with its respective membrane surface, the concentration just inside the membrane surface can be related to the concentrations in the adjacent region by the following partitioning expressions:

$$PC = \frac{C_{m(0)}}{C_{(0)}} \text{ at } x = 0$$

$$PC = \frac{C_{m(h)}}{C_{(h)}} \text{ at } x = h$$

where

PC = partition coefficient of the drug in the mem-brane material

C_m = drug concentration at the inside surface of the membrane

C = drug concentra-tion at the out-side surface of the membrane adjacent to C_m

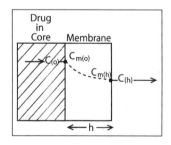

h = thickness of the membrane (i.e., the diffusional pathway length)

When x = 0, the drug has not begun to leave the reservoir and move through the membrane. Here the par-tition coefficient is between the reservoir and the material on the inner surface of the membrane. When x = h, the drug has passed from the reservoir, crossed the mem-brane, and is leaving the delivery system altogether. The partition coefficient is between the membrane material and the biological fluid outside of the delivery system.

Assuming that D and PC are constant, the equation for Fick's first law can be integrated and simplified to give:

$$J = \frac{DPC\Delta C}{h}$$

where

ΔC = concentration difference across the membrane

Since $C_{m(0)} \gg C_{m(h)}$ and is approximately equal to the saturation solubility of the drug in the membrane ma-terial (C_s), the equation can be written as:

$$J = \frac{DPC}{h} C_s$$

The geometry of any delivery system will influence the diffusion rate. The simplest system to consider is the rectangular slab, in which the drug is released from only one surface. With this geometry, the rate of drug release is:

$$\frac{dM_t}{dt} = \frac{DPCS}{h} C_s$$

where

M_t = mass of drug released (M) after time t

S = surface area of the membrane

Plots of the cumulative amount of drug re-leased from the delivery system versus time show a linear relationship.

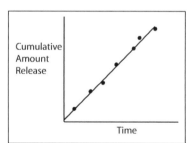

Table 22.4 shows drug release equations for more complex geometric-shaped delivery systems.

The equation predicts a constant *zero order release rate* if all the parameters on the right side of the equation remain constant. As seen with membrane dissolution

TABLE 22.4: DRUG RELEASE RATE EQUATIONS FOR MORE COMPLEX DELIVERY SYSTEMS

Geometry	Rate of Drug Release	Schematic Drawing	Parameters
Cylinder	$\frac{dM_t}{dt} = \frac{2\pi h DPC}{\ln(r_o / r_i)} C_s$		h = height of cylinder r_o = outside radius r_i = inside radius
Sphere	$\frac{dM_t}{dt} = \frac{4\pi r_o r_i DPC}{r_o = r_i} C_s$		

systems, these factors never truly remain constant. A common problem is that some membrane materials tend to swell when they are in contact with biological fluids. This swelling behavior changes the membrane diffusion coefficient, surface area, thickness, and solubility properties. For example, the increased membrane thickness will increase the length of the *diffusional pathway*. The summation of these changes results in delivery systems that typically approximate first order drug release.

Equations have been developed to predict these first order release profiles. For the geometry of a rectangular slab with diffusion through only one side, such an equation is

$$\frac{dM_t}{dt} = \frac{DPCSC_o}{h} \; e^{-\frac{DPCS}{V_1 h} t}$$

where

C_o = initial concentration of drug in device

V_1 = volume of "drug containing material" (i.e., volume of the drug core)

Similar first order equations have been developed for the deliveries shown in Table 22.4 Additional equations have been developed for all geometries if the membrane material is porous—i.e., has openings between 200 and 500 Å (1 angstrom = 1.0×10^{-10} meters).

The magnitude of the partition coefficient can be useful in predicting if the delivery system will be effective. The coefficient represents the concentration of drug in the membrane relative to that in the core. So if PC is greater than 1, this indicates that the core will be depleted of drug rapidly, and thus the system will be ineffective as a constant release delivery system. If PC is less than 1, the drug will tend to stay in the core and only enter the membrane slowly, which would be the desired outcome for an effective delivery system. The formulation strategy of having two times the solubility concentration of the drug in the core also ensures that PC will be less than 1.

Membrane diffusion systems also exhibit *lag times* and *burst effects*. Lag time depends on how much time has elapsed between manufacture and use. If the system is used relatively soon after construction, there may be a lag time before the drug release rate stabilizes. This is because little or no drug is in the membrane itself; and the lag time is when the drug is diffusing across and saturating the membrane.

Burst effects occur if a large initial release rate is seen before the release rate stabilizes. This means that the delivery system has been stored for some time and the drug has had time to diffuse across and saturate the membrane. Once the drug's diffusion is controlled by the membrane, the accelerated release rate will subside.

Membrane diffusion delivery systems usually are made by two processes, depending on the size of the drug containing unit. If particles are to be coated, microencapsulation techniques are used. If a larger unit such as a tablet is being coated, a tableting machine capable of placing a membrane around a drug core is used. Membrane materials that have been used include gelatin, methylcellulose, ethylcellulose, hydroxypropyl cellulose, polyhydroxymethacrylate, polyvinyl acetate, and various waxes such as carnauba wax. Often these are used in combinations to achieve the desired membrane properties —thickness, hardness, permeability, and so on. Table 22.5 gives examples of membrane diffusion drug delivery products.

TABLE 22.5: EXAMPLES OF MEMBRANE DIFFUSION DRUG DELIVERY PRODUCTS

Product Name	Manufacturer	Active Ingredient
Ocusert Pilo – 20®	Alza	Pilocarpine
Progestasert®	Alza	Progesterone
Transderm – Nitro®	Novartis	Nitroglycerin
Transderm – Scop®	Novartis	Scopolamine
Catapres – TTS®	Boehringer Ingelheim	Clonidine
Estraderm®	Novartis	Estradiol

Matrix Diffusion (Monolithic)

In the matrix diffusion, or monolithic, delivery system, the drug is dispersed homogenously throughout a matrix and the diffusion of the drug through the matrix to the outside is the rate limiting step. The matrix does not dissolve or erode during the intended life of the system. When the system is expended of drug, the matrix device will be excreted with the feces (if orally administered) or will have to be removed from the patient. Most of these systems do not produce a constant zero order release rate, but they can produce very slow release rates that in many applications are indistinguishable from zero order.

In the matrix, the drug adjacent to the biological fluid dissolves first and diffuses out of the matrix. The fluid then penetrates into the vacated space in the matrix and dissolves more drug, which diffuses out. The process continues until all of the drug is expended from the system. For the system to be matrix diffusion controlled, the rate of drug dissolution within the matrix must be faster than the diffusion rate of dissolved drug leaving the matrix. As the drug leaves the matrix, a *depletion*

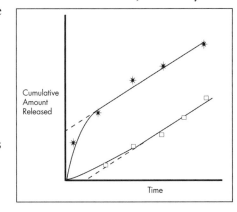

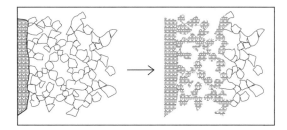

zone forms and increases with time. This zone adds to the length of the diffusional pathway that the drug must traverse to reach the outside of the system.

Deriving a mathematical model to describe such a system with an ever increasing depletion zone involves the following assumptions:

• The total amount of drug present in the matrix exceeds the saturation solubility of the drug in the matrix material.

• The biological fluid exhibits sink conditions at all times.

• The diameter of the drug particles is smaller than the length of the diffusional pathway.

• The diffusion coefficient of the drug in the matrix material remains constant.

• The matrix material and the drug have no interaction.

The following equation is based on the release of drug from a rectangular slab with the release occurring at only one surface.

$$\frac{dM}{dh} = C_o - C_s/2$$

where

    dM = change in the amount of drug released per unit area

    dh = change in the thickness of the depletion zone

    C_o = total amount of drug in a unit volume of the matrix

    C_s = solubility of the drug in a unit volume of the matrix

Using the equation that describes membrane diffusion from a rectangular slab and letting $D_m = DKS$:

$$dM = \frac{D_m C_s}{h} dt$$

If the two equations above are equated, solved for h, and that value of h is substituted back into the integrated form of the equation above, an equation for M (the amount of drug per unit area) can be derived.

$$M = [D_m C_s(2C_o - C_s)t]^{1/2}$$

When the amount of drug in the system exceeds the saturation concentration (i.e., $C_o \gg C_s$), this equation can be simplified to:

$$M = (2D_m C_s C_o t)^{1/2}$$

which indicates that the amount of drug released from the system will be a function of the square root of time. If a plot is constructed of the cumulative amount of drug release from a system versus (time)$^{1/2}$, a straight line will result and the release rate can be determined from the slope of the line.

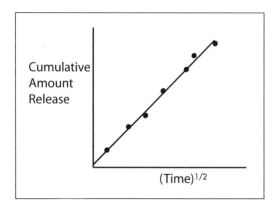

This drug release versus (time)$^{1/2}$ equation describes the release rate from a system in which the drug occupies 0%–5% of the volume of the matrix. Here it is thought that the volume of the vacated space in the depletion zone will not influence the overall release rate of the drug and that the release rate still will be governed by diffusion of the drug through the matrix material. As the drug volume increases (e.g., 15%–20%), porosity and tortuosity have to be considered because the increased volume of the vacated space (porosity) will impact the diffusional pathway length of the drug (tortuosity). The larger vacated space also allows more biological fluid to penetrate farther into the system and the release rate of the drug becomes controlled by diffusion through the fluid-filled vacated space, not through the matrix material.

An equation to describe the drug release from such a "porous" system is:

$$M = [D_s C_a \tfrac{\epsilon}{T} 2C_o - \epsilon C_a)t]^{1/2}$$

where

    ϵ = porosity of the matrix material

    T = tortuosity in the matrix material

    C_a = solubility of the drug in the biological fluid

    D_s = constant equal to the diffusion coefficient of the drug through the biological fluid, the partition coefficient of the drug between the matrix material and the biological fluid, and the volume of the biological fluid

Note that D_s and C_a represent factors that pertain to the interaction of the drug and the biological fluid, and not the matrix material.

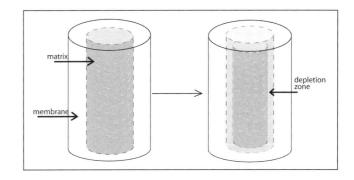

The most common method of preparing matrix diffusion tablets is to mix the drug with the matrix material and then compress the mixture. With waxy materials, the wax first is melted and the drug then is added. The mixture is allowed to congeal, and it then is granulated, sized, and compressed. If an immediate release portion of the dose is necessary, it generally is incorporated into a coating that is placed on the matrix.

Three types of materials are commonly used in matrix diffusion delivery systems:

1. Plastic matrices are made from methyl acrylate—methyl methacrylate copolymers, polyvinyl chloride, and polyethylene; the Gradumet® tablet (Abbott Laboratories) is the primary example of this type of matrix material.

2. Many of the celluloses (methylcellulose, hydroxypropylmethyl cellulose, carboxymethylcellulose), as well as Carbopol 934 also have been used.

3. Carnauba wax and glyceryl tristearate are examples of waxy substances that have been investigated as suitable matrix materials.

Table 22.6 gives examples of matrix diffusion drug delivery products.

TABLE 22.6: EXAMPLES OF MATRIX DIFFUSION DRUG DELIVERY PRODUCTS

Product Name	Manufacturer	Active Ingredient
Desoxyn® Gradumet®	Abbott	Methamphetamine hydrochloride
Fero-Gradumet®	Abbott	Ferrous sulfate
PBZ-SR®	Novartis	Tripelennamine hydrochloride
Procanbid®	Monarch	Procainamide hydrochloride
Nitro-dur®	Key	Nitroglycerin
Deponit®	Schwarz Pharma	Nitroglycerin
Estring®	Pharmacia & Upjohn	Estradiol

Membrane–Matrix Hybrids

It should not be surprising that some delivery systems are combinations of membrane and matrix systems. One variation is a matrix diffusion drug core encased with a non-eroding membrane that has a lower permeability to the drug. When the drug first begins to be released (i.e., when the depletion zone is small), the rate of release is influenced predominantly by diffusion through the encasing membrane. As the depletion zone becomes larger, the length of the diffusional pathway through the increasing depletion zone will have the predominant influence on release. Such a delivery system slows and extends drug release further than could be accomplished with the

matrix diffusion system alone. In some cases, the release rate approximates zero order.

Another type of hybrid system is a matrix diffusion core in which the matrix both erodes and dissolves. The complexity of this system arises from the fact that the diffusional pathway length is changing radically during the drug release process. A zero order release can occur only if the material erosion does not change the surface area. This is best accomplished by using flat slabs in which diffusion and erosion occur on only one surface. The inherent advantage of such a system is that the matrix is removed endogenously through dissolution and does not have to be removed physically. Some examples of membrane–matrix hybrid products are given in Table 22.7.

TABLE 22.7: EXAMPLES OF MEMBRANE-MATRIX DRUG DELIVERY PRODUCTS

Product Name	Manufacturer	Active Ingredient
Mirena®	Berlex	Levonorgestrel
NuvaRing®	Organon	Etonogestrel, ethinyl estradiol

A third type of hybrid system places the drug in a matrix material that swells when hydrated. When the system comes in contact with biological fluids, the material begins to hydrate and a gel forms around the surface of the system. As fluid permeates farther into the matrix, the gel layer becomes thicker. When the gel layer becomes fully hydrated, the outer surface of the layer begins to erode. The drug release rate is controlled by a series of steps. The biological fluid must enter the swollen matrix, move through the gel, move through the unhydrated matrix material, and then dissolve the drug. In turn, the drug must diffuse back through the same series of barriers. Valrelease® (Roche) is a matrix tablet with a resulting bulk density less than one, so it is buoyant in the gastric fluid. This provides a novel mechanism for extending the residence time of the drug in the gastrointestinal tract.

In these systems, the release rate is highly dependent on the material swelling rate, drug solubility, and fraction of the drug that is soluble in the material. These systems usually minimize burst effects because the matrix material must swell before the drug is released. Requirements of a suitable matrix material are that:

- the material must hydrate and form the gel layer rapidly enough to establish control over the penetrating rate of the biological fluids;
- the viscosity of the gel layer must be such that the drug can diffuse through it at a useful rate; and
- the material must have some aqueous solubility so it will erode.

The most commonly used matrix materials that meet these criteria are the hydrophilic cellulose polymers such as hydroxypropylmethyl cellulose.

As drug release proceeds, the surface area of this system and the thickness of the diffusion layer will not remain constant. The gel layer does not form all at one time but, instead, achieves its steady state thickness some time after drug release has started. The surface area of the device also will change with time as the gel layer continues to erode and the biological fluid penetrates farther. Therefore, these delivery systems are not expected to provide a constant zero order release rate. Rather, an extended release is expected to occur as a result of a slow first order release rate.

Microreservoirs are systems that have drug crystals suspended in solution that are inside of a water permeable membrane. These microreservoirs are interspersed in a matrix that may or may not have an outer encasing membrane. The biological fluid penetrates the outer membrane (if present), through the matrix material and through the water permeable membrane before it can dissolve the suspended drug crystals. The dissolved drug then diffuses back through the same barriers. The transdermal delivery device Nitro-Disc uses this technology in its *Microseal Drug Delivery System®*, in which nitro-

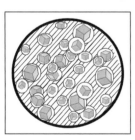

glycerin and lactose are suspended in a 40% polyethylene glycol 400 solution and the solution is dispersed in a mixture of isopropyl palmitate (a dispersing agent) and silicone elastomer. The resulting dispersion then is molded into the transdermal patch device.

Research continues to produce an array of novel hybrid delivery systems. For example, one experimental system has been shown to be sensitive to the amount of a marker compound in the vicinity of the delivery system. The outer hydrogel membrane contained urease in cross-linked bovine serum albumin. The inner drug matrix contained hydrocortisone (the acid drug) in an n-hexyl half ester of methyl vinyl ether:maleic anhydride copolymer. Urea was the marker compound that surrounded the delivery system. As the urea concentration was

increased, the rate of hydrocortisone release also was increased. The urea penetrated into the outer hydrogel membrane and was converted enzymatically to NH_4HCO_3 and NH_4OH, which increased the pH in the membrane. The inner drug matrix dissolution was sensitive to changes in pH, so as the pH increased, the dissolution of the matrix also increased with the subsequent release of more hydrocortisone.[1]

Osmotic Pressure

In these systems, osmotic pressure provides the driving force for drug release. In one type of osmotic drug delivery system (OROS® system), a core made up of the active drug and an "osmotically active" agent (e.g., KCl) is surrounded by a semipermeable membrane having a single laser-drilled hole.

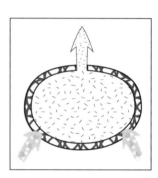

When the system is administered, biological fluid penetrates the semipermeable membrane into the core and dissolves or suspends the drug in solution. Because the membrane is not permeable to the drug, as the osmotic pressure increases inside, the system begins to force the drug solution through the delivery orifice. The rate of fluid influx and the delivery of drug solution depends on the osmotic gradient between the contents of the core and the biological fluid. Drug delivery is essentially constant as long as this gradient remains constant. Excess drug is placed in the core to ensure that the constant delivery rate will extend through the intended life of the system.

The system operates essentially independent of the administration environment. Oral osmotic systems are not affected by gastrointestinal acidity, feeding conditions, or gastrointestinal motility. The drug release rate may be altered by changing the size of the system, the thickness or composition of the semipermeable membrane, or the diameter of the drug delivery orifice. Materials that have been used as the semipermeable membrane include polyvinyl alcohol, polyurethane, cellulose acetate, ethylcellulose, and polyvinyl chloride.

The drug release rate can be determined from the following derivation:

$$\frac{dV}{dt} = \left(\frac{kS}{h}\right)(\Delta\pi = \Delta P)$$

where

$\frac{dV}{dt}$ = volume flow rate of biological fluid into the system

k = membrane permeability

S = membrane surface area

h = membrane thickness

$\Delta\pi$ = osmotic pressure difference between the core and the biological fluid

ΔP = hydrostatic pressure difference

If the delivery orifice is of sufficient size, the hydrostatic pressure difference will be small compared to the osmotic pressure difference, and the equation simplifies to:

$$\frac{dV}{dt} = \left(\frac{kS}{h}\right)\Delta\pi$$

Thus, the volume flow rate of biological fluid into the system is determined predominantly by the permeability, surface area, and thickness of the membrane. Because the volume imbibed into the system will equal the volume leaving the system, the ~~delivery~~ rate $\frac{dM_t}{dt}$ will be the product of the volume flow rate multiplied by the drug concentration C_s.

$$\frac{dM_t}{dt} = \frac{dV}{dt}\, C_s$$

Several types of osmotic delivery systems have been developed. The systems are categorized into two groups: *elemental osmotic pumps* and *miniosmotic pumps*. The elemental pumps have no movable partitions inside the system; i.e., the drug and osmotic agent are in the same reservoir (OROS system). Mini pumps have two compartments—one for the drug reservoir and another for the osmotic agent, with a movable partition between them. The movable partition may be a non-collapsible membrane that crosses some portion of the system, or it may be a collapsible sac that is compressed as the osmotic pressure increases. This illustration shows a mini pump osmotic system (GITS® system). Table 22.8 gives some examples of products that are based on an osmotic delivery system.

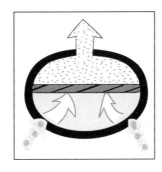

Both types of osmotic pump delivery systems have several variations. The COER® (Controlled Onset Extended Release) delivery system delays drug release

4 to 5 hours. A layer of erodible polymer is applied to the outer surface of the semipermeable membrane, which slowly erodes and delays the onset of drug release. The OROS-CT® (Colon Targeted) delivery system is a miniosmotic pump with an enteric coating. The system is designed especially to deliver the drug in the colon.

Ion Exchange

Ion exchange systems are advantageous when masking the unpleasant taste of a drug or if attempting to protect the drug from enzymatic degradation. Ion exchange resins are water insoluble, cross-linked polymers that have repeating salt-forming functional groups along their framework. The resins contain the active drug and release the drug as it is exchanged for ions present at the site of administration. The administration sites require a high concentration of endogenous ions, so oral, intramuscular, and subcutaneous administrations are typically used.

To prepare an ion exchange delivery system, the resin is loaded with drug by exposing the resin to the drug in a chromatographic column or in a solution. The drug will exchange for the resin salt ions and therefore will be retained on the resin framework. The resin then is dried and sized to form particles or beads that subsequently can be tableted, encapsulated, or suspended in solution. Resins are available with either cationic or anionic groups; the charge is selected to be opposite that of the drug. The exchange reactions that will load the resin might be depicted as follows:

$Resin$–$SO_3^-H^+$ + H_2N–$Drug$ →
      $Resin$–$SO_3^{-+}H_3N$–$Drug$ (basic drug)

$Resin$–$NH_3^+OH^-$ + $HOOC$–$Drug$ →
      $Resin$–$NH_3^{+-}OOC$–$Drug$ + H_2O (acidic drug)

When the delivery system is administered, the reverse type of reaction occurs. Ions that are resident at the site of administration will exchange for the drug, freeing it to diffuse out of the resin. This exchange reaction depends on the ionic environment (i.e., pH) and the resident ions present and their concentrations. With oral administration, the resident ions in the stomach are H^+ and Cl^- from HCl. In the intestine the ions are Na^+ and Cl^- from NaCl. The exchange reaction might be depicted as follows:

In the stomach:

$Resin$–$SO_3^{-+}H_3N$–$Drug$ + H^+ → $Resin$–$SO_3^-H^+$ + ^+H_3N–$Drug$

In the intestine:

$Resin$–$NH_3^{+-}OOC$–$Drug$ + Cl^- → $Resin$–$NH_3^+Cl^-$ + ^-OOC–$Drug$

TABLE 22.8: EXAMPLES OF OSMOTIC BASED DRUG DELIVERY PRODUCTS

Product Name	Manufacturer	Active Ingredient
Glucotrol XL®	Pfizer (GITS System)	Glipizide
Covera–HS®	Searle (COER System)	Verapamil hydrochloride
Procardia XL®	Pfizer (GITS System)	Nifedipine

Once released from the resin, the drug must diffuse out of the resin. This usually is the rate limiting step and is controlled by the area of diffusion, the porosity and length of the diffusional pathway inside the resin, and the extent of cross-linking in the resin (i.e., structural rigidity). Another factor influencing the drug release process is the amount of fluid contained inside the resin. Increasing the cross-linking of the resin will extrude fluid from inside the resin, which will limit the flow of ions toward the drug and the drug through and away from the resin.

A variation of the traditional ion exchange resin system is to apply a coating to the drug resin complex and place the beads in a matrix diffusion shell. An example of this technology is the *PennKinetic® system*. In this system, the drug resin complex is granulated into beads and coated with polyethylene glycol 4000 (PEG 4000). The PEG interpenetrates the resin and prevents it from swelling. These coated granules then are placed in a matrix diffusion system, so when the system is administered, biological fluid and ions must penetrate the matrix, diffuse through the PEG, enter the resin, and exchange

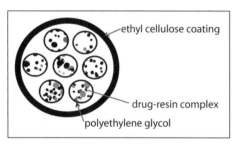

for the drug. Then the drug diffuses through the resin, the PEG, and the matrix material before being released from the system.

Another coating may be added on the matrix diffusion material to act as yet another barrier to drug release.

Resins used in these systems generally are copolymers of polystyrene. Polistirex is a divinyl benzene sulfonic acid–polystyrene copolymer that in used in the Penn-Kinetic system. The several drugs formulated in this delivery system include dextromethorphan (Delsym), chlorpheniramine, phentermine, and hydrocodone. Another copolymer, Polacrilex, is used in Nicorette gum. The gum contains buffers to maintain an increased pH and protect the stability of nicotine. A polystyrene–trimethylbenzyl ammonium chloride copolymer is the resin in cholestyramine (Questran) that is used in treating hypercholesterolemia.

Parenterals

Extended duration of action can be obtained in parenterally administered delivery systems. Modified release may be achieved in a number of ways, including the use of crystal or amorphous drug forms having prolonged dissolution characteristics, slowly dissolving chemical complexes of the drug, solutions or suspensions of the drug in slowly absorbed carriers or vehicles, increased particle size of the drug in suspension, or injection of slowly eroding microspheres of the drug.

The sites of administration used most commonly for modified release drug delivery systems are subcutaneous and intramuscular administration. When a delivery system is administrated in a liquid formulation, a "depot" or repository forms inside the tissue and serves as a drug reservoir. The rate of drug release from this depot depends on many factors such as the nature of the vehicle used, the physicochemical characteristics of the drug, the interaction between the drug and vehicle with the tissue, the depth of injection, and the local blood supply.

Release of a drug from an aqueous solution can be reduced by increasing the viscosity. The increased viscosity also localizes the injection volume. Thus, the absorptive area is reduced, which contributes to decreasing the rate of drug release. Examples of viscosity enhancing agents used in these systems are methylcellulose, sodium carboxymethylcellulose, and polyvinyl pyrrolidone.

Aqueous suspensions often are used as parenteral delivery systems because dissolution is the predominant rate limiting parameter. One common approach to decrease the dissolution rate is to increase the particle size of the drug. Another approach is to increase the viscosity of the suspension. Probably the most common strategy used to decrease the dissolution rate is to decrease the solubility of the drug. This is accomplished by using a less soluble salt form or polymorphic crystal form of the drug.

Table 22.9 gives examples of modified release aqueous suspensions.

TABLE 22.9: EXAMPLES OF AQUEOUS SUSPENSIONS WITH MODIFIED RELEASE

Product Name	Manufacturer	Active Ingredient
Crysticillin AS®	Apothecon	Penicillin G procaine
Wycillin®	Wyeth-Ayerst	Penicillin G procaine
Depo-Provera®	Pharmacia & Upjohn	Medroxyprogesterone acetate
Depo-Medrol®	Pharmacia & Upjohn	Methylprednisolone acetate
Aristospan®	Fujisawa	Triamcinolone hexacetonide
Celestone Soluspan®	Schering	Betamethasone sodium phosphate, betamethasone acetate
Semilente Iletin I®	Eli Lilly	Insulin
Lente Iletin I®	Eli Lilly	Insulin
Ultralente Iletin I®	Eli Lilly	Insulin

When oil solutions are used to reduce the release rate of the drug, the rate determining step is the partitioning of the drug out of the oil and into the surrounding biological fluid. Some oils that have been used for intramuscular injection are sesame, olive, maize, cottonseed, and castor oil. If the drug is suspended in an oil, the drug first must dissolve in the oil phase and then partition into the surrounding fluid. As expected, the duration of action obtained from oil suspensions is longer than from oil solutions.

Some drug products suspended in oil to achieve modified release are given in Table 22.10.

TABLE 22.10: EXAMPLES OF OLEAGINOUS SUSPENSIONS WITH MODIFIED RELEASE

Product Name	Manufacturer	Active Ingredient
Prolixin Decanoate®	Apothecon	Fluphenazine decanoate in sesame oil
Deca-Durabolin®	Organon	Nandrolone decanoate in sesame oil
Depo-Testosterone®	Pharmacia & Upjohn	Testosterone cypionate in cottonseed oil
Solganal®	Schering	Aurothioglucose in sesame oil

Both w/o and o/w emulsions have been used to modify drug release after parenteral administration. Four types of delivery systems are possible depending on the combinations of emulsion types and where the drug is predominantly located in the emulsion (i.e., in the oil phase or in the aqueous phase). If the drug is in the internal phase of the w/o emulsion, the partition behavior between the internal and external phases and the partitioning out of the oil phase will influence the release of the drug. A w/o emulsion delivery system does not offer an advantage over an oil solution system if the drug is in the external phase. One additional variation is to suspend the drug in the internal phase, where its release then will depend on dissolution of the drug in the aqueous internal phase, partitioning into the oleaginous external phase, and then partitioning out of the emulsion. Analogous situations exist for o/w emulsions.

With each of the formulations mentioned above (i.e., solutions, suspensions, emulsions) the drug also may be complexed with some other component (e.g., a macromolecule) to further modify the release rate. Macromolecules used as complexing agents in parenteral delivery systems include biological agents such as antibiotics and proteins, or synthetic polymers such as methylcellulose, sodium carboxymethylcellulose, or polyvinyl pyrrolidone. Complexes also can be formed between drugs and small molecules (e.g., caffeine). In this case, the entire complex undergoes absorption, so the physicochemical properties of the complex are what affect the release rate.

Liposomes

Liposomes typically are made by dispersing phospholipids in aqueous media. The phospholipids hydrate, swell and spontaneously form multilamellar (many layers), concentric bilayer vesicles with aqueous media between the lipid bilayers. These systems, commonly referred to as multilamellar vesicles (MLVs), have diameters in the range of 0.5–5 microns. When MLVs are sonicated or diluted, they will produce small unilamellar

(i.e., one layer) vesicles (SUVs) with diameters in the range of 0.02–0.1 microns that have an aqueous media core.

The phospholipids used in making liposomes are amphiphilic—having both a hydrophilic part and a hydrophobic part. The hydrophobic portion is composed of fatty acids containing 10 to 24 carbon atoms. The hydrophilic portion may contain phosphoric acid or lecithin. Because of their unique structure, liposomes can be used as a delivery system for both hydrophilic and hydrophobic compounds. Hydrophilic compounds reside in the aqueous portion of the vesicles, and the hydrophobic compounds remain in the lipid portion. The drug is incorporated into the liposome by making an aqueous solution of the drug and then mixing in the other liposomal ingredients.

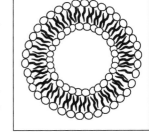

The physical characteristics and stability of liposomes depend on pH, ionic strength, the presence of divalent cations, and the nature of the phospholipids used. In general, these vesicle systems have low permeability to ionic and polar substances, but this varies greatly with the liposome composition. Positively charged phospholipids, however, tend to be impermeable to cations, and negatively charged liposomes are permeable to cations. Positively and negatively charged liposomes are both readily permeable by anions. An increase in temperature will alter the liposomal permeability markedly by causing the lipids to undergo a phase transition to a less ordered, more fluid configuration. Also, the liposomal permeability can be changed by some proteins (e.g., cytochrome-C, serum high density lipoproteins) that penetrate the vesicles. Cholesterol commonly is added to most liposome formulations to prevent this protein penetration by forming a more closely packed bilayer system.

The liposomal entrapment efficiency of drugs varies among the different types of liposomes. MLVs have modest efficiency in trapping drugs, whereas SUVs have limited efficiency. But SUVs tend to be more homogenous in size and more consistent in producing the desired size than MLVs. In reaching a compromise between size and entrapment efficiency, large unilamellar vesicles (LUVs) have been developed. LUVs seem to be three to four times more efficient than SUVs in trapping water soluble drugs, but they tend to be less stable.

As mentioned, hydrophilic drugs are trapped in the aqueous portion and lipophilic drugs are found in the lipid portion of the liposome. Hydrophilic drugs will be released only when the bilayer structure is disrupted or when the drug can diffuse out of the system. Lipophilic drugs will be released only when the bilayer structure is disrupted. Usually liposomes cannot release their drug component without interacting with cells. These cellular interactions can occur in several ways, and more than one may be occurring in any given interaction.

- Endocytosis by phagocytic cells such as macrophages and neutrophils: The entire content of the liposome is made available to the cell.

- Adsorption to the cell surface: The drug must diffuse through the lipids of the liposome and the cell membrane.

- Fusion with the plasma cell membrane: The lipid portion of the vesicle becomes part of the cell membrane.

- Liposomal lipid exchange to cellular or subcellular membranes.

Liposomes are administered intravenously and may remain in the body for hours or days, depending on their physical composition, size, and surface charge. Typical half lives range from minutes to several hours. The larger liposomes (MLVs and LUVs) are taken up by the reticuloendothelial system (RES), predominately in the liver and spleen. Though the SUVs have a broader tissue distribution, they, too, are taken up by the RES organs. The uptake effectively removes liposomes from the systemic circulation but provides an opportunity to target the delivery system for organs such as the liver, spleen, bone marrow, and lymphoid organs.

Several strategies have been employed to limit the RES uptake of liposomes.

1. The use of antibodies bound to the liposome. The antibody directs the liposome system to a specific antigenic receptor on a specific cell type surface.

2. The use of carbohydrate determinants that are glycoprotein or glycolipid cell surface components involved in cell-to-cell recognition, interaction, or adhesion.

3. The making of "stealth" liposomes; these polyethylene glycol coated liposomes are not taken up by the RES organs and have a systemic circulation time of up to 55 hours.

Advantages of these systems include the ability to deliver hydrophilic and hydrophobic drugs, to target the delivery, and to alter the delivery by changing the physical composition, size, and surface charge of the liposome. Liposomes with extended circulation times (stealth liposomes) can deliver drugs that normally are degraded rapidly. Liposomes have inherent disadvantages in the areas of stability and uniformity of size production. Some examples of products based on liposome technology are given in Table 22.11.

TABLE 22.11: EXAMPLE OF MODIFIED RELEASE PRODUCTS BASED ON LIPOSOME TECHNOLOGY

Product Name	Manufacturer	Active Ingredient
Abelcet Injection®	Elan	Amphotericin B
Amphotec®	Intermune	Amphotericin B cholesteryl sulfate
DaunoXome®	Gilead Sciences	Daunorubicin citrate
Doxil®	Alza	Doxorubicin hydrochloride

NOTES

1. Concepts and System Design (chapter 1) in *Novel Drug Delivery Systems*, 2nd edition, edited by Chien, Y. W. Volume 50: Drugs and the Pharmaceutical Sciences. Marcel Dekker, New York, NY, 1992, pp. 1–42.

ADDITIONAL READING

Fundamentals of Rate-Controlled Drug Delivery (chapter 2) in *Novel Drug Delivery Systems*, 2nd edition, edited by Y. W. Chien, Volume 50: Drugs and the Pharmaceutical Sciences. Marcel Dekker, New York, NY, 1992, pp. 43–137.

Jantzen, G. M., and Robinson, J. B. Sustained- and Controlled-Release Drug Delivery Systems (chapter 15) in *Modern Pharmaceutics*, 4th edition, edited by G. S. Banker and C. T. Rhodes, Volume 121: *Drugs and the Pharmaceutical Sciences*. Marcel Dekker, New York, NY, 2002, pp. 501–528.

Compounded Modified Release Formulations

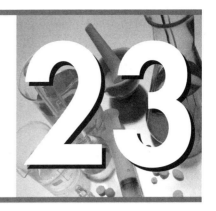

MANY TYPES OF MANUFACTURED PRODUCTS HAVE modified release delivery systems. With *extemporaneously* compounded preparations, only capsules and suppositories use such strategies. The development of modified release compounded formulations has been slow because few prescriptions call for such preparations, and the published research is limited.

Modified Release Capsules

The release rate of an active drug from a capsule depends on the drug itself and the other excipients inside the capsule. When capsules are placed in aqueous environments, water dissolves the capsule shell and begins to penetrate the capsule's contents. If this penetration is rapid, the release rate of the drug is enhanced. If the penetration is slow, the release rate is retarded.

Rapid Release

The two methods to increase the release rate of a drug from a capsule are to

1. use hydrophilic excipients, and
2. pierce holes in the capsule.

As water enters the capsule's contents, hydrophilic excipients will quickly dissolve, freeing the drug contained within the capsule contents. Adding a small quantity of sodium bicarbonate and citric acid to the excipient mixture will produce carbon dioxide, which also will help the capsule to open sooner. Adding sodium lauryl sulfate allows water to penetrate the capsule faster and speeds dissolution. If an extremely rapid release is desired, piercing holes in the capsule with a straight pen will allow even faster penetration of the gastrointestinal fluids into the capsule.

Slow Release

Modified release capsules also can be prepared using hydroxypropylmethyl cellulose products (Methocel® A, E, F, and K).[1,2] Hydroxypropylmethyl cellulose is a cellulose derivative that is used as a hydrophilic matrix material. When hydroxypropylmethyl cellulose hydrates, it forms a gel of such consistency that drug diffusion through the gel can be controlled. A *hydrophilic matrix modified release system* is a dynamic system in which polymer wetting, polymer hydration, and polymer dissolution all occur simultaneously. At the same time, other soluble excipients or drugs will also wet, dissolve, and diffuse out of the matrix and insoluble materials will be held in place until the surrounding polymer erodes or dissolves.

Initially the surface becomes wet and the hydroxypropylmethyl cellulose starts to partially hydrate, forming a gel layer on the surface of the capsule. As water continues to permeate the capsule, the gel layer becomes thicker, and soluble drug begins to diffuse out through the gel layer. Ultimately, water will dissolve the capsule shell and continue to penetrate the drug core. Therefore, release is controlled by dissolution of soluble drug into the penetrating water and diffusion across the gel layer. A successful hydrophilic matrix modified release system will wet and hydrate to form a gel layer fast enough to protect the interior of the capsule from dissolving and disintegrating during the initial wetting and hydration phase. If the polymer is too slow to hydrate, gastric fluids may penetrate to the capsule core, dissolve the drug substance, and allow the drug to diffuse out prematurely.

Among the hydroxypropylmethyl cellulose products, the rate at which the polymers hydrate differs significantly. This is because of the varying proportions of the two chemical substituents attached to the cellulose backbone: hydroxypropoxyl and methoxyl substitution. The methoxyl substituent is a relatively hydrophobic component and does not contribute as much to the hydrophilic nature of the polymer and the rate at which it will hydrate. The hydroxypropoxyl group does contribute greatly to the rate of polymer hydration. As a result, Methocel K products are the fastest to hydrate (see Table 23.1) because they have the lower amount of the hydrophobic methoxyl substitution and a higher amount of the hydrophilic hydroxypropoxyl substitution.

Increasing the concentration of the polymer in a matrix system increases the viscosity of the gel that forms on the capsule surface. Therefore, an increase in the concentration of the polymer used will generally decrease the drug diffusion and drug release. The

TABLE 23.1: PERCENTAGE OF CHEMICAL SUBSTITUTION IN METHOCEL PRODUCTS

Product	% Methoxyl	% Hydroxypropoxyl	Relative Rate of Hydration
Methocel A	27.5–31.5	0	Slowest
Methocel E	28–30	7–12	Next Fastest
Methocel F	27–30	4–7.5	Slow
Methocel K	19–24	7–12	Fastest

increase in the concentration of polymer also tends to accelerate gel formation since wetting is achieved more readily.

Sodium alginate also has been used as a gel forming excipient to slow drug release from capsules. This is a polysaccharide extracted from brown seaweeds using dilute alkali. It consists mainly of the sodium salt of alginic acid, which is a polyuronic acid. Sodium alginate is slowly soluble in water and forms a viscous colloidal solution that can be converted into a gel with the addition of divalent cations or by a reduction in pH.

Delayed Release

A delayed release capsule can be accomplished by coating the capsule with materials such as stearic acid, shellac, casein, cellulose acetate phthalate, and natural and synthetic waxes. These coating materials are acid insoluble but are soluble in alkaline environments. Applying these coating materials extemporaneously requires skill and additional equipment. Three methods of coating capsules have been described.[3]

Modified Release Suppositories

Modified release formulations have been developed for suppositories. Pluronic polyols retarded the release of riboflavin[4] and alginic acid has been indicated as another ingredient that can be used to slow the release rate from a suppository.[5] Given the success of using hydroxypropylmethyl cellulose in capsules, the same effect on the release rate would be expected in suppositories, although no data are available to support this strategy.

One report details a hollow-type suppository formulation being used to enhance the release of diazepam.[6] The release of diazepam from this suppository was faster than from conventional suppositories made with the same base or polyethylene glycols.

Demonstration of Modified Release from Capsules

Most pharmacists are not able to determine the rate of modified release from any compounded formulation because they lack the proper equipment. This demonstration

of data, however, is to show that such experiments are straightforward and can be carried out if the proper equipment is available.

℞

Salicylic Acid	4 mg
Methocel E4M	qs
Lactose	qs
Mft.	Modified Release Capsules

Methocel E4M is the hydrophilic matrix material in the formulation. To achieve a modified release, 40% of the capsule volume should be Methocel. The remaining 60% can be the active drug, or a combination of the active drug and lactose acting as a filler. Capsules made with 4 mg of salicylic acid and q.s. to 350 mg with lactose are used as a control. The total material content in the modified release capsules is to be 350 mg, so 40% of 350 mg or 140 mg will be Methocel E4M, salicylic acid will be 4 mg of the capsule contents, and lactose must be 206 mg. If Methocel E4M is not available, Methocel K100 (30%) can be used. The amounts of the remaining ingredients will have to be adjusted accordingly.

The procedure for measuring drug release is as follows:

1. Put 100 ml of 0.01N HCl in each of two 250 ml beakers.

2. Put one modified release capsule in one beaker, and one "control" capsule in the other beaker. Stagger the times of placement by about 5 minutes.

3. Begin stirring the solutions (at a modest speed) and continue to stir throughout the experiment. Ensure that the spinning rates are as equal as possible.

4. At selected time points, remove 3 ml of sample from the beaker and place in a cuvette. Replace the volume withdrawn with the equal volume of fresh 0.01N HCl. Replace the volume removed as quickly as possible (have fresh 0.01N HCl in a beaker). The samples do not have to be read immediately.

5. Try to take a sample every 15 minutes with a clean syringe. Taking the sample exactly every 15 minutes is not critical, but knowing when the sample was taken is critical (e.g., 16 minutes, 14.5 minutes). Be sure to record the time on the data sheet as soon as possible. Stagger the sampling times between the control capsule and the modified release capsule by approximately 5 minutes.

6. Read the absorbance at 310 nm using 0.01N HCl for a blank. From a Beer's Law plot, calculate the amount of drug released.

7. The data obtained dictate when to stop the experiment. In the sample control capsule data in Table 23.2 (experiment conducted in water), the repeated

TABLE 23.2: SAMPLE DATA OF SALICYLIC ACID RELEASE FROM CONVENTIONAL AND MODIFIED RELEASE CAPSULES

Conventional Capsule					Modified Release Capsule				
Clock Time	Run Time	Absorb.	Conc.	Amount Released	Clock Time	Run Time	Absorb.	Conc.	Amount Released
2:40	0	0.000	0.0	0.0	2:35	0	0.000	0.0	0.0
2:55	15	0.005	0.0010	0.10	2:50	15	0.012	0.0015	0.15
3:10	30	0.016	0.0017	0.17	3:05	30	0.031	0.0027	0.27
3:25	45	0.031	0.0027	0.27	3:20	45	0.059	0.0044	0.44
3:40	60	0.048	0.0037	0.37	3:35	60	0.089	0.0063	0.63
3:55	75	0.065	0.0048	0.48	3:50	75	0.123	0.0084	0.84
4:10	90	0.592	0.037	3.75	4:05	90	0.160	0.011	1.07
4:25	105	0.609	0.039	3.85	4:20	105	0.194	0.013	1.28
4:40	120	0.610	0.039	3.86	4:35	120	0.240	0.016	1.56
4:55	135	0.614	0.039	3.88	4:50	135	0.287	0.019	1.85
5:10	150	0.612	0.039	3.87	5:05	150	0.302	0.019	1.95

TABLE 23.3: DEMONSTRATION DATA OF SALICYLIC ACID RELEASE FROM CONVENTIONAL AND MODIFIED RELEASE CAPSULES INTO 0.01N HCl

Conventional Capsule					Modified Release Capsule				
Clock Time	Run Time	Absorb.	Conc.	Amount Released	Clock Time	Run Time	Absorb.	Conc.	Amount Released
2:20	0	0.000	0.0	0.0	2:15	0	0.000	0.0	0.0
2:35	15	0.301	0.014	1.38	2:30	15	0.030	0.00044	0.044
2:50	30	0.808	0.039	3.87	2:45	30	0.176	0.0076	0.76
3:05	45	0.815	0.039	3.90	3:00	45	0.368	0.017	1.71
3:20	60	0.822	0.039	3.94	3:15	60	0.516	0.024	2.48
3:35	75	0.800	0.038	3.83	3:30	75	0.637	0.030	3.03
3:50	90	0.800	0.038	3.83	3:45	90	0.740	0.035	3.54
4:05	105	0.804	0.039	3.85	4:00	105	0.814	0.039	3.90

absorbance value was around 0.600, indicating that all of the salicylic acid that was going to be released had been released. Therefore, the modified release capsule sampling would have to be continued until the absorbance reaches about 0.600. The data showed that after 2.5 hours, salicylic acid was still being released from the modified release capsule.

The demonstration data experiment was conducted in 0.01N HCl (as instructed), and the data are given in Table 23.3.

The *rate of release* is determined by plotting the Amount Released versus some function of time. For matrix diffusion controlled release, adaptations of the Higuchi equation are used; time is expressed as the square root of time and has units of minutes$^{1/2}$. A linear trend line is fit through the points that occur after a lag time or before any asymptotic values are reached.

The release of salicylic acid in 0.01N HCl is illustrated in Figure 23.1. The data show that the conventional

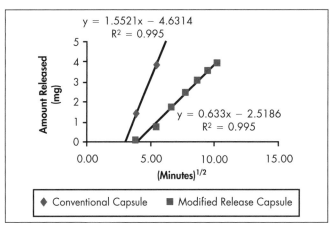

FIGURE 23.1 RELEASE OF SALICYLIC ACID INTO 0.01N HCl

capsule apparently released all of its contents by 30 minutes because after that time the amount released remained constant. The release rate of 1.55 mg/minutes$^{1/2}$ was almost three times as fast as seen with the modified release capsule. More important, the modified release capsule released the drug continuously for hours, whereas the conventional capsule released all the drug within 30 minutes.

NOTES

1. Timmons, E. D., and Timmons, S. P. Custom Compounded Micronized Hormones in a Slow Release Capsule Matrix. *International Journal of Pharmaceutical Compounding* 6:378–379, 2002.

2. Bogner, R. H., Szwejkowski, J., and Houston, A. Release of Morphine Sulfate from Compounded Slow Release Capsules: The Effect of Formulation on Release. *International Journal of Pharmaceutical Compounding* 5:401–405, 2001.

3. Allen, L. V., Jr. Capsules (chapter 10) in *The Art, Science, and Technology of Pharmaceutical Compounding*, 2nd edition. American Pharmaceutical Association, Washington, DC, 2002, p. 133–159.

4. Anderson, D., Amigi, M. M. Preparation and Evaluation of Sustained Drug Release from Pluronic Polyol Rectal Suppositories. *International Journal of Pharmaceutical Compounding* 5:234–237, 2001.

5. Allen, L. V., Jr. Morphine Sulfate Slow-Release Suppositories. *International Journal of Pharmaceutical Compounding* 1:32–33, 1997.

6. Kaewnopparat, N., Kaewnopparat, S., Rojanarat, W., and Ingkatawornwong, S. Enhanced Release of Diazepam from Hollow-Type Suppositories. *International Journal of Pharmaceutical Compounding* 8:310–312, 2004.

CHAPTER TWENTY-FOUR

Sterile Compounded Formulations: Routes of Administration

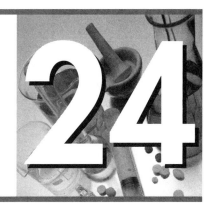

SOME ROUTES OF ADMINISTRATION DEMAND THAT products be free of microbial contamination as they enter the body. This is required because some routes of administration bypass the body's natural defense mechanisms, or some tissues or organs are so sensitive and vital that such contamination causes serious damage.

All of these "sterility demanding" routes are parenteral routes, but not all parenteral routes are sterility demanding. The term *parenteral* means "next to or beside the enteral." *Enteral* refers to the alimentary tract, so parenteral means sites that are outside of or beside the alimentary tract. The enteral routes of administration are oral, buccal, sublingual, and rectal, so any other route is considered a parenteral administration site. Topical administration is a parenteral route that does not require sterile formulations.

Parenteral routes of administration have the following advantages:

1. They are indicated when a drug is poorly absorbed following oral administration or is degraded by gastric acid or gastrointestinal enzymes.

2. They are preferred when a rapid and highly predictable drug response is desired, as in an emergency situation.

3. They are useful when a patient is uncooperative, unconscious, or unable to take the drug via an enteral route.

4. They are used when localized drug therapy is desired.

5. They provide a predictable and nearly complete bioavailability.

The major disadvantages are the following:

1. They are more expensive than enteral route formulations.

2. They require sterile formulations.

3. They require administration by a skilled or trained person.

4. The dose is difficult to remove after it has been administered.

Injection Dependent Routes of Administration

Several of the sterility demanding routes require that a needle (or catheter) and some type of propelling device (syringe, pump, gravity feed bag) be used to place the formulation in the desired anatomical site. These routes can be said to be *injection dependent* routes.

Injection dependent routes have several characteristics in common. The formulations that can be used with injectables are limited to solutions, suspensions, and emulsions. Also, many of the routes are limited in the volume of formulation that can be injected because excessive volumes will cause pain and cell necrosis.

Intravenous Route

Several sites on the body are used to administer drugs intravenously: the veins of the antecubital area (in front of the elbow), the back of the hand, and some of the larger veins in the foot. On some occasions a vein must be exposed by a surgical cut-down.

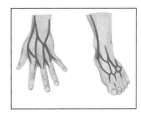 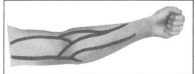

Intravenous administration provides the most rapid onset of action of any parenteral route because there is no barrier to absorption and the drug is completely available to the body. Drugs that are too irritating for intramuscular or subcutaneous administration (such as chemotherapy agents) can be given by this route. Many different types of catheters (indwelling soft tubes) or needles are used to administer intravenous formulations. Placement of these devices is crucial to avoid problems of extravasation or infiltration.

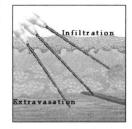

Among the several complications that can arise from intravenous administration are the following:

- *Thrombosis.* Thrombus formation can result from many factors: extremes in solution pH, particulate material, irritant properties of the drug, needle or catheter trauma, and selecting a vein that is too small for the volume of solution injected.

- *Phlebitis.* Phlebitis, or inflammation of the vein, can be caused by the same factors that cause thrombosis.

- *Air emboli.* Air emboli result from air introduced into the vein. Although the human body is not harmed by small amounts of air, a good practice is to purge all air bubbles from the formulation and administration sets before using them.

- *Particulate material.* Particulate material usually consists of small pieces of glass that chip from the formulation vial, or rubber that comes from the rubber closure on injection vials. Although great care is taken to eliminate particulate material, placing a final filter in the administration line just before it enters the venous system is a typical precaution.

The intravenous formulation that is administered most commonly is the solution. Solutions usually are aqueous but also may contain glycols, alcohols, or other non-aqueous solvents. Injectable suspensions are difficult to formulate because they must possess syringeability and injectability. *Syringeability* refers to the ease at which the suspension can be withdrawn from a container into a syringe. *Injectability* refers to the properties of the suspension while being injected such as evenness of flow and freedom from clogging. Intravenously administered *emulsions* are heterogeneous formulations that contain both aqueous and nonaqueous components. Fat emulsions and total parenteral nutrition (TPN) emulsions are used to provide triglycerides, fatty acids, and calories for patients who cannot absorb them through the gastrointestinal tract.

Intramuscular Route

The intramuscular route of administration is considered less hazardous and easier to use than the intravenous route. The onset of action typically is longer than with intravenous administration but shorter than with sub-cutaneous administration. More pain is associated with intramuscular administration than with intravenous administration.

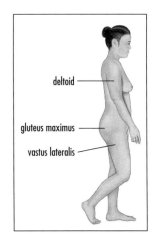

Intramuscular (IM) injections enter the striated muscle fibers under the subcutaneous layer of the skin. The needles used for these injections are 1 inch to 1.5 inches long and 19 to 22 gauge in size. The principal sites of injection are the gluteal (buttocks), deltoid (upper arm), and vastus lateralis (thigh) muscles.

When administering intramuscular injections into the gluteus maximus, the size of the needle must be considered carefully. If the needle length is too short to penetrate the muscle tissue, the injection will be made in the lipomatous (fatty) tissue. Women tend to have more fat in the gluteal region than men do, so longer needles should be used with female patients. Obese patients also require longer needles.

If a series of injections is to be given, the injection site is varied or rotated. Generally, only limited injection volumes can be administered by intramuscular injection: 2 ml in the deltoid and thigh muscles, and up to 5 ml in the gluteus maximus.

The site of injection should be as far as possible from major nerves and blood vessels, to avoid neural damage and accidental intravenous administration. To ensure that the needle has not entered a blood vessel, the syringe should be aspirated slightly after needle insertion and before injection to see if blood enters the syringe. Other injuries that can occur following intramuscular injection are abscesses, cysts, embolisms, hematomas, skin sloughing, and scar formation.

The Z-tract injection technique is useful for medications that stain upper tissue (e.g., iron dextran injection) or drugs that irritate tissues (e.g., diazepam). The skin is laterally displaced prior to injection, the needle is inserted, and the injection is performed. The needle then is withdrawn and the skin released. This creates a "Z" pattern that blocks infiltration of the drug into the subcutaneous tissue. These injections are generally 2 to 3 inches deep.

Intramuscular injections typically result in lower but more sustained blood concentrations than intravenous administration. This is partly because intramuscular injections require an absorption step that delays the time to peak concentrations. When a formulation is injected, a *depot* forms inside the muscle tissue, which acts as a repository for the drug. The absorption rate from this depot depends on many physiological factors such as muscle exercise, depth of injection, and local blood supply.

The absorption rate from the depot is influenced by many formulation factors:

- Aqueous solutions typically provide the fastest absorption possible from the depot.

- Oleaginous solutions provide slightly slower absorption than aqueous solutions. To further alter the absorption rate from oleaginous solutions, drugs are formulated as suspensions or colloids in aqueous and oleaginous solvents, or as oil-in-water (o/w) emulsions and water-in-oil (w/o) emulsions.

- Different salt forms of the drug may be used to take advantage of a slower dissolution rate or a lower solubility inherent with the salt.

- O/W emulsions are formulated such that large particles of the drug are contained in the oil phase. In this case, the drug dissolves slowly but also diffuses slowly out of the oil phase and still requires more time to diffuse through the water phase of the emulsion. Thus, three processes influence the absorption rate of this type of formulation.

Combinations of these factors can be used to achieve the desired absorption rate. For example, for a very slow absorption rate, a low solubility salt form could be placed as a suspension in an oleaginous solvent. Here the salt dissolves slowly because of its limited solubility and then diffuses slowly through the oleaginous solvent.

Intradermal Route

The *dermis* is the more vascular layer of the skin just beneath the epidermis. The usual site for intradermal injections is the anterior surface of the forearm. Needles are generally 3/8 inches long and 25 to 26 gauge. For this route of administration, 0.1 ml of solution is the maximum volume that can be administered.

Drugs that are injected intradermally are agents for diagnostic determinations, desensitization, or immunization. During injection, a *wheal* or raised blister-like area forms on the skin surface as the solution is injected. The drug will be absorbed from this depot into the dermis.

Subcutaneous Route

The subcutaneous (SC, SQ) route is one of the most versatile routes of administration in that it can be used for both short-term and long-term therapies. The drug is injected into or a device is implanted beneath the surface of the skin in the loose interstitial tissues of the upper arm, the anterior surface of the thigh, or the lower portion of the abdomen. The upper back also can be used as a site of subcutaneous administration.

The site of injection usually is rotated when injections are given frequently. The maximum volume of medication that can be injected subcutaneously is about 2 ml. Needles are generally 3/8 to 1 inch in length and 24 to 27 gauge.

Absorption of drugs from the subcutaneous tissue is influenced by the same factors that determine the rate of absorption from intramuscular sites: slowly soluble salt forms, suspensions versus solutions, differences in particle size, viscosity of the injection vehicle, and so forth. The vascularity in the subcutaneous tissue, however, is less than that of muscle tissue and, therefore, absorption may be slower than after intramuscular administration but

more rapid and predictable than after oral administration.

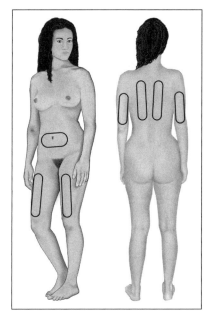

The absorption rate can be changed in the following ways:

- Applying heat or massaging the site increases the absorption rates of many drugs.
- Co-administration of vasodilators or hyaluronidase increases the absorption rates of some drugs.
- Administering epinephrine decreases blood flow, which can decrease the absorption rate.

Many different solution and suspension formulations are administered subcutaneously. Heparin, insulin, and enoxaparin are the most common drugs routinely administered by this route. Drugs that are administered by this route must be soluble and potent in small concentrations because only a small volume can be injected.

Despite the advantages of this route of administration, some precautions are in order:

- Drugs that are irritating and those in highly viscous (thick) suspensions may produce induration, sloughing, or abscess formation, and may be painful to the patient.
- Irritating drugs and vasoconstrictors can lead to abscesses or necrosis.
- If frequent injections are required, the injection sites must be rotated.

One of the most obvious ways to achieve very long-term drug release is to place the drug in a delivery system or device that can be *implanted* into a body tissue. The subcutaneous tissue is the ideal site for implanting these devices. Implantation often requires a surgical procedure or a specialized injection device. The fact that the device will be in constant contact with the subcutaneous tissue requires that the device materials be biocompatible and do not promote infection or sterile abscess. Another advantage is that the device can be removed easily if necessary.

Many devices are used in subcutaneous implantation. Some of the devices provide drug release for months or years. For example, Viadur™ DUROS® implants are made from a titanium alloy and are capable of delivering the drug for up to 1 year. Norplant II® systems are able to provide drug release for up to 5 years. Other devices include degradable microspheres, vapor pressure devices for morphine release, osmotic pressure devices to deliver insulin, and magnetically or ultrasonically activated pellets. Sometimes ports 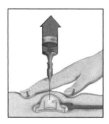 and pumps are placed in the subcutaneous space and a delivery catheter is placed in a vein, a cavity, or an artery.

Epidural Route

The brain and spinal cord are covered by three protective membranes called *meninges,* the outermost of which is the *dura mater*. The spinal cord is protected from injury as it goes down the back by passing through the central cavities of the vertebrae in the vertebral column. The *epidural space* is the space in the central cavities between the dura mater and the vertebral column.

Epidural administration is an effective means of controlling chronic pain. It is commonly used in the labor and delivery settings, as well as postoperative settings. The advantage of this route of administration is that effective drug dosages generally are much lower than dosages administered by other routes and typically produce fewer side effects. Studies have shown that epidural administration produces longer-lasting pain relief, more alert patients, and earlier ambulation.

When epidural administration will be temporary or short-term, a catheter is inserted into the epidural space 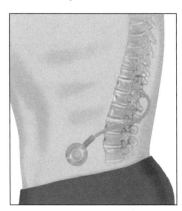 but usually is not sutured in place. The catheter exits from the insertion site on the back. If the administration will be permanent or long term, the catheter is "tunneled" and exits on the side of the body or on the abdomen. A variation of the technique is to implant a Port-a-Cath® subcutaneously and connect that device to the indwelling catheter. The necessity of sterile compounded formulations is obvious for this route of administration. Preservatives are strictly contraindicated in epidural formulations to prevent nerve damage.

Intrathecal Route

The *arachnoid mater* is the innermost meninge. Intrathecal injections place formulations in the subarachnoid space underneath the arachnoid mater. This space is filled with the cerebral spinal fluid that circulates around the spinal cord and the brain. Intrathecal injections allow dosages about one-tenth those in epidural administration.

Intrathecal administration, however, carries a greater risk and consequence of bacterial contamination than epidural administration because the cerebral spinal fluid is a good medium for the growth of bacteria. These injections also may cause "spinal headaches" when the needle puncture does not seal off and cerebral spinal fluid continually leaks into the epidural space.

Intrathecal administration often is the route selected to give single injections of narcotics for postoperative pain management. Implantable infusion pumps are used to chronically administer medications to the intrathecal space. These administration techniques allow for very low doses of medications to be given in a controlled manner and reduce the incidence of side effects. The reservoirs in these pumps typically hold between 18 and 50 ml of solution; therefore, the solution concentrations will be high. Formulating high concentration solutions may entail problems with solubility, pH, buffering, and so forth.[1] Also, to avoid nerve damage, these solutions must not contain preservatives.

Needle Gauge Size

There are different types of injection dependent formulations, but each requires a needle or some type of access device to accomplish the administration. Recommendations are summarized in Table 24.1.

Injection Independent Routes of Administration

The demand for sterility to protect sensitive and vital tissues or organs is most evident with the intranasal, inhalation, and ophthalmic routes of administration. These are considered *injection independent*, as a needle or catheter is not required to administer formulations via these routes.

Intranasal Route

The adult nasal cavity has a capacity of about 20 ml— a very large surface area for absorption and a very rich blood supply. Intranasal administration typically is used to administer drugs to the upper respiratory tract. The absorption of some drugs, however, gives rise to blood concentrations similar to concentrations when the drug is administered intravenously. Because of this favorable absorption, intranasal administration has been investigated as a possible route of systemic administration for drugs such as insulin, glucagon, progesterone, propranolol, and narcotic analgesics—to mention just a few.

The drug can be lost following intranasal administration by three mechanisms:

1. *Metabolism in the nasal mucosa.* The nasal mucosa is an enzymatically active tissue, and some drugs

TABLE 24.1: ACCESS DEVICE GAUGE RECOMMENDATIONS FOR VARIOUS INJECTION DEPENDENT ADMINISTRATIONS

Gauge	Appropriate Uses	Comments
16–18	IV infusion • In adults and adolescents • Of viscous fluids and large volumes • At rapid infusion rates	Large vessel required Insertion may be painful
19–20	IV infusion • In adults, adolescents, and older children • Of blood products and other viscous fluids IM injection	Large vessel required Insertion may be painful
21	IV injection or infusion • In most ages IM injection	
22–23	IV infusion • In all ages including infants and elderly • Of non-viscous fluids • At slow to moderate infusion rates IM injection	Suitable for small or fragile veins Infusion control devices may be required Insertion through tough skin may be difficult
24–27	IV infusion • In all ages including infants, toddlers, and elderly • Of non-viscous fluids • At slow to moderate infusion rates Subcutaneous (SC) injection Intradermal (ID) injection (25–26 gauge)	Especially useful for very small veins Infusion control devices may be required Insertion through tough skin may be difficult

are degraded significantly when administered by this route.

2. *Mucous flow and ciliary movement.* The normal physiology of the nasal cavity is designed to move mucus and inhaled contaminants up and away from the lungs and toward the orifice of the nose. Some of the drug will be lost, then, as the drug is swept outward by these processes.

3. *Swallowing.* Intranasal administration can cause the drug to be swallowed, and in some cases enough drug will be swallowed to equal an oral dose. This may lead to a systemic effect from the drug even though it is administered intranasally.

Compounded formulations used for intranasal administration include solutions, suspensions, and gels. The liquids typically are sterile, isotonic, weakly buffered, and preserved so as not to interfere with the nasal cilia. The buffered products have a pH between 4 and 8, and optimally at the pH of maximum stability of the active drug if it is in that range. Although isotonicity is 300 mOsmol/L, osmotic pressures ranging from 200 to 600 mOsmol/L are acceptable for intranasal administration.

Generally, solutions and suspensions are administered as drops. Solutions also can be administered as a fine mist from a nasal spray bottle. Nasal sprays are preferred to drops because drops are more likely to drain into the back of the mouth and throat and be swallowed. Nasal sprays also can be administered with the aid of a *metered dose inhaler (MDI)*, which will better control the volume of spray dispensed with each actuation.

If the drug is sufficiently volatile, it should be administered as a *nasal inhaler.* The inhaler is a cylindrical 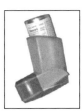 tube with a cap that contains fibrous material impregnated with a volatile drug. The cap is removed and the inhaler tip is placed just inside the nostril. As the person inhales, air is pulled through the tube, pulling the vaporized drug into the nasal cavity. Gels usually are dispensed in small syringes containing the required dosage for one application.

If drops or sprays are used, the quantity of drug administered in each drop or each spray should be calibrated. To calibrate a dropper:

1. Drop the formulation into a small graduated cylinder (5 ml or 10 ml), using the same dropper the patient will use.

2. Count the number of drops required to dispense 3 ml of solution.

3. Divide the number of drops by 3 to give the number of drops per ml.

4. Calculate the number of drops needed to dispense the volume of formulation in one dose.

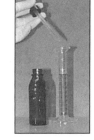

To calibrate a spray bottle:

1. Weigh the spray bottle when filled with the formulation.

2. Prime the bottle, and then deliver 10 sprays into a plastic bag.

3. Re-weigh the spray bottle.

4. Divide the difference in the two weights by 10 to give the volume delivered with each spray.

5. Calculate the number of sprays needed to dispense the volume of formulation in one dose (assume specific gravity = 1).

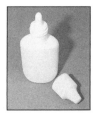

Keep in mind that the patient's manner of squeezing the spray bottle will be different. The pharmacist may want to observe while the patient carries out the spray bottle calibrate procedure.

HOW TO USE INTRANASAL DROPS

1. Blow your nose gently to clear the nostrils.
2. Wash your hands with soap and warm water.
3. Lie down on a bed with your head tilted back and your neck supported (allow your head to hang over the edge of the bed or place a small pillow under your shoulders). Tilt your head back so it is hanging lower than your shoulders. Note: If putting drops into the nose of a child, lay the child on his/her back over your lap, with the head tilted back.
4. Draw up a small amount of medication into the medicine dropper.
5. Breathe through your mouth.
6. Place the tip of the medicine dropper just inside nostril (about 1/3 inch). Avoid touching the dropper against the nostril or anything else.
7. Place the directed number of drops into the nostril.
8. Repeat steps 3–7 for the other nostril if directed to do so.
9. Remain lying down for about 5 minutes so the medication has a chance to spread throughout the nasal passages.
10. Replace the medicine dropper in its container, and close the bottle tightly.
11. Wash your hands.

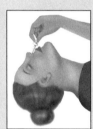

TIPS

- Some of the solution may drain down into your mouth. If the taste is unpleasant, cough out the excess solution into a tissue.
- Have someone help instill the nose drops if that is easier.

HOW TO USE INTRANASAL SPRAYS OR PUMPS

1. Blow your nose gently to clear the nostrils.
2. Wash your hands with soap and warm water.
3. Hold your head in an upright position.
4. Close one nostril with one finger.
5. With your mouth closed, insert the tip of the spray or pump into the open nostril. Sniff in through the nostril while quickly and firmly squeezing the spray container or activating the pump.
6. Hold your breath for a few seconds, then breathe out through your mouth.
7. Repeat this procedure for the other nostril only if directed to do so.
8. Rinse the spray or pump tip with hot water, and replace the cap tightly on the container.
9. Wash your hands.

Inhalation Route

Inhalation dosage forms are intended to deliver drugs to the lungs to affect pulmonary function or treat allergic symptoms. Examples of drugs administered by inhalation are adrenocorticoid steroids (e.g., beclomethasone), bronchodilators (e.g., isoproterenol, metaproterenol, albuterol), and antiallergics (e.g., cromolyn).

The lungs have a large surface area and a rich blood supply to the alveolar epithelium, both of which favor rapid absorption. But the absorption of drugs from the lungs varies considerably, so this route is not considered an alternative to intravenous administration. Administering drugs via this route is dependent on factors that involve the formulation, the administration device, and the anatomy of the lungs.

Compounded inhalation formulations consist generally of solutions, suspensions, and powders. Several delivery devices are used to administer compounded inhalation formulations. Figure 24.1 shows these devices.

Atomizers are devices that break up a liquid into an aerosol. A squeeze bulb is used to blow air into the device. The air causes the drug solution to rise in a small dip tube and vaporizes the liquid in the air stream. To produce even smaller droplets, the air stream is directed into a baffle or bead, which breaks the droplets as they collide with the device. The air and liquid then exit the atomizer.

A *nebulizer* contains an atomizing unit within a chamber. When the rubber bulb is depressed, the medication solution is drawn up a dip tube and aerosolized by the passing air stream. Baffles or beads also may be present in the chamber. The fine droplets exit the nebulizer, and the larger droplets collect on the chamber and fall back into the reservoir, where they can be used again.

Vaporizers produce a fine mist of steam. Volatile medication is added to the water in the vaporizer or to the special medication cup that some models have. The medication volatilizes and is inhaled as the patient breathes.

Insufflators are used to administer powders not only to the mouth but also to the nose and ear. Squeezing the rubber bulb of an insufflator causes turbulence within

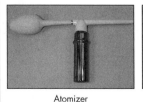
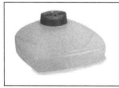
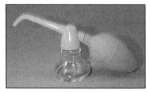
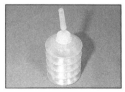

| Atomizer | Nebulizer | Vaporizer | Insufflator | Puffer |

FIGURE 24.1: INHALATION DRUG DELIVERY DEVICES

the powder reservoir, which forces some of the powder into the air stream and out of the device.

Puffers are similar to insufflators in that they are used to administer powders. A puffer is a plastic accordion-shaped container with a spout on one end. The powder is placed inside the container, and the puffer is actuated by squeezing the device. A portion of the powder is ejected from the spout.

Commercial inhalation products are either a metered dose inhaler (MDI) or a dry powder inhaler. Commercial aerosols typically are MDIs that deliver a fixed dose in a spray with each actuation of the device. These inhalers are devices in which liquid or suspension droplets constitute the internal phase and a gas constitutes the external phase.

Coordination is required on the part of the patient between breathing in (inspiration) and activating the MDI. Extender devices or *spacers* are available to assist

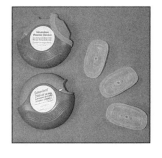

patients who cannot coordinate these two activities. The spacer goes between the MDI's mouthpiece and the patient's mouth. The spacer allows the patient to separate activation and inspiration by 3 to 5 seconds.

Dry powder inhalers are contained in manufactured cartridges or disks. When the patient administers a dose, the device first is activated by some mechanical motion and the dry powder becomes ready for inspiration. Then the patient inhales through the mouthpiece of the device and draws the powder into the pulmonary tract along with the inspired air. These devices have overcome a major problem of inhalation therapy—synchronizing deep inspiration with administration of the drug. Some of these devices are Diskhaler®, Turbuhaler®, Diskus®, and Rotahaler®.

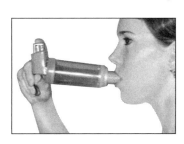

Regardless of the formulation or the administration device, inhalation therapy also depends on the coordination, the breathing patterns, and the respiration depth of the patient at the time of administration. Upon actuation, inhalation devices produce either liquid droplets or powder particles. There is a strong correlation between the inspired particle size and its final deposition inside the lungs. Large particles (about 20 microns) impact at the back of the mouth and throat and eventually are swallowed rather than inhaled. Particles from 1 to 10 microns reach the terminal bronchioles and are more available for local therapy. Smaller particles (0.6 micron) penetrate to the alveolar sacs, where absorption is most rapid but

retention is minimal because a large fraction of the dose is exhaled. The particles that reach the alveolar sacs and remain there are responsible for providing systemic effects.

Ophthalmics

Drugs are administered to the eye for local effects such as miosis, mydriasis, anesthesia, or reduction of intra-ocular pressure (i.e., glaucoma). Formulations that are used include aqueous solutions, aqueous suspensions, ointments, and implants. Every ophthalmic product must be sterile in its final container, and the pH, buffer capacity, viscosity, and tonicity of the formulation must be carefully controlled.

Following ophthalmic administration, a drug can be lost in three unique ways:

1. *Immediate loss because of spillage.* The normal volume of tears in the eye is estimated to be 7 microliters, and if blinking occurs, the eye can hold up to 10 microliters without spilling. The normal commercial eyedropper dispenses 50 microliters of solution; thus, more than half of the dose will be lost from the eye by overflow. The ideal volume of drug solution to administer would be 5 to 10 microliters; however, microliter dosing eyedroppers generally are not available to patients.

2. *Lacrimal drainage.* Tears wash the eyeball as they flow from the lacrimal gland across the eye and drain into the lacrimal canalicula. In humans, the rate of tear production is approximately 2 microliters per minute; thus, the entire tear volume in the eye turns over every 2 to 3 minutes. This rapid washing and turnover also accounts for loss of an ophthalmic dose in a relatively short time.

3. *Drug absorption into the conjunctiva.* The conjunctiva has a large blood supply that can remove the drug from the ocular tissues rapidly.

Ophthalmic administration delivers a drug onto the eye, into the eye, or onto the conjunctiva. Transcorneal transport (drug penetration into the eye) is not effective because only an estimated one-tenth of a dose penetrates the eye. Following ophthalmic administration, systemic effects are possible. Drugs can enter the systemic circulation in two ways:

1. Drugs that enter the lacrimal canalicula are emptied into the gastrointestinal tract, where they can be absorbed into the circulation.

2. Drugs can be absorbed through the conjunctiva of the eye directly into the circulation.

Most compounded ophthalmic solutions and suspensions are packaged in eyedropper bottles called *droptainers,* which are easier to handle than dropper bottles.

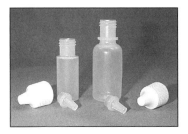

Patients should be shown how to instill the drops into their eyes properly, and every effort should be made to emphasize the need to instill only one drop, not two or three, per administration.

In an effort to maintain longer contact between the drug and the surrounding tissue, suspensions, ointments, and inserts have been developed. When aqueous suspensions are used, the particle size is kept to a minimum to prevent irritation of the eye. After administration of this dosage form, it is possible to find particles adhering to the conjunctiva.

Ointments tend to keep the drug in contact with the eye longer than suspensions do. Most ophthalmic ointment bases are a mixture of mineral oil and white petrolatum and have a melting point close to body temperature. Ointments, however, tend to blur the vision as they remain viscous and are not removed easily by the tear fluid. Therefore, ointments are used most often at night as adjunctive therapy to eyedrops, which are used during the day. Ophthalmic ointment tubes typically are small, holding approximately 3.5 g of ointment and fitted with narrow gauge tips that permit the extrusion of narrow bands of ointment.

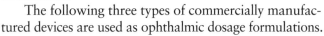

The following three types of commercially manufactured devices are used as ophthalmic dosage formulations.

1. Special *hydrogel contact lenses* can be placed in a solution containing a drug (e.g., an antibiotic), and the hydrophilic nature of the lenses will absorb some of the drug. When the lenses are worn, the drug will be released from the lenses over a period of time. Although this may be a convenient method of drug administration for people who customarily wear contact lenses, introduction of the drug into the lens may change the refractive qualities.

2. Ocusert® is a nonerodible *ocular insert* designed to deliver pilocarpine at a controlled rate for up to 7 days. The insert is placed in the cul-de-sac between the eyeball and the eyelid. Patients who wear the insert use a fraction of the dose of pilocarpine that they would with drop therapy. The biggest disadvantage of the insert is its tendency to float on the eyeball, particularly upon arising in the morning.

3. Soluble *ophthalmic drug inserts* are dried polymeric solutions that have been fashioned into a film or a rod. These solid inserts are placed in the cul-de-sac between the eyeball and the eyelid. As they absorb tears, they slowly erode. Lacrisert® is an insert used in treating moderate to severe dry eye syndrome.

HOW TO USE OPHTHALMIC DROPS

1. Wash your hands thoroughly with soap and warm water.

2. If the product container is transparent, check the solution before using it. If it is discolored or has changed in any way since it was purchased (e.g., particles in the solution, color change), don't use the solution.

3. If the product container has a depressible rubber bulb, draw up a small amount of medication into the eyedropper by first squeezing, then relieving pressure on the bulb.

4. Tilt your head back with your chin up, and look toward the ceiling.

5. With both eyes open, gently draw down the lower lid of the affected eye with your index finger.

6. In the "gutter" formed, place one drop of the solution. Hold the dropper or administration tip as close as possible to the lid without actually touching your eye. Do not allow the dropper or administration tip to touch any surface.

7. If possible, hold your eyelid open, and don't blink for 30 seconds.

8. Press your finger against the inner corner of your eye for one minute. This will keep the medication in your eye.

9. Cap the bottle tightly.

TIPS

- Keep in mind that this is a sterile solution. Contamination of the dropper or eye solution can lead to a serious eye infection.

- If irritation persists or increases, discontinue use immediately.

- Avoid eye make-up while using eye solutions.

- Use a mirror when applying the drops, or have someone help instill the eye drops.

HOW TO USE AN OPHTHALMIC OINTMENT

1. Wash your hands carefully with soap and warm water.

2. Hold the ointment tube in your hand for a few minutes to warm and soften the ointment.

3. Before applying the ointment, gently cleanse the affected eyelid with warm water and a soft cloth.

4. In front of a mirror, with the affected eye looking upward, gently pull the lower eyelid downward with your index finger to form a pouch.

5. Squeeze a thin line (approximately ¼–½ inch) of the ointment along the pouch. Be careful when applying this ointment. Do not allow the tip of the ointment tube to touch the eyelid, eyeball, finger, or any surface.

6. Close the eyelid gently and rotate the eyeball to distribute the ointment. Blink several times to spread the ointment evenly.

7. Replace the cap on the ointment tube.

TIPS

- After application, your vision may be blurred temporarily. Don't be alarmed. This will clear up shortly, but don't drive a car or operate machinery until your vision has cleared.

- This is a sterile ointment. Avoid contamination of the tip or the cap of the tube, which could lead to a serious eye infection.

- If irritation persists or increases, discontinue use immediately.

- Generally avoid eye make-up while using eye ointments.

- Have someone help apply your eye ointment.

Otic

The external ear consists of the pinna (part of the ear lobe), the auricle (opening to the ear), and the external auditory canal. The external auditory canal starts at the auricle and ends at the tympanic membrane. The auricle contains many nerves, which can be quite painful when inflamed. As the external auditory canal proceeds toward the tympanic membrane, the skin becomes thicker and contains both apocrine and exocrine glands along with hair follicles. *Cerumen* is the waxy material commonly called ear wax that is formed when the oily secretions from the exocrine glands mix with the fatty fluid from the apocrine glands. Cerumen normally moves outward toward the auricle when the jaw moves, as when talking or chewing. Therefore, the external auditory canal is self-cleaning.

Compounded otic preparations that are used to treat common ear problems include solutions, suspensions, gels, ointments, and powders. Otic solutions and suspensions are instilled into the ear. These solutions are used to remove ear wax, purulent discharges from an infection, or foreign bodies from the external auditory canal. Suspensions are expected to provide a longer drug effect, or they may be required because of insolubility of the drug.

Otic gels and ointments are semisolid preparations applied to the auricle. Any ointment base can be used in their preparation, and they typically contain antibacterial, antifungal, or corticosteroid ingredients. Fine powders used as insufflations might contain antibacterial or antifungal agents. However, these can form a powder–ear wax buildup in the external auditory canal, and therefore are not used often.

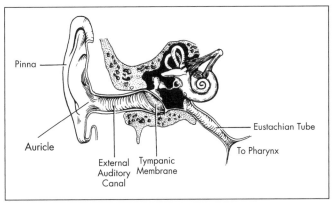

"Human Ear" by Hans F. E. Wachtmeister and L. J. Scott, Chapter 31 in General Biology Laboratory Manual: Encounters with Life, *7th edition (Denver, CO: Morton Publishing Company, 2006), p. 288.*

NOTES

1. Vidrine, E. Compounding Intrathecal Medications. *International Journal of Pharmaceutical Compounding* 4:24–25, 2000.

ADDITIONAL READING

Allen, L.V., Jr. Ophthalmic, Otic, and Nasal Preparations (chapter 20). In *The Art, Science, and Technology of Pharmaceutical Compounding*, 2nd edition. American Pharmaceutical Association, Washington, DC, 2002, pp. 325–351.

Roberts, R., Moore, E. Sterile Compounding of Respiratory Inhalation Solutions. *International Journal of Pharmaceutical Compounding* 6:415–17, 2002.

Allen, L.V., Jr. Basics of Compounding for Disorders of the External Ear. *International Journal of Pharmaceutical Compounding* 8:46–48, 2004.

CHAPTER TWENTY-FIVE

Sterile Compounding–Part 1: Equipment, Devices, and Processes

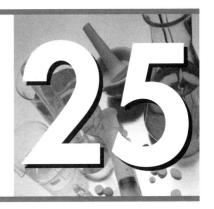

PHARMACISTS HAVE BEEN PROVIDING STERILE COMpounding services for decades. These services have included parenteral therapies, infusion services, and utilization of complex infusion administration devices and supplies. In the past two decades, however, compounding sterile formulations and providing administration services have expanded beyond the patient care institution. These additional areas include home care agencies, infusion service agencies, outpatient clinics, and community pharmacies. Pharmacists also are providing patient and caregiver assessments, education, and skills training, and are taking the responsibility for coordinating patient care through an interdisciplinary team.

Pharmacists compound a wide variety of sterile formulations in these different settings. The formulations include products administered by injection (intravenous, intramuscular, subcutaneous, intradermal, intrathecal, epidural) or inhalation, intranasal, ophthalmic, and otic routes of administration.

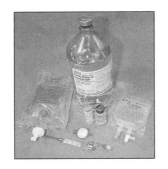

Requirements of Sterile Formulations

Sterile formulations for either institutional or home care use must adhere to a number of special requirements involving

- sterility
- particulate material
- pyrogen-free
- stability
- pH
- osmotic pressure.

Sterility means freedom from bacteria and other microorganisms. *Sterile* is not a relative term. An item is either sterile or not sterile. If the sterile formulation is a solution, it must be free of all visible *particulate material*

—the mobile, undissolved substances unintentionally present in parenteral products. Examples of particulate materials are cellulose, glass, rubber cores from closures, cloth or cotton fibers, metal, plastic, rust, diatoms, and dandruff. Sterile suspensions and ointments may contain particulate material, but these usually are the active drug or an ingredient, and not contaminants.

Potential sources of particulate material are

1. the product itself,
2. manufacturing processes and variables such as the environment, equipment, and personnel,
3. the packaging components,
4. the administration sets and devices used to administer the product, and
5. the manipulations and environment of the product at the time of administration.

The USP/NF chapter <788> Particulate Matter in Injections sets limits on the number and size of particulates that are permissible in parenteral formulations.[1] For large volume parenterals, the limit is not more than 12 particles/ml that are equal to or larger than 10 microns and not more than 2 particles/ml that are equal to or larger than 25 microns. For small volume parenterals, the limit is 3,000 particles/container that are equal to or larger than 10 microns and not more than 300/container that are equal to or larger than 25 microns. Particles measuring 50 microns or larger can be detected by visual inspection. Specialized equipment is needed to detect particles smaller than 50 microns in size.

Sterile formulations must be *pyrogen-free*. Pyrogens are metabolic byproducts of living microorganisms. If pyrogens are detected in a sterile product, this indicates that bacteria have proliferated somewhere during the formulation process. In humans, pyrogens cause significant discomfort but rarely are fatal. Symptoms include fever and chills, cutaneous vasoconstriction, higher arterial blood pressure, increased heart workload, pupillary dilation, decreased respiration, nausea and malaise, severe diarrhea, or pain in the back and legs.

The *stability* of drugs in sterile formulations is an important consideration. In institutional settings, most admixtures are prepared hours before they are to be administered and generally are utilized within a short period of time. In home health care settings, admixtures are prepared days in advance of when they are to be administered and generally are utilized over longer periods of time than in the clinical setting.

Physiological pH is about 7.4, and an effort should be made to provide sterile formulations that do not vary significantly from that normal pH. Of course, in some situations this becomes a secondary consideration because acidic or alkaline solutions may be needed to solubilize drugs or to be used as a therapeutic treatment themselves.

Osmotic pressure is a characteristic of any solution that has dissolved particles in the solution. Blood has an osmolarity of approximately 300 milliosmoles per liter (mOsmol/L) and, ideally, any sterile solution would be formulated to have the same osmolarity. The most commonly used large volume parenteral solutions have osmolarities similar to that of blood—for example, 0.9% sodium chloride solution (308 mOsmol/L). Intravenous solutions that have larger osmolarity values (hypertonic) or smaller osmolarity values (hypotonic) may damage red blood cells and cause pain and irritation of tissues. In some therapeutic situations, however, it may be necessary to administer hypertonic or hypotonic solutions. In these cases the solutions usually are given slowly through large veins to minimize the reactions.

Types of Sterile Dosage Forms

There are many types of sterile dosage forms. The actual product selected for a given drug depends on the nature of the drug itself, the nature of the product formulation, the route of administration, and therapeutic considerations. Table 25.1 shows that solutions are administered

TABLE 25.1: FORMULATIONS USED IN VARIOUS ROUTES OF ADMINISTRATION

Intravenous, intramuscular, intradermal	Solutions	Intranasal	Solutions
	Suspensions		Suspensions
	Emulsions		Sprays
Subcutaneous	Solutions		Aerosols
	Suspensions		Inhalers
	Emulsions		Powders
	Implants	Inhalation	Solutions
Ophthalmic	Solutions		Aerosols
	Suspensions		Powders
	Ointments		
	Inserts		
Otic	Solutions		
	Suspensions		
	Gels		

in all routes, that suspensions and emulsions are used in most routes, and that specific products are used as needed for the unique characteristics of each route of administration.

Parenterals

Liquid formulations that are intended to be injected into the systemic circulation are called *injections*. These formulations generally are aqueous but might be mixtures of water with glycols, alcohol, or other non-aqueous solvents. Injected emulsions are used to administer subcutaneous allergenic extracts, modified release depot intramuscular injections, and intravenous nutrients emulsions.

Parenterals are labeled as *Injections* with the following conventions:

- [Drug] Injection—liquid preparations of the active drug
- [Drug] for Injection—dry solids that when reconstituted meet the standards of [Drug] Injection
- [Drug] Injectable Suspension—liquid preparations of solids suspended in a suspension medium
- [Drug] for Injectable Suspension—dry solids that when reconstituted meet the standards of [Drug] Injectable Suspensions
- [Drug] Injectable Emulsion—liquid preparations of the active drug dispersed in an emulsion medium.

Solutions, suspensions, and emulsions intended for injection are prepared in the same general manner as all solutions and dispersed systems, but they have the following differences:

- Solvents or vehicles used must meet standards that assure their safety when injected.
- The use of added substances such as buffers, stabilizers, and microbial preservatives is restricted in certain parenteral products; the use of coloring agents is strictly prohibited.
- The products must be sterile and pyrogen-free.
- The products must meet compendial standards for particulate matter.
- The products are prepared in environmentally controlled areas by trained personnel.
- The products are packaged in hermetically sealed containers of high quality.
- Each container has a slight excess of formulation, which permits withdrawal of the labeled volume.
- There are limitations on the types of containers (single dose or multiple dose) that may be used for certain injections.

The same physicochemical and therapeutic considerations taken with non-parenteral liquid formulations are applied to parenteral liquid formulations. For example, if a drug is unstable in solution, it might be prepared as a dry powder for reconstitution or as a suspension. If a drug is insoluble or unstable in water, it might be formulated in a vehicle that will partially or totally replace water. Drugs that are dissolved in aqueous vehicles and are soluble in body fluids are expected to have a more rapid onset of action than drugs in oleaginous solutions. Drugs in aqueous suspensions are expected to have a more rapid onset of action than drugs in oleaginous suspensions.

One critical factor is unique to parenteral injections: These formulations are administered through needles having an internal diameter of 300 to 600 microns. Thus, the flow properties of syringeability and injectability are crucial. *Syringeability* refers to the characteristics of manipulating an injection in a syringe and includes factors such as ease of withdrawal from a container into the syringe, clogging and foaming tendencies, and accuracy of dose management. *Injectability* refers to the properties of the injection while it actually is being administered and includes factors such as pressure or force required for injection, evenness of flow, aspiration qualities, and freedom from clogging.

Solvents

Some injections are used as solvents to reconstitute lyophilized powders or as diluents in the manufacturing process. Water for Injection USP is the most widely used solvent for large scale manufacturing. This water is purified by distillation or by the reverse osmosis of Purified Water USP and must meet the same standards for total solids as Purified Water USP. Water for Injection USP may not contain added substances. Although Water for Injection USP is not required to be sterile, it must be pyrogen-free. The water is intended to be used in the manufacture of injectable products that are sterilized after their preparation.

Sterile Water for Injection USP is Water for Injection USP that has been sterilized and packaged in single dose containers of less than 1 liter. It also must be pyrogen-free and may not contain added substance. This water may contain slightly more total solids than Water for Injection USP because of the possible leaching of glass constituents into the product during the sterilization process. This water cannot be directly administered intravenously because it has no tonicity.

Bacteriostatic Water for Injection USP is Sterile Water for Injection USP containing one or more antimicrobial agents. It is packaged in prefilled syringes or in vials containing not more than 30 ml. This size limitation is intended to prevent the administration of large quantities of bacteriostatic agents that could cause toxicity. If volumes greater than 5 ml of solvent are required, Sterile Water for Injection USP is the preferred solvent. Bacteriostatic Water for Injection USP is employed as a sterile

vehicle in the preparation of small volumes of injectable products.

The USP regulations require that the labeling state, "Not for Use in Newborns." This labeling statement was the result of problems encountered in neonates and the toxicity of the bacteriostatic agent benzyl alcohol. Toxicity reports in the early 1980s showed that neonates who received Bacteriostatic Water for Injection USP experienced a "gasping syndrome," which included metabolic acidosis, respiratory distress, central nervous system dysfunction, apnea, seizure, coma, intraventricular hemorrhage, hepatic and renal failure, and eventual cardiovascular collapse and death. Some neonates died from an injection of as little as 11 ml/kg/day of Bacteriostatic Water for Injection USP.

Sodium Chloride Injection USP is a sterile isotonic solution of sodium chloride in Water for Injection USP. It contains no antimicrobial agents. The solution is used as a sterile vehicle and as a catheter or intravenous line flush to maintain patency. Usually 3 ml is used to flush the line after each use, or every 8 hours if the line is not used.

Bacteriostatic Sodium Chloride Injection USP is a sterile isotonic solution of 0.9% sodium chloride in Water for Injection USP that contains antimicrobial agents. Similar to Bacteriostatic Water for Injection USP, this solvent must be packaged in not more than 30 ml containers and must carry specific labeling as to the nature of the antimicrobial agents. Bacteriostatic Sodium Chloride Injection USP also is used to flush a catheter or IV line to maintain patency. It, too, carries the "Not for Use in Newborns" warning.

Although an aqueous vehicle generally is preferred for injections, it may not be possible because of limited water solubility or aqueous stability of the active drug. A non-aqueous solvent or a co-solvent system may be necessary to overcome these problems with stability or solubility. Among the non-aqueous solvents used are fixed vegetable oils, glycerin, polyethylene glycol 300, ethyl alcohol, and propylene glycol.

The USP restricts the use of fixed vegetable oils in parenteral products.

- These oils are not to be used for intravenous administration but must be reserved for intramuscular injections because the oils could interrupt normal blood flow.
- The oils must remain clear when cooled to 10°C to ensure the stability and clarity of the injectable product upon refrigeration.
- The oils must not contain mineral oil or paraffin, as these materials are not absorbed.
- Because the fluidity of an oil depends upon the proportion of unsaturated fatty acids to saturated acids, the oils must meet specific requirements of iodine number and saponification number.

Some oils may be quite irritating when injected even though they have relatively low toxicities. Because some patients exhibit allergic reactions to specific oils, the label must state the specific oil present in the product. The fixed oils used most commonly are corn oil, cottonseed oil, peanut oil, palm oil, and sesame oil. Sesame oil is the preferred oil for most of the injections because of its stability (except in light).

Water miscible solvents are widely used in parenterals to enhance drug solubility and to serve as stabilizers. A common example of an injectable product formulated with non-aqueous solvents is intravenous diazepam, which contains 40% propylene glycol and 10% ethanol. Mixed solvent systems do not exhibit many of the disadvantages associated with fixed oils but also may be irritating or increase toxicity, especially when present in large amounts or in high concentrations.

Added Substances

The USP permits certain substances to be added to injections to maintain stability, ensure sterility, or aid in administration. Clearly these substances must be non-toxic in the amounts administered, must not interfere with therapeutic efficacy, and must not interfere with specified assays and tests. These substances include antimicrobial agents, buffers, chelating agents, inert gases, solubilizing agents, protectants, substances for adjusting tonicity, and antioxidants.

Antibacterial Preservatives A suitable preservative system is required in all multiple dose parenteral products, to inhibit the growth of microorganisms that are introduced accidentally during withdrawal of individual doses. Preservatives may be added to nonsterile single dose parenteral products as a sterility assurance measure. The chosen preservative system must be free of interactions with other components of the formulation. For example, proteins can bind thimerosal, reducing its efficacy. In another example, the partitioning of a preservative into a micellar phase or an internal oil phase of an emulsion can reduce the concentration of preservative available for activity.

Buffers Many drugs require a certain pH range for maximum stability. In addition, drug solubility is highly dependent on the pH of the solution. Therefore, buffers of sufficient buffer capacity are added to maintain the pH of the injection. The pH of a formulation can be influenced by the degradation of the drug or other added substances, container and stopper effects, diffusion of gases into the formulation through the closure, or gases dissolved in the product or in the container headspace.

Chelating Agents Chelating agents are added to complex and thereby inactivate metals such as copper, iron, and zinc. These metals often are catalysts for oxidative degradation reactions. Metal contamination can be caused by material impurities, solvents, containers and stoppers, and manufacturing equipment. The most widely used chelating agents are edetic acid (EDTA) derivatives and their salts.

Inert Gases For formulations that are unstable in oxygen, the air in the solution or in the container headspace is displaced with nitrogen or argon.

Solubilizers Solubilizing agents are used to increase the solubility of the active drug in the formulation. Typical agents include ethyl alcohol, glycerin, polyethylene glycol, and propylene glycol. The agents also can be used alone as non-aqueous solvents or in co-solvent systems to improve solubility. Surfactants also are used as solubilizers. They are used most often in suspensions to wet powders and improve syringeability, and for solubilizing fat soluble vitamins in parenteral nutrition solutions.

Protectants A protectant is an added substance that prevents the loss of drug activity because of the manufacturing process or adsorption to equipment or packaging materials. For example, active drugs can be adsorbed to filters and silicone tubing during the manufacturing process or adsorb to rubber closures and other polymeric materials used in the packaging process. During administration, the drug can adsorb to polymeric administration sets and equipment.

Cryoprotectants and lyoprotectants are used to inhibit loss of integrity of the active drug resulting from freezing and drying. Polyethylene glycol protects lactate dehydrogenase and phosphofructokinase from freezing damage, and glucose and trehalose protect both proteins from drying damage. Human serum albumin (HSA) is commonly used as a protectant. The albumin is present in the formulation container at a higher concentration than the active drug, and it is preferentially adsorbed, thereby preventing adsorption of the drug. Protectants are used primarily in protein and liposomal formulations.

Substances to Adjust Tonicity Many intravenous injections have to be isotonic to prevent hemolysis or crenation of red blood cells. Dextrose, sodium chloride, and potassium chloride are commonly used to achieve isotonicity in a parenteral formulation.

Antioxidants Antioxidants are preferentially oxidized, compared to the active drug, and become consumed over time. Salts of sulfur dioxide including bisulfite, metasulfite, and sulfite are the most common antioxidants used in aqueous injections. The appropriate antioxidant concentration to use in a formulation depends on the reactivity of the drug, the type of container, whether the container is single or multiple dose, the presence of inert gases, and the length of time the product is to be protected.

Classification of Parenterals

One useful categorization of injections is based on the size of the final product packaging. Parenteral solutions are packaged as *Large Volume Parenteral (LVP)* solutions or *Small Volume Parenteral (SVP)* solutions.

Large Volume Parenteral (LVP) Solutions

LVP solutions typically are bags or bottles holding 100 ml or more of solution. The three types of containers are: glass bottle with an air vent tube, glass bottle without an air vent tube, and plastic bags. LVP solutions typically are used (1) for correcting disturbances in electrolyte and fluid balance, (2) for parenteral nutrition, and (3) as a vehicle for administering other drugs.

Plastic bags have advantages over glass bottles in that they do not break, they weigh less, they take up less

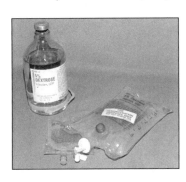

storage space, and they take up much less disposal space. Some drugs, however, adsorb to the plastic. Also, some drugs and solutions leach plasticizer out of the plastic that was added to keep the plastic pliable. Newer plastics are minimizing some of these problems.

Plastic bags are available in different sizes, the most common of which are 250, 500, and 1,000 ml. Graduation marks on the front of the bag marked at 25 ml to 100 ml intervals indicate the volume of solution used. The plastic bag system collapses as the solution is administered so a vacuum is not created inside the bag.

At one end of the bag are two ports of about the same length.

1. The *administration set port* has a plastic cover to maintain the sterility of the bag; the cover is easily removed. Solution will not drip out of the bag through this port because of a plastic diaphragm about ½ inch inside the port. When the spike of the administration set is inserted into the port, the diaphragm is punctured and the solution will flow out of the bag into the administration set. This inner diaphragm cannot be resealed once it is punctured.

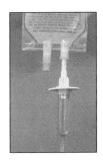

2. The *medication port* is covered by a protective rubber tip. Drugs are added to the solution through this port, using a needle and syringe. There is an inner plastic diaphragm about ½ inch inside the port, just like the administration set port. This inner diaphragm will not reseal when punctured by a needle, but the

protective rubber tip prevents solutions from leaking from the bag once the diaphragm is punctured.

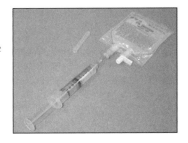

Because of the advantages of plastic bags, glass LVP solution bottles are not used often. The major advantage of glass bottles is to administer drugs that are incompatible with plastic bags. Glass intravenous bottles are packaged with a vacuum, sealed with a solid rubber closure, and held in place by an aluminum band. Graduation marks along the sides of the bottle usually are spaced every 20 ml to 50 ml.

Solutions in either the plastic bag or the glass bottle flow from the container to the patient through an *administration set*. But for solutions to flow out of a glass container, air must be able to enter the container to relieve the vacuum as the solution leaves. In some bottles, air tubes are built into the rubber closure for this purpose. Other bottles do not have these, in which case an administration set with a filtered airway in the spike must be used.

Small Volume Parenteral (SVP) Solutions

Small volume parenteral (SVP) solutions usually are 100 ml or less and are packaged in different ways de-

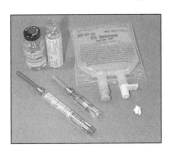

pending on the intended use. If the SVP is a liquid used primarily to deliver medications, it is packaged in a small plastic *minibag* of 50–100 ml. SVPs also can be packaged as *ampules*, *vials*, and *prefilled syringes*. Liquid drugs are supplied in sealed ampules, vials sealed with a rubber closure, or prefilled syringes. Powdered drugs are supplied in vials that must be constituted before being added to any solution. SVPs typically are added to a minibag or an LVP, but they also may serve as the final container in ready-to-mix systems. The term *admixture* denotes a solution in which an SVP has been incorporated into a minibag or an LVP.

Ampules An ampule is a sealed glass container with an elongated neck that must be broken off before using. Most ampules are weakened around the neck for easy breaking, and these have a colored band. If the ampule is not weakened, it must be scored with a file before opening. It is useful to wrap an alcohol wipe or small piece of gauze around the top of the ampule before breaking it, to provide some protection if the ampule shatters and possibly releases glass splinters into the air.

A 5 micron filter needle should be used when drawing the contents of an ampule into a syringe, as glass particles may have fallen inside the ampule when the top was snapped off. The filter needle should be removed and replaced with the regular needle before injecting the drug into any solution.

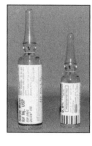

Vials Drugs and other additives are packaged in vials as either liquids or lyophilized powders. Vials are made of glass or plastic and are sealed with a rubber stopper. A needle is used to add contents to or withdraw contents from the vial. Before withdrawing contents from a vial, an equal volume of air usually is injected into the vial to pressurize the vial and aid in withdrawing the contents. Some medications, however, are packaged under pressure or may produce gas (and therefore pressure) upon reconstitution. In these situations, air should not be injected into the vial before withdrawing the solution.

Dry powder formulations are lyophilized or freeze-dried powders that must be reconstituted with some suitable diluent to make a liquid formulation before being withdrawn from the vial. Several diluents might be used to reconstitute the dry powders; the appropriate diluent is indicated in the product information insert. Common diluents are Sterile Water for Injection USP, Bacteriostatic Water for Injection USP, and Sodium Chloride Injection USP.

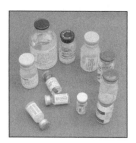

Vials may be designated for *single dose* or *multiple dose* use. Single dose vials do not contain preservatives and should be discarded after one use. Multiple dose vials contain a preservative to inhibit bacterial contamination once the vial has been used. Also, the rubber closure on multiple dose vials will reseal. This allows for a number of doses of variable volume to be withdrawn.

Prefilled Syringes There are two varieties of prefilled syringes:

1. A cartridge type package is a single syringe and needle unit that is placed in a special holder before use. The syringe and needle unit is discarded after use, but the holder is used again with a new unit.

2. A prefilled glass tube closed at both ends with rubber stoppers is placed into a specially designed syringe that has a needle attached to it. After use, all of the pieces are discarded.

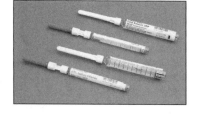

Ready-to-Mix Systems Ready-to-mix systems consist of a specially designed minibag with an adapter for attaching a drug vial. The admixing takes place inside the bag just prior to administration. Major advantages of ready-to-mix systems are a significant reduction in waste and a lower potential for medication error because the drug vial remains attached to the minibag and can be rechecked as needed. These systems do cost more, and they have the potential of not activating properly, so the patient could receive only the diluent or a partial dose of drug. Examples of these systems are Mix-O-Vial® (Upjohn-Pharmacia), ADD-Vantage® (Abbott), and Monovial Safety Guard® (Becton Dickinson).

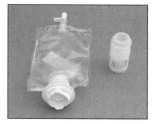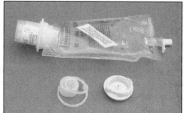

Dry Powders

Many drugs are too unstable in aqueous medium to be formulated as a solution, suspension, or emulsion for injection. In these cases, the drug is formulated as a dry powder that is to be reconstituted with a suitable diluent before administration. The reconstituted powder usually will be an aqueous solution, but occasionally it may be in aqueous suspension.

Dry Powders for Reconstitution Dry powders for reconstitution may be produced by several methods including

- putting the formulation into vials as a liquid and then freeze-drying,
- crystallization followed by vial filling, and
- spray drying followed by vial filling.

1. *Lyophilization (freeze-drying)*. The advantages of producing these powders are that: (a) water can be removed at low temperatures, which protect heat labile materials; (b) the powder will have a rapid rate of solution because of the resulting large surface area of the powder; and (c) vials can be filled rapidly and more accurately as a solution compared to filling vials with a powder, which minimizes airborne particulate matter. Lyophilization, however, may degrade some protein molecules and might cause a drug to convert to a less stable crystalline form.

To begin the freeze-drying process, vials are filled with a solution containing the active drug and the other ingredients of the formulation. When the vial is filled, a special slotted stopper is inserted partially into the neck of the vial and the vials are placed in the chamber of the lyophilizer. The solution is frozen in the vials as the temperature in the chamber is reduced to about −40°C.

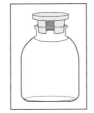

When the solution has solidified, the pressure in the chamber is reduced to less than the vapor pressure of ice at that temperature and heat is applied. Water is removed by *sublimation* of the ice in this primary drying period. Additional drying (i.e., secondary drying) may be required to remove water that remains associated with the ingredients. The vapor pressure of ice at various temperatures is shown in Table 25.2.

TABLE 25.2: VAPOR PRESSURE OF ICE AT VARIOUS TEMPERATURES USED IN LYOPHILIZATION

Temperature (°C)	Vapor Pressure (mm Hg)
−40	0.096
−30	0.286
−20	0.776
−10	1.950
0	4.579

"Parenteral Products," by J. C. Boylan and S. L. Nail, (chapter 12) in Modern Pharmaceutics, 4th edition (New York: Marcel Dekker, Inc., 2002), pp. 381–414.

2. *Crystallization.* Aseptic crystallization is used primarily to produce sterile aqueous suspensions. The crystallization is achieved by first dissolving the active drug (and other ingredients) in a suitable solvent, then filter sterilizing that solution, and then adding another solvent to the filtered solution in which the drug is not soluble. This causes the solute to crystallize and precipitate from solution. The crystals are collected and transferred to vials. The major disadvantage of this method is that the crystal precipitate can vary in size and shape from batch to batch.

3. *Spray drying.* The process of spray drying is similar to crystallization in that the active drug is dissolved in a solvent that is filter sterilized. The solution then is passed through an atomizer that creates an aerosol of the filtered solution. The aerosol comes in contact with a stream of hot sterile gas (usually air), which evaporates the solvent and causes hollow spheres to form. The spheres are collected and transferred to vials. The major disadvantage of this method is the requirement to maintain sterile conditions in the gas, the spray dryer, and the transfer of the spheres to the vials.

Dry Powders for Injection Independent Routes of Administration Dry powders are administered by inhalation using devices such as metered dose inhalers or dry powder inhalers. These devices deliver micronized particles of active drug in metered quantities. In addition to the active drug, the aerosols contain inert propellants and other ingredients that ensure the desired flow properties, metering uniformity, and protection from the package environment. The powders are contained in small cartridges or disks.

Other Sterile Dosage Forms

Many of the other parenteral dosage forms actually are sterile *dosage devices*. Examples of these devices are subcutaneous implants, infusion pumps, and Port-A-Cath®. More traditional dosage forms are the ophthalmic inserts and ointments. These products vary in their design and manufacturing process, but they all share the requirement of sterility. These devices and dosage forms are described in other chapters.

Equipment and Devices Used in Sterile Compounding

Many different devices and specialized equipment are used in sterile compounding. Many of the devices are sterile before they are used, to help maintain sterility of the final product. Most of the equipment is designed to produce an ultra clean environment in which to use the devices. Laminar flow hoods are the primary example of such specialized equipment.

Laminar Flow Hoods

The preparation of parenteral products requires that products and devices that are already sterile or pyrogen-free not be contaminated during the compounding process. Contamination can come from the environment in which the product is being prepared, as well as from the person preparing it. The best way to reduce the environmental risk is to use a laminar flow hood, which establishes and maintains an ultra clean work area.

Laminar flow hoods (either vertical or horizontal) used in sterile compounding must be Class 100 (under 100 particles of 0.5 micron size per cubic foot). In a *horizontal laminar flow hood*, as shown in Figure 25.1, room air is drawn into the hood through a prefilter to remove relatively large contaminants such as dust and lint. The air then is channeled through a HEPA (high efficiency particulate air) filter that removes 99.97% of the particles larger than 0.3 microns. The filtered air then flows out over the entire work surface at a uniform velocity (e.g., laminar flow) of 80–100 ft/min. The constant flow of air out of the laminar flow hood removes contaminants introduced into the work area by material or personnel and prevents room air from entering the work area. Laminar flow hoods, however, do not protect personnel or the environment from the hazards of the drug being compounded within the hood.

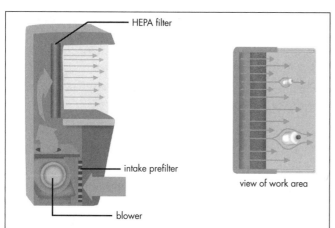

Hoods take up room air and channel it through the HEPA filter. The air crosses the work area in a horizontal direction and exits the hood. The illustration above shows a design where room air enters the hood through the bottom. Other models have room air entering from the back or top of the hood.

FIGURE 25.1: HORIZONTAL LAMINAR AIR FLOW HOOD

In *vertical laminar flow hoods*, the filtered air enters at the top of the work area and moves downward. In some models the air moves downward all the way through the work area before it is returned to the room air. In other models the air moves downward initially but then turns inside the work area and exits from the hood through the opening at the front of the hood.

Laminar air flow can be easily disrupted, which will increase the risk of contamination. Sneezing, coughing, talking directly into a hood, and breezes from open doors or windows can disrupt the air flow sufficiently to contaminate the work area.

Positioning of material and working inside a hood requires training, practice, and attention to details. Because laminar flow air begins to mix with outside air near the edge of the hood, all the work should be done at least 6 inches inside the hood to derive the benefits of the laminar air flow. A direct, open path must be maintained between the filter and the area inside the hood. Air downstream from nonsterile objects, such as solution containers or the operator's hands, becomes contaminated from particles blown off these objects. Large objects such as solution containers should not be placed at the back of the work area next to the filter. These objects contaminate everything downstream in addition to disrupting the laminar flow pattern of the air (see Figure 25.1).

Because laminar flow hoods blow air toward the operator, *biological safety cabinets* are preferred when protection for both the personnel and the environment is desired. Biological safety cabinets are designed differently than laminar flow hoods. They take air into the cabinet through a prefilter and channel it through a HEPA filter located in the top of the cabinet. The air flow is directed downward toward the work surface, just as with a vertical laminar flow hood. As the air approaches the work surface, however, it is pulled through vents at the front, back, and sides of the cabinet. The air is channeled so a major portion is recirculated back into the cabinet and a minor portion is passed through another HEPA filter before being exhausted into the room.

There are two types of biological safety cabinets:

- Class 2, type A (just described), represents the minimum recommended environment for preparing chemotherapy agents.

- Class 2, type B, cabinets have greater intake flow velocities and are vented outside the building rather than back into the room.

Biological safety hoods should be used only when preparing chemotherapy drugs because these hoods protect both the personnel and the environment from contamination. Laminar flow hoods should not be used because they blow air across the work surface toward the operator and into the work environment.

Maintaining laminar flow hoods and biological safety cabinets is essential. Changing prefilters and HEPA filters, non-routine cleaning of the hood, and any other maintenance should be done according to the manufacturer's recommendations and time schedules. A quality control standard operating procedure (SOP) should be developed and followed for each hood, to ensure that maintenance is done when required and to document that maintenance indeed has been done. A sample document has been published.[2]

Clean Rooms

In a pharmacy, laminar flow hoods and biological safety hoods generally are housed in an area that is isolated from the main traffic. These areas are commonly referred to as *clean rooms*. Originally, clean room facilities varied significantly between pharmacies, but the USP/NF <797> regulations now state that clean room facilities

- must be a designated area in the pharmacy,

- should be in a section of the facility where traffic is limited,

- must have unrestricted air flow,

- must allow only designated personnel to enter the space, and only for the purpose of aseptic preparation,

- should be large enough to accommodate all the necessary equipment such as the laminar flow hoods (or safety cabinets) needed for aseptic compounding, and

- should provide for the proper storage of drugs and supplies.

There should be an additional room adjacent to the clean room (the anteroom), where gowning and handwashing take place.

The regulations also state that clean rooms must have flow properties where the air quality, temperature, and humidity are highly regulated, to greatly reduce the risk of cross-contamination. The air in a clean room must be filtered repeatedly to remove dust particles, particulates, and other impurities. The clean room usually has only one door, which should remain closed when not in use. It should have positive pressure, which means that when the door is open, the air will flow out of the clean room.[3]

Filters

Filters are used to remove particles from solutions. These particles might be particulate matter, or they might be microorganisms. The two types of filters are:

1. *depth filters*, which trap particles by passing the solution through tortuous channels, and
2. *membrane filters*, more commonly used, consisting of materials with pores of a uniform size; the pores retain particles larger than their size.

Both the depth filter and the membrane filter are available in a wide range of pore sizes. Common pore sizes are 0.22, 0.45, 1.2, 5.0, and 10.0 microns. Filters are packaged in a variety of ways. Membrane filters often are packaged in a round plastic holder that can be easily attached to the end of a syringe. Some filters are attached to administration sets and serve as "final filters," (e.g., a Pall filter), which filters the solution immediately before it enters the patient's vein. In some administration sets, filters are built into the set already.

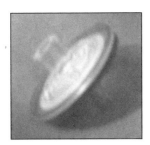 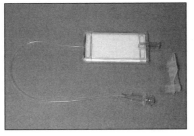

Filters also can be placed inside of needles; these are called *filter needles*. Double ended filter needles comprise a simple unit that has a filter between two needles. This allows the solution to be transferred directly from one container to another container and eliminates the need for using a syringe to transfer the

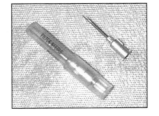

solution. Filters also are supplied as single units to be used in specialized filtration apparatus.

The depth filter is rigid enough so a solution can be filtered either by pulling it into or expelling it from a syringe. Pulling the drug solution into the syringe requires the following steps:

1. Attach the filter needle to the syringe.
2. Pull the solution into the syringe.
3. Remove air bubbles from the syringe.
4. Remove the filter needle.
5. Attach a new needle to the syringe.
6. Expel the solution from the syringe into the next container.

A new needle is required before pushing the solution out of the syringe into the next container. If the solution is pushed back through the same filter needle, the solution will be recontaminated.

Membrane filters are intended to filter a solution only as it is expelled from a syringe. The steps are as follows:

1. Attach a regular needle to the syringe.
2. Pull the solution into the syringe.
3. Remove air bubbles from the syringe.
4. Remove the needle from the syringe.
5. Attach a membrane filter to the syringe.
6. Place a regular needle on the other end of the filter.
7. Eliminate air from the filter chamber by holding the syringe in a vertical position so the needle is pointing upward. Air must be expelled before the filter becomes wet; otherwise, the air will not pass through the filter.
8. Once air has been expelled, apply pressure slowly and continuously to push the solution from the syringe, through the filter, and into the next container.

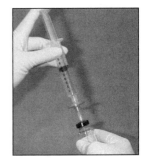

Syringes

The basic parts of a syringe are

- the *barrel*, a tube that is open at one end and tapers into a hollow tip at the other end,
- the *plunger*, a piston-type rod with a slightly cone-shaped top that moves inside the barrel of the syringe, and
- the *tip of the syringe*, which provides the point of attachment for a needle.

The volume of solution inside a syringe is indicated by *graduation lines* on the barrel. Graduation lines may be expressed in milliliters or in fractions of a milliliter, depending on the capacity of the syringe. The larger the capacity, the larger is the interval between graduation lines.

The three common types of hypodermic syringe tips are Slip-Tip®, Luer-Lok®, and eccentric. Slip-Tips® allow the needle to be held on the syringe by friction. The needle is reasonably secure, but it may come off if it is not attached properly or if considerable pressure is applied. Luer-Lok® tips incorporate a collar with grooves that lock the needle in place. Eccentric tips, which are off-center, are used when the needle must be parallel to the plane of injection, such as an intradermal injection.

Syringes are available in different sizes ranging from 1 to 60 ml. As a rule, the syringe should have a capacity the next size larger than the volume to be measured. For example, a 3 ml syringe should be selected to measure 2.3 ml and a 5 ml syringe to measure 3.8 ml. In this way, the graduation marks on the syringe will be in the smallest possible increments for the volume measured. Syringes should not be filled to capacity because the plunger can be dislodged easily.

Liquids are drawn into the syringe by pulling back on the plunger. The tip of the syringe must be submerged fully in the liquid to prevent air from being drawn into the syringe. Generally, an excess of solution is drawn

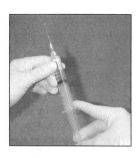

into the syringe so any air bubbles may be expelled by holding the syringe tip up, tapping the syringe until the air bubbles rise into the hub, and depressing the plunger to expel the air. This ensures that the hub will be filled completely with solution and the volume of delivery will be accurate.

When many repetitions of filling a syringe to the same volume are needed, the Cornwall syringe is used. This manual device has a two-way valve attached to both the syringe and the solution to be drawn into the syringe. Each time the grip is released, the syringe fills with solution. Each time the grip is compressed, the syringe volume is expelled. This basic design concept has electronic versions.

Needles

A needle has three parts:

1. the *hub*, which is at one end of the needle and is the part that attaches to the syringe,
2. the *shaft*, which is the long, slender stem of the needle, and
3. the *bevel*, which is the tapered point at the tip.

The hollow bore of the needle shaft is known as the *lumen*. Disposable needles always should be used when preparing admixtures, as they are presterilized and wrapped individually to maintain sterility.

Needle size is designated by length and gauge. The length of a needle is measured in inches from the juncture of the hub and the shaft to the tip of the point. Needle lengths range from $\frac{3}{8}$ inch to $3\frac{1}{2}$ inches, and some special use needles are even longer. The gauge of a needle, used to designate the size of the lumen, ranges from 27 (the finest) to 13 (the largest).

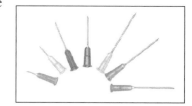

When choosing a needle size, the two considerations are

1. the viscosity of the solution, and
2. the nature of the rubber closure on the parenteral container.

Needles with larger lumens should be used for viscous solutions. Smaller gauge needles are preferred if the rubber closure can be cored easily. *Coring* occurs when a needle punctures or tears a piece of the rubber closure and the piece then falls into the container and contaminates the particulate material. To prevent coring:

1. Place the parenteral to be punctured on a flat surface and position the needle point on the surface of the rubber closure so the bevel is facing upward and the needle is at about a 45-degree angle to the closure surface.
2. Place downward pressure on the needle while gradually bringing the needle up to an upright position. Just before penetrating the closure, the needle should be at a vertical (90-degree) angle.

Administration Devices

Administration devices can be thought of as the connection between the patient and a parenteral formulation. Some formulations are administered quickly, but most are administered over some period of time, which could be as short as 0.5 hour and as long as 24 hours. Administration devices are used to provide access to the patient and control the rate of administration of the formulation into the patient.

Administration Set

The basic method to administer a LVP solution is to use an *administration set*. The set contains a spiked plastic device to pierce the administration set port on the LVP container. This connects to a *volume control* or *drip chamber* that may be used to set the flow rate. Drip

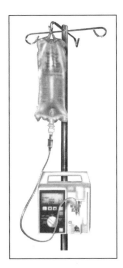

chambers control the flow rate by regulating the drop size. Another way to control the flow rate is to use a clamp that pinches the tubing.

A controller also may be used to regulate the flow rate. Most controllers use a photoelectric sensor to compare the actual gravity flow rate to a programmed flow rate, and relax or constrict the IV tubing to increase or decrease the flow rate. Beyond the flow rate controlling device, the line leads to a rubber injection port with a needle that is placed in the patient.

Piggybacks

Medications often are administered with *piggybacks* that are SVPs with 50–100 ml of fluid. Piggybacks can be connected directly to an administration set at a *y-injection* port, or may be connected directly to an infusion pump, where it is mixed with the primary LVP fluid. Piggybacks typically are infused over 30 to 60 minutes.

Heparin Locks

In some instances a patient does not have a primary LVP solution, yet must receive piggyback medications. This is done through a *heparin lock*, which is a short piece of tubing attached to a needle or an intravenous catheter. When the tubing is not being

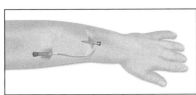

used for the piggyback, heparin is used to fill the tubing and that prevents blood from clotting in the tube.

Positive Pressure Infusion Devices (Pumps)

Positive pressure infusion devices generate a pressure that will cause fluid to flow through tubing into the patient's vascular system. These devices overcome minor occlusions and resistance associated with an intravenous system, viscous solutions, and vascular back pressure. Most pumps have operating pressures in the 2–12 pounds per square inch (psi) range. Pressures around 2 psi are used to keep the vascular access open, whereas arterial access requires pressures about 10–12 psi.

Combination Controllers and Pumps

Combination controllers and pumps provide both the safety of low infusion pressures and the availability of

positive pressure in one device. The user selects whether to use the device as a controller or as a pump.

Types of Positive Pressure Pumps

Positive pressure pumps include peristaltic pumps, cassette pumps, syringe pumps, and pumps with elastomeric reservoirs.

Peristaltic Pumps

Peristaltic pumps infuse solutions in "micropulses" produced by a massaging action on the IV tubing. Special infusion sets are used because the tubing has been reinforced with a silastic insert at the point of contact with the peristaltic mechanism. This reinforcement keeps the tubing from stretching and deforming, which would lead to variations in the flow rate. A linear peristaltic pump has finger-like projections that occlude the tubing in a successive manner in a rippling, wave-like motion. Rotary peristaltic pumps compress the tubing against a rotor housing with rollers mounted on it. As the rotor turns, the rollers occlude the tubing and force the fluid to flow toward the patient while drawing new fluid from the IV bag.

Cassette Pumps

Cassette pumps often are used as ambulatory pumps because many are about the size of a hand, allowing freedom of movement for the patient. In this type of pump, a cassette acts as a reservoir and fits into the pump housing. Tubing connects the cassette to the patient. The pump makes the cassette fill and then empty in two separate, sequential cycles to deliver a measured volume of fluid.

Syringe type cassette pumps move a motor-driven plunger into and out of a fluid-filled chamber. In a piston activated diaphragm cassette pump, a flexible diaphragm is mounted near a moving piston. Each inward stroke of the piston compresses the diaphragm, directing solution to the patient. Each outward stroke allows the diaphragm to relax and refills the chamber. Multiple chamber pumps allow one chamber to refill while the other chamber directs fluid to the patient.

Syringe Pumps

In a syringe pump, the syringe is attached to a pump that expels solution from the syringe by advancing either the plunger or the barrel of the syringe at a predetermined rate. Syringe pumps commonly are used for the infusion of intermittent medications such as antibiotics, antineoplastic drugs, analgesics, and anesthetics. Because they can deliver solutions at very low and precisely controlled flow rates, they are especially useful for neonatal, infant, and critical care applications where small volumes have to be given over extended periods of time.

Pumps with Elastomeric Reservoirs

A pump with an elastomeric reservoir is a tennis ball sized pump with a balloon-like reservoir surrounded by a rigid, protective outer shell. The elastic reservoir is filled with a solution that exerts a constant positive pressure, forcing the solution through the tubing into the patient. The combination of the pressure and dimensions of the tubing determines the pump's flow rate. The fill volume and the flow rate are design factors of the individual pump. Fill volumes, however, range from 50–400 ml, and flow rates from 2–200 ml/hr. These are single use pumps.

Processes

In a general sense, a *process* is any mechanism or activity that establishes a high degree of assurance that specific objectives are being achieved. Concerning sterile dosage forms, the objective is to produce products that consistently meet predetermined specifications and quality attributes. Sterile products are required to be sterile, pyrogen-free, and within limits with respect to particulate matter. Thus, many processes are included both in the compounding and the quality assurance of sterile dosage forms. Several of these processes are detailed below.

Sterilization

Sterilization is the process of killing or removing all viable microorganisms from materials. The USP/NF chapter <1211> Sterilization and Sterility Assurance of Compendial Articles describes sterilization by five processes:[4]

1. steam (moist heat)
2. dry heat
3. ionized radiation
4. gas
5. filtration

Steam

The most common and dependable method of sterilization is steam, or moist heat. This method employs water under pressure and elevated temperature. When water is heated to 121°C (which requires a pressure of approximate 30 psi), it is converted to saturated steam. When the steam makes contact with a cooler object, it condenses back to water and transfers heat to the object. Therefore, materials being sterilized by this method must contain water or permit saturated steam to penetrate and make contact with all surfaces to be sterilized.

The moist heat causes bacteria or spore cellular proteins to coagulate, which leads to cell death. The sterilization of materials requires 15 minutes at 121°C and typically is done in an autoclave. Most autoclaves have air exhaust systems so air can be removed and replaced with steam. Moist heat is the desired method of sterilization for any item that can withstand high temperatures. Common materials that are sterilized by moist heat include

- aqueous solutions or suspensions,
- glassware (Pyrex),
- surgical dressings,
- rubber articles,
- sealed glass ampules, and
- high density plastic tubing.

Dry Heat

Dry heat sterilization is used when materials cannot be steam sterilized (i.e., surfaces that cannot be wetted by steam). Dry heat also is used to depyrogenate glass and other inert surfaces, but the temperatures required are much higher than needed for sterilization. The sterilization process is carried out in a convection oven (either gas heated or electric heated). Dry heat is less efficient than moist heat, so longer exposure times and higher temperatures are required. The various heating cycles that can be used are

- 180°C (360°F) for 45 minutes
- 170°C (340°F) for 60 minutes
- 160°C (320°F) for 120 minutes
- 150°C (300°F) for 150 minutes
- 140°C (285°F) for 180 minutes

Table 25.3 lists chemicals and containers that are dry heat sterilized.

TABLE 25.3: CHEMICALS AND MATERIALS THAT CAN BE DRY HEAT STERILIZED

Chemicals That Must Be Dry Heat Sterilized	Containers That Can be Dry Heat Sterilized If Not Heat Labile
Bulk powders	Glassware (flasks, bottles, test tubes, funnels)
Petrolatum	Ampules
Oils	Petri dishes
Greases	Ointment jars
Waxes	

Ionized Radiation

Radiation sterilization is the method of choice for materials that cannot withstand high temperatures. Because of the cost and requirements of producing the radiation, this method generally is used only for large scale applications. The two types of radiation are

1. particulate radiation (protons, neutrons, etc.), and
2. electromagnetic radiation such as X-rays, gamma radiation, and ultraviolet light.

Electromagnetic radiation is less costly to produce than particulate radiation and has better penetrating power. Gamma radiation is used to sterilize plastic bottles, bags, syringes, and intravenous administration sets.

Gas

Materials that cannot withstand high temperatures, moisture, or radiation sterilization can be gas sterilized. The ideal gas must be able to penetrate materials, yet be removed completely at the end of the cycle. The only viable sterilizing gas is ethylene oxide. Newer agents being utilized include chlorine dioxide, peracetic acid, and vapor phase hydrogen peroxide.

Ethylene oxide alkylates the DNA and RNA of microorganisms and is effective at a concentration of 250 to 1,500 mg/Liter. A typical cycle would use a temperature of 30°–65°C, 30%–60% relative humidity, and an exposure time between 4 and 8 hours. Ethylene oxide has the disadvantage of being highly flammable and leaving a toxic reside (ethylene glycol, ethylene chlorohydrin) on treated materials.

Filtration

Filtration does not destroy microorganisms but, rather, removes them from the product. Filtration is not a *terminal sterilization procedure* as are the other methods. Filtration will sterilize the product, but after filtration, the sterile product is aseptically combined with its packaging. Filtration is used for materials that are chemically or physically unstable if sterilized by heat, gas, or radiation.

Depth filters are not used for filtration sterilization. They are constructed of randomly oriented fibers or particles (diatomaceous earth, porcelain, asbestos) that have been pressed, wound, or otherwise bonded together to form a tortuous pathway for flow. Because the random structure of material inside the filter creates fluid flow pathways that can vary from extremely narrow to very wide, microorganisms could pass through a depth filter and not be removed from the formulation being filtered. Filter materials also can break off or come loose during filtration, and appear in the filtrate.

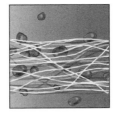

Membrane filters have a continuous uniform structure that consists of fixed size pores. Particles that are larger than the pore openings cannot pass through the filter and are retained on the surface of the filter. The amount of material a membrane filter retains is limited by the surface area of the filter. A pore size of 0.22 microns is required to render solutions free of microorganisms.

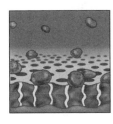

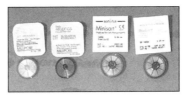
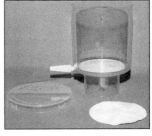

Membrane filters are available commercially as sheets or circles of the filter material that are placed in specially designed holders or platforms. They also are available ready assembled in holders or platforms.

Membrane filters used in an administration set will eliminate the risk of air embolism. Once a membrane filter is wet, air cannot pass through it unless the "bubble point pressure" of the filter is exceeded. Bubble point pressures for a 0.22 micron membrane filter are approximately 55 psi, a pressure that will not occur during parenteral administration. Therefore, any air that enters the administration set will be stopped at the filter surface and not allowed to enter the patient's body.

The same bubble point pressure is used in another way: After a filter is used, the integrity of the filter can be determined if the wetted filter is exposed to a gas under high pressure. If the filter is intact, the appearance of bubbles on the filter surface should occur when the gas pressure is about 50–55 psi. If the filter integrity has been compromised, however, the bubble point pressure will be much lower.

When selecting a membrane filter, several parameters must be considered. Hydrophilic filters are easily wetted and are used for aqueous solutions. Hydrophobic filters repel water but allow solvents such as alcohol and air to pass, so these filters would be used to sterilize solutions that contain alcohol or isopropyl alcohol, or as air filters. Other considerations include the filter's volume capacity, how much pressure can be applied to the filter without damaging its integrity, and the filter's compatibility or adsorption profile for the material being filtered.

The material to be filtered also requires consideration. Viscous oils can be filtered, but this is a time-consuming process. Heating the oil reduces its viscosity and makes filtration easier. Some powders also can be filtration sterilized by first dissolving the powder in a solvent and filtering the resulting solution, then evaporating the solvent under aseptic conditions.

Combinations of Sterilization Methods

Sterilization methods can be combined. For example, a sterile suspension can be prepared by heat sterilizing the powder ingredients, filtration sterilizing the vehicle, and then aseptically combining the two sterile phases.

Consideration also must be given to the sterilization of containers, closures, and apparatus. A nonsterile surface that comes in contact with a sterilized product will render the product nonsterile. These contact surfaces also must be pyrogen-free. The temperatures and times necessary for depyrogenation are substantially greater than those for sterility. It probably will be necessary to depyrogenate containers, closures, and apparatus separately from the formulation, and then aseptically combine them.

Several references have listed the procedural details for sterility testing.[5] Of the two general types of tests, one involves the use of culture medium and the other uses biological indicators. When using culture medium, the test sample can be introduced directly into the medium or the sample can be filtered and the filter transferred to the culture medium.

The preferred method of verifying sterility is to use biological indicators. A *biological indicator* is a preparation of a specific microorganism that is resistant to a particular sterilization process. The microorganisms are embedded either on paper or on plastic strips and are included with the materials being sterilized. The microorganisms used for the different sterilization methods are shown in Table 25.4.

TABLE 25.4: BIOLOGICAL INDICATORS FOR STERILIZATION METHODS

Method of Sterilization	Biological Indicator
Moist heat, ethylene oxide	*Bacillus stearothermophilus*
Dry heat	*Bacillus subtilis*
Ionizing radiation	*Bacillus pumilus, Bacillus stearothermophilus, Bacillus subtilis*

Sterility Testing

According to the USP/NF chapter <797>, sterile products that are produced from nonsterile components should be tested for the presence of microbial contaminants and pyrogens. Procedures for sterility testing are described in chapter <71>[6] and chapter <1211>. Routine sterility tests of compounded formulations are performed by inoculating culture medium and checking for signs of microbial growth by counting colony forming units (CFU) on the solid medium, or using turbidimetry of broth cultures.[7] Further identification of microorganisms is accomplished using various biochemical tests and is recommended by USP for natural products, oral and topical solutions, and suspensions. These testing processes allow for the conditional release of the product before completing the sterility test; however, the pharmacy must implement methods for recall if the product is found to be contaminated.

Media Fills

The "Validation" section of the chapter <797> describes an evaluation procedure commonly referred to as *media fills*. The evaluation involves an operator manipulating microbial growth medium (usually soybean casein digest medium) according to a prescribed procedure. The procedure requires multiple aseptic transfers to multiple containers. It is recommended that the validation procedure be done at peak periods of fatigue, stress, and pacing demands (e.g., immediately after normal production activity).

The premise behind medium fills is that the growth medium will support the growth of the contaminating microbe and that this growth can be detected. The other requirement of the validation is that the medium must be manipulated using the same aseptic techniques actually being evaluated. This validation is not intended to be a one-time evaluation. The USP recommends that competent operators be challenged quarterly. Other references suggest that 40 validation samples should be prepared for each 800 admixtures prepared, or that 10 validation samples be prepared each month.[8] Regardless of the frequency, a competent sterile compounder will have to be evaluated on a regular and ongoing basis.

Other Methods

A sterility testing process might involve routinely sending formulations to a contract analytical laboratory. Analysis of drug content, sterility, and pyrogenicity can be done using randomly selected samples. Or the process could consist of observing and testing formulation variables such as color, clarity, uniformity of dispersion, odor, consistency, pH, specific gravity, and so forth.

The process also could consist of documenting adherence to formulation records, policies and procedures, SOPs using compounding records, or techniques or procedures. Some example forms for home infusion pharmacies have been published.[9] Sample documentation forms for routine techniques and procedures are provided at the end of this chapter. These examples would be modified as necessary for each individual pharmacy.

Depyrogenation

Pyrogens are organic compounds that are soluble in water and are not removed by filtration. They usually are *endotoxins*, which are lipopolysaccharides produced by gram-negative bacteria. Pyrogens are introduced into formulations through water, glassware, equipment, or chemicals, especially chemicals crystallized or precipitated from contaminated water. Pyrogens tend to be stable over a long time.[10]

A formulation can be tested to be pyrogen-free using a rabbit test, which involves injecting rabbits with the product and then determining the degree of rise in their body temperature. Obviously, this test is not practical in a pharmacy, but there is a Limulus Amebocyte Lysate (LAL) reagent. The procedure for detecting endotoxins or pyrogens is described in the chapter <85> Bacterial

Endotoxins Test.[11] LAL contains a clottable protein in the presence of endotoxins. The detection endpoints are the formation of a gel in the gel-clot method, or turbidity or a chromogenic substance in the spectrophotometric method. The quantity of endotoxin is expressed in USP Endotoxin Units (USP-EU) and is estimated from a parallel serial dilution of the sample, as well as reference endotoxin in the gel-clot method, or extrapolated from a calibration curve in the spectrophotometric method.

Depyrogenation (the destruction or elimination of pyrogens or endotoxins) is achieved using a variety of methods: heat, acid and base hydrolysis, liquid hydrogen peroxide, radiation, ultrafiltration, and affinity chromatography. Many of these methods cannot be done by a compounding pharmacist. What can be done is to rinse rubber stoppers and plastic materials with copious amounts of Sterile Water for Injection. Equipment can be depyrogenized by heating it at 250°C for 45 minutes. Because this extreme heat will effect most formulations, the equipment must be treated before compounding begins, and aseptic techniques must be used during the compounding procedure to prevent the introduction of pyrogens.

Particulate Matter

Particulate matter consists of the mobile, undissolved substances unintentionally present in parenteral products. The USP requires that every final container of an injection be inspected visually. Injection production lots are inspected manually under good light against a black and white background. This inspection will reveal particulate matter about and above 50 micron in size. A SOP for a compounding pharmacy has been published.[12]

Testing for particulate matter below 50 microns is carried out using electronic imaging systems that count and measure the size of particles by means of a shadow cast by the particles as they pass through a high-intensity light beam. If the product is not a clear, colorless solution or if it exceeds the limits specified for the light obscuration test, it is submitted for a microscopic count test.

Effectiveness of Preservatives

Preservatives such as antioxidants, antimicrobials, and antifungals often are added to formulations to improve the stability of the product or to protect it from microbial contamination. The USP/NF chapter <51> addresses testing of the effectiveness of antimicrobial protection.[13] Typical dosage forms that must demonstrate antimicrobial effectiveness include ophthalmics, nasal, dialysis, and otic products and formulations.

Incompatibilities

Incompatibility refers to physicochemical phenomena such as concentration dependent precipitation and acid–base reactions that result in a visually evident change in the product. These changes might include precipitation, cloudiness or haziness, color change, viscosity change, effervescence (evolution of a gas), or the formation of immiscible layers.[14,15] Factors that cause incompatibilities include pH, solubility, concentration, complexation, and light. Incompatibilities occur when two or more drugs are mixed together, or between a drug and its vehicle or container. Most incompatibilities are found when the drug is dissolved or dispersed in a vehicle, not when the drug is in powder form.

The most important factor responsible for incompatibility is a change in the acid–base environment, as pH is a critical parameter in a drug's solubility and its stability. Although profiles of pH solubility and pH degradation rate are determined early in a drug's development, these two rates may not be directly related. For example, increasing the pH might increase the solubility of a drug but would cause it to degrade faster. The acid–base environment can be altered when diluting, adding another drug or ingredient, or changing the type of container. Temperature also has an effect on pH.

Incompatibilities expected when a drug is placed into an aqueous solution can be different than those expected if the drug is dissolved in a non-aqueous solvent. Non-aqueous solvents may have very different viscosities than water. Some drugs must be formulated in co-solvent mixtures for dissolution, and the effect of that environment might be difficult to predict. Some of these non-aqueous solvents are alcohol, propylene glycol, glycerin, polyethylene glycols, and oils such as corn, cottonseed, and peanut.

Some drug products are stable and compatible at selected concentrations but not at other concentrations. Generally, the more concentrated a drug solution, the greater is the likelihood that an instability or incompatibility will occur, although this rule has exceptions.

Light-sensitive drugs generally are packaged by the manufacturer in appropriate light-resistant containers. The incompatibility comes when the drug is removed from that container and placed in a new environment that does not afford the necessary light protection.

Another type of incompatibility is called *leaching*, in which a substance is removed from, or leached out of, something else. Most commonly a solution will leach a chemical out of the container in which it is stored. Several preparations and drugs are known to leach the plasticizer di-2-ethylhexl phthalate (DEHP) from polyvinyl chloride bags. DEHP is a known carcinogen. Therefore, these formulations are packaged in ethylene-vinyl acetate containers.

Suggestions for minimizing incompatibilities are the following:

- Use only freshly prepared solutions.
- Follow an established order of mixing, and mix the formulation thoroughly after adding each ingredient.

Do not shake products vigorously unless indicated in the labeling. Rotate or swirl products to minimize foaming and the formation of air bubbles.

- Use as few additives as possible.
- Dilute any problem additive.
- Develop an incompatibility table or file for frequently compounded formulations. Information can be obtained from published resources. (This information is valid only for the specific drug and concentration, the manufacturer, the container, and so on.)
- If the solution is filtered, ensure that any removed particulate matter is not the active drug. Have information about the "sorption" tendency of the drug and selected filter system.

If an incompatibility cannot be corrected or prevented, consider the following administration techniques:

- Administer the drugs separately at staggered times.
- Flush the administration line or set between drug administrations, and use normal saline, not heparin.
- Use an alternative site of administration.

Concentrations Commonly Used in Parenteral Solutions

The drug concentration in a parenteral solution may be stated in a variety of ways. Each method of expressing the concentration is related to a specific property of the solution. The common concentrations and their units are:

- International Units (activity per volume)
- Percentage (weight per volume, volume per volume, weight per weight)
- Molecular Weight (molecules per volume)
- Equivalents (valence per volume)
- Osmolarity (dissolved particles per volume)

Because the potency and purity of drugs from biological sources vary depending on the source, they are measured by units of activity rather than by weight. Drugs commonly measured in units include penicillin, insulin, heparin, and some vitamins.

Percentage concentrations refer to the drug's weight per 100 ml if the drug is a solid, or the drug's volume per 100 ml if the drug is a liquid and the vehicle is a liquid. For example, a 5% dextrose solution contains 5 grams of dextrose (a solid) in 100 ml of solution (weight/volume). A 5% acetic acid solution (common household vinegar) contains 5 ml of acetic acid (a liquid) per 100 ml of solution (volume/volume). Percentage

concentrations are applied to vehicles other than liquids. A 10% zinc oxide ointment would have 10 g of zinc oxide (a solid) in 100 g of ointment (weight/weight).

The measurement of molecules per volume or the number of moles per volume is expressed as molarity. A mole is the number of grams of a drug numerically equal to its molecular weight. The molecular weight is the sum of the atomic weights of all of the atoms that make up the drug. For example, potassium chloride (KCl) has a molecular weight of 74.6. One mole of potassium chloride would be 74.6 grams.

Most often, parenteral concentrations are expressed as mole/liter (written as mol/L, or M). Thus, a 1 M solution of potassium chloride would have 74.6 grams of the drug in 1,000 ml (1 liter) of solution. Some molarity concentrations are expressed as millimole/L. A millimole is one-thousandth of a mole, which would be 74.6 mg in 1,000 ml of solution.

When determining the molecular weight of a drug, it is critical to take into account the salt form of the drug and the "waters of hydration." Drugs come in different salt forms for a variety of reasons. For example, chloride is found as sodium salt, potassium salt, and calcium salt. The waters of hydration are water molecules that become associated with drug molecules. For example, calcium chloride ($CaCl_2$) exists in three different hydration forms —anhydrous (no associated waters), the dihydrate with two associated waters, and the hexahydrate with six waters of hydration. The dihydrate form is the one used in making parenteral solutions.

Another expression of concentration is the equivalent (Eq). This is the way concentrations of common electrolytes, such as potassium chloride, sodium chloride, and sodium acetate, are expressed. An equivalent weight is equal to the molecular weight of the drug divided by the valence of the ions that form when the drug is dissolved in solution. The valence of the ions is either the number of positive charges *or* the number of negative charges, not both.

When an electrolyte dissolves in solution, it divides into ions. For example, potassium chloride (KCl) splits into one potassium ion (K^+) and one chloride ion (Cl^-); therefore, the valence of KCl is 1 because there is either one positive charge on the potassium ion or one negative charge on the chloride ion. Anhydrous calcium chloride ($CaCl_2$) dissociates into one calcium ion (Ca^{++}) and two chloride ions (Cl^-). Its valence is equal to 2 because there are either two positive charges on the single calcium ion or one negative charge on two chloride ions. An equivalent weight of KCL would be 74.6 g divided by 1, or 74.6 g. An equivalent weight of $CaCl_2$ would be 111.0 g divided by 2, or 55.5 g. Equivalent solutions are expressed as Eq/liter (written as Eq/L). Thus, a 1 Eq solution of potassium chloride would have 74.6 g in

1,000 ml (1 liter) of solution. Some equivalent concentrations are expressed as milliequivalents/L. A milliequivalent is one-thousandth of an equivalent weight.

The other common expression for concentration is the osmole (Osmol). An osmole is equal to the molecular weight of the drug divided by the number of ions formed when a drug dissociates in solution. Potassium chloride forms two ions when it dissolves in solution. Therefore, 1 Osmol of potassium chloride would be its molecular weight (74.6 g) divided by 2 (1 Osmol = 37.3 g). Anhydrous calcium chloride forms three ions when it dissolves in solution; 1 Osmol would be its molecular weight (111.0 g) divided by 3 (1 Osmol = 37.0 g). Most Osmol solutions are expressed as Osmol/liter (written as Osmol/L). Some concentrations are expressed as mOsmol/L. A milliosmole is one-thousandth of an osmole.

NOTES

1. <788> Particulate Matter in Injections: The United States Pharmacopeia 29/National Formulary 24, The United States Pharmacopeial Convention, Inc., Rockville, MD, 2005, pp. 2722–2729.

2. Allen, L.V., Jr. Standard Operating Procedure for Maintenance of a Horizontal Laminar Air Flow Hood. *International Journal of Pharmaceutical Compounding* 1:344–345, 1997.

3. <797> Pharmaceutical Compounding—Sterile Preparations: The United States Pharmacopeia 29/National Formulary 24, The United States Pharmacopeial Convention, Inc., Rockville, MD, 2005, pp. 2735–2751.

4. <1211> Sterilization and Sterility Assurance of Compendial Articles: The United States Pharmacopeia 29/National Formulary 24, The United States Pharmacopeial Convention, Inc., Rockville, MD, 2005, pp. 3041–3046.

5. Hagman, D. E. Sterilization (chapter 40) in *Remington: The Science and Practice of Pharmacy*, 21st edition. Lippincott Williams & Wilkins, Philadelphia, PA, 2006, pp. 776–801.

6. <71> Sterility Tests: The United States Pharmacopeia 29/National Formulary 24, The United States Pharmacopeial Convention, Inc., Rockville, MD, 2005, pp. 2508–2513.

7. <81> Antibiotics—Microbial Assays: The United States Pharmacopeia 29/National Formulary 24, The United States Pharmacopeial Convention, Inc., Rockville, MD, 2005, pp. 2513–2520.

8. Schneider, P. J. Process Validation (chapter 16) in Buchanan, E. C, McKinnon, B. T., Scheckelhoff, D. J, and Schneider, P. J. *Principles of Sterile Product Preparation*. American Society of Health-System Pharmacists, Inc., Bethesda, MD, 1995, pp. 121–124.

9. Lima, H. A. Required Documentation for Home Infusion Pharmacies—Compounding Records. *International Journal of Pharmaceutical Compounding* 2:354–359, 1998.

10. Akers, M. J. Sterilization and Depyrogenation: Principles and Methods. *International Journal of Pharmaceutical Compounding* 3:263–269, 1999.

11. <85> Bacterial Endotoxins Test: The United States Pharmacopoeia 29/National Formulary 24, The United States Pharmacopeial Convention, Inc., Rockville, MD, 2005, pp 2521–2524.

12. Tran, T., Kupiec, T. C., and Trissel, L. A. Quality-Control Analytical Methods: Particulate Matter in Injections: What is it and What are the Concerns? *International Journal of Pharmaceutical Compounding* 10:202–204, 2006.

13. <51> Antimicrobial Effectiveness Testing: The United States Pharmacopoeia 29/National Formulary 24, The United States Pharmacopeial Convention, Inc., Rockville, MD, 2005, pp. 2499–2500.

14. Lima, H. A. Drug Stability and Compatibility: Special Considerations for Home Health Care. *International Journal of Pharmaceutical Compounding* 1:301–305, 1997.

15. Allen, L. V., Jr. Parenteral Admixture Incompatibilities: An Introduction. *International Journal of Pharmaceutical Compounding* 1:165–167, 1997.

ADDITIONAL READING

Caputo, R. A., Huffman, A., and Reich, R. USP Chapter <797>: Practical Solutions for Microbiology, Sterility and Pyrogen Testing. *International Journal of Pharmaceutical Compounding* 9:11–13, 2005.

Dawson, M. F. Basics of Compounding: Application of the USP Bacterial Endotoxins Test to Compounded Sterile Preparations. *International Journal of Pharmaceutical Compounding* 10:36–39, 2006.

Rice, S. P., and Markel, J. A. A Review of Parenteral Admixtures Requiring Select Containers and Administration Sets. *International Journal of Pharmaceutical Compounding* 6:120–122, 2002.

McGuire, J., and Kupiec, T. C. Quality-Control Analytial Methods: The quality of Sterility Testing. *International Journal of Pharmaceutical Compounding* 11:52–55, 2007.

DOCUMENTATION OF PROCESS VALIDATION

Handwashing Technique

Procedure	YES	NO
Removes all jewelry, watches, etc., up to elbow	☐	☐
Starts water and adjusts to appropriate temperature	☐	☐
Avoids unnecessary splashing during process	☐	☐
Scrubs hands starting with fingernails first, using appropriate scrub brush	☐	☐
Uses sufficient antimicrobial cleanser and scrubs thoroughly for at least 30 seconds	☐	☐
Cleans all four surfaces of each finger	☐	☐
Cleans all surfaces of hands, wrists, and arms up to the elbows, using a circular motion	☐	☐
Does not touch sink, faucet, or other objects that may contaminate hands during the process	☐	☐
Rinses off all soap residue	☐	☐
Rinses hands holding them upright and allowing water to drip down to elbow	☐	☐
Does not turn off water until hands are completely dry	☐	☐
Turns off water with a clean, dry, lint-free paper towel	☐	☐
Does not touch faucet or sink while turning off water	☐	☐

Place a checkmark (✔) in the appropriate column while observing the personnel.

Evaluator:

Date Evaluated:

DOCUMENTATION OF PROCESS VALIDATION

Cleaning a Horizontal Laminar Flow Hood

Procedure	YES	NO
Follows proper handwashing procedure and uses proper technique	☐	☐
Wears appropriate apparel as required by institution (gown, gloves, etc.)	☐	☐
Knows that hood should be left running continuously	☐	☐
If hood was turned off, turns it on and lets run for a least 30 minutes prior to use	☐	☐
Selects clean gauze and 70% isopropyl alcohol to clean hood	☐	☐
Does not spray alcohol inside hood	☐	☐
Cleans IV pole first, if applicable	☐	☐
Cleans sides of hood second, beginning at the top and working in a vertical motion from back to front of hood with overlapping strokes	☐	☐
Cleans work surface of hood last, beginning in back and working in a horizontal motion from side to side with overlapping strokes	☐	☐
Does not contaminate previously cleaned surfaces at any time during processes	☐	☐
Stands outside the hood properly, allowing only the head to enter inside the hood	☐	☐
Does not contaminate hood by coughing, sneezing, chewing gum, or excessive talking	☐	☐
Knows that hood certification is every 6 months, if moved, or if filter damage is suspected	☐	☐
Knows that prefilter should be changed monthly	☐	☐

Place a checkmark (✔) in the appropriate column while observing the personnel.

Evaluator: _____

Date Evaluated: _____

DOCUMENTATION OF PROCESS VALIDATION

Vial Reconstitution and Transfer to IV Bag

Procedure	YES	NO
Performs all required calculations prior to drug preparation	☐	☐
Follows proper handwashing procedure and uses proper technique	☐	☐
Wears appropriate apparel as required by institution (gown, gloves, etc.)	☐	☐
Cleans laminar flow hood following proper procedure and technique	☐	☐
Brings the correct drugs (correct strength/concentrations) into the hood for preparation	☐	☐
Brings the correct supplies into the hood before beginning the procedure	☐	☐
Inspects all products for particulate matter, contamination prior to use, expiration date	☐	☐
Removes dust cover from drugs and supplies before placing them in the hood	☐	☐
Cleans rubber diaphragm on vial correctly with alcohol prep pad	☐	☐
Assembles syringe and needle correctly in hood	☐	☐
Inserts needle correctly into vial to prevent coring	☐	☐
Adds desired volume of diluent to the vial and withdraws proper volume of air to prevent vial from aspirating	☐	☐
Allows drug to completely dissolve before withdrawing any liquid	☐	☐
Injects appropriate amount of air for fluid being withdrawn	☐	☐
Correctly measures amount of liquid to withdraw	☐	☐
Cleans the medication port of IV bag before injecting contents of syringe	☐	☐
Does not core or puncture side of medication port when adding drug to IV bag	☐	☐
Properly mixes contents of IV bag	☐	☐
Properly seals medication port of IV bag	☐	☐
Inspects final product contents for contaminants, particulate matter	☐	☐
Does not block air flow from HEPA filter with hands or other objects inside hood	☐	☐
Does not take hands out or leave hood during preparation	☐	☐
Does not use outer 6 inches of hood opening or work too close to side/back of hood	☐	☐
Does not contaminate hood by coughing, sneezing, chewing gum, or excessive talking	☐	☐
Properly discards all waste including sharps	☐	☐

Place a checkmark (✓) in the appropriate column while observing the personnel.

Evaluator: _____

Date Evaluated: _____

DOCUMENTATION OF PROCESS VALIDATION

Ampule Withdrawal and Transfer to IV Bag

Procedure	YES	NO
Performs all required calculations prior to drug preparation	☐	☐
Follows proper handwashing procedure and uses proper technique	☐	☐
Wears appropriate apparel as required by institution (gown, gloves, etc.)	☐	☐
Cleans laminar flow hood following proper procedure and technique	☐	☐
Brings the correct drugs (correct strength/concentrations) into the hood for preparation	☐	☐
Brings the correct supplies into the hood before beginning the procedure	☐	☐
Inspects all products for particulate matter, contamination prior to use, expiration date	☐	☐
Removes dust cover from drugs and supplies before placing them in the hood	☐	☐
Cleans ampule neck with alcohol swab before breaking	☐	☐
Wraps ampule neck with alcohol swab or gauze before breaking	☐	☐
Breaks ampule away from the body, HEPA filter, and other sterile products	☐	☐
Assembles filter needle/straw and syringe correctly in the hood	☐	☐
Withdraws fluid from ampule without spilling contents	☐	☐
Removes filter needle/straw and changes to a new needle to inject fluid into IV bag	☐	☐
Correctly measures amount of fluid to inject into IV bag	☐	☐
Cleans medication port of IV bag before injecting contents of syringe	☐	☐
Does not core or puncture side of medication port when adding drug to IV bag	☐	☐
Properly mixes contents of IV bag	☐	☐
Properly seals medication port of IV bag	☐	☐
Inspects final product contents for contaminants, particulate matter	☐	☐
Does not block air flow from HEPA filter with hands or other objects inside hood	☐	☐
Does not take hands out or leave hood during preparation	☐	☐
Does not use outer 6 inches of hood opening or work too close to side/back of hood	☐	☐
Does not contaminate hood by coughing, sneezing, chewing gum, or excessive talking	☐	☐
Properly discards all waste including sharps	☐	☐

Place a checkmark (✔) in the appropriate column while observing the personnel.

Evaluator: _____

Date Evaluated: _____

Sterile Compounding— Part 2: Aseptic Techniques

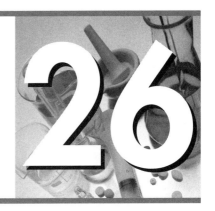

THE USP/NF CHAPTER <797> PHARMACEUTICAL COMpounding—Sterile Preparations[1] makes the point that sterile compounding requires cleaner facilities, specific training and testing of personnel in principles and practices of aseptic manipulations, air quality evaluation and maintenance, and knowledge of sterilization and solution stability principles and practices.[1] Other chapters in this book have covered facilities, air quality, sterilization, and stability. Aseptic techniques are detailed in this chapter.

Chapter <797> requires that sterile compounding be conducted in a laminar flow hood of ISO Class 5 (Class 100). The hoods are to be located in an ISO Class 8 (Class 100,000) clean room. Working in a specified laminar flow hood, however, is not sufficient to ensure sterility of the compounded formulation. The hood provides an ultra clean work area but does not provide sterility. Products that are placed in the hood for assembly or compounding are either sterilized beforehand or will be sterilized by filtration while in the hood. Personnel carrying out these procedures must use techniques to minimize potential contamination (by microorganisms, particulate material, pyrogens) during these manipulations.

Aseptic techniques are the sum total of methods and manipulations required to minimize the contamination of sterile products from the environment in which the formulation is being prepared or from the person preparing it. Aseptic techniques include everything from proper handwashing and gowning, to working in a laminar flow hood, to knowing how to manipulate vials, ampules, bags, syringes, needles, and filters inside a laminar flow hood, to proper inspection of the prepared formulation.

Working in a Laminar Flow Hood

The following are considered the minimum requirements for good aseptic technique. A much more extensive list of procedures has been published.[2]

1. Maintain a designated "clean" area around the hood. For example, cardboard cartons are notorious dust generators and should not be in the immediate vicinity of the hood.

2. Conduct all manipulations inside a properly maintained and certified laminar flow hood. Allow the laminar flow hood to operate for at least 30 minutes before use. Clean the laminar flow hood in accordance with an established procedure.

3. Assemble all necessary supplies and check each for packaging damage, expiration dates, and particulate material. Squeeze plastic solution containers to check for leaks. Use only sterilized needles, syringes, and filters; check the protective covering of each to verify that it is intact. Remove dust coverings.

4. Wear lint-free garments or clothing covers, head and facial hair covers, and a mask. Wear sterile gloves when working in the laminar flow hood or biological safety cabinet.

5. Remove all jewelry, and scrub hands and arms to the elbows with a suitable antibacterial agent, following an established procedure.

6. Place supplies in the hood with smaller supplies closer to the HEPA filter and larger supplies farther from the HEPA filter. Arrange supplies to maximize laminar flow. Plan the work area to be at least 3 inches from the back of the hood, and 6 inches inside the front of the hood.

7. Swab all surfaces that require entry (puncture) with an alcohol wipe. Avoid excess alcohol or lint that might be carried into the solution.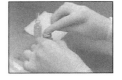

8. Give close attention to hand position and the direction of air flow over injection ports or objects being manipulated. Minimize hand movements within the hood.

9. Do all manipulations at least 6 inches inside the outer edge of the hood. Do not remove the hands from the hood until the compounding procedure is complete and the final inspection of the formulation has been done.

10. When using syringes, do not touch the syringe plunger with the fingers when the syringe will be used for multiple dilutions or manipulations.

11. Examine all completed formulations before removing them from the hood.

12. Return excess solutions to their original vial, an empty vial, or some other suitable, closed container before discarding them.

13. Place all syringes, needles, ampules, vials, and pre-filled syringes in puncture-proof containers, and dispose of them according to institutional procedures. In many health care facilities, these containers often are labeled "Sharps," indicating objects that might puncture or cut the skin of anyone who handles them.

Aseptically Transferring Drug From a Vial

Two types of parenteral vials are used in making admixtures: (1) a vial that already has the drug in solution, and (2) a vial requiring that a lyophilized powder be dissolved in a diluent to make a solution. In either case, a needle will be used to penetrate the rubber closure on the vial. *Coring* occurs when a needle punctures or tears a piece of the rubber closure and the piece then falls into the container and contaminates the vial with particulate material. To prevent coring:

1. Place the parenteral to be punctured on a flat surface, and position the needle point on the surface of the rubber closure so the bevel is facing upward and the needle is at about a 45-degree angle to the closure surface.

2. Place downward pressure on the needle while gradually bringing the needle up to an upright position. Just before penetrating the closure, the needle should be at a vertical (90-degree) angle.

If the drug is already in solution, the aseptic transfer technique is as follows:

1. Draw into the syringe a volume of air equal to the volume of drug solution to be withdrawn.

2. Place the vial on the work surface and penetrate the vial without coring. Inject the air.

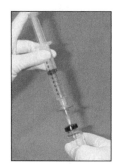

3. Invert the vial. Use one hand to hold the vial and the barrel of the syringe and the other hand to hold the syringe plunger.

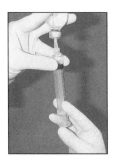

4. Withdraw the drug solution.

5. Fill the syringe to a slight excess of the drug solution. Remove all air bubbles from the syringe by

tapping the syringe. Once air bubbles have been removed, push the excess solution back into the vial.

6. Withdraw the needle from the vial.

7. Transfer the solution in the syringe into a final container, again minimizing coring.

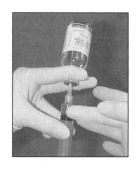

If the drug is a lyophilized powder in a vial, it will have to be reconstituted before it can be withdrawn. First determine the correct volume of suitable diluent to use. This information will be in the drug product information. Then follow these steps:

1. Perform steps 1–6 above to draw the correct volume of diluent into a syringe.

2. Transfer the diluent into the vial containing the lyophilized powder, minimizing coring.

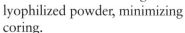

3. Once the diluent is added, remove a volume of air from the vial equal to slightly more than the volume of diluent added. This will create a negative pressure in the vial and decrease the likelihood that aerosol droplets will be sprayed when the needle is withdrawn.

4. Withdraw the needle.

5. Swirl the vial until the drug is dissolved.

6. Using a new needle and syringe, perform steps 1–6 again to withdraw the correct volume of reconstituted drug solution into the syringe.

7. Transfer the reconstituted drug solution in the syringe into a final container, again minimizing coring.

Aseptically Transferring Drug From an Ampule

Ampules have a colored stripe around the neck if they are pre-scored, to indicate that the manufacturer has weakened the neck to facilitate opening. Some ampules are not pre-scored by the manufacturer, so the neck first must be weakened (scored) with a fine file. The ampule always is broken open at the neck.

To open an ampule:

1. Hold the ampule upright and tap the top to remove solution from the headspace.

2. Swab the neck of the ampule with an alcohol swab.

3. Wrap the neck with an alcohol pad or gauze, and grasp the top with the thumb and index finger of

one hand. With the other hand, grasp the bottom of the ampule.

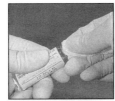

4. Quickly snap the ampule, moving the hands away and outward. Do not open the ampule toward the HEPA filter or any other sterile supplies in the hood. If the ampule does not snap easily, rotate it slightly and try again.

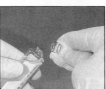

5. Inspect the opened ampule for any particles of glass that might have fallen inside.

To transfer the drug solution from an opened ampule:

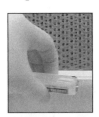

1. Hold the ampule at about a 20-degree down angle.

2. Insert a needle/straw into the ampule, taking care not to touch the ampule neck where it is broken.

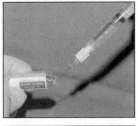

3. Position the needle in the shoulder area of the ampule, beveled edge down. This will avoid pulling glass particles into the syringe.

4. Withdraw the solution, but keep the needle submerged to avoid drawing air into the syringe.

5. Withdraw the needle from the ampule and remove all air bubbles from the syringe.

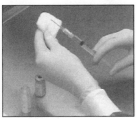

6. Transfer the solution to the final container, using a filter needle or membrane filter.

Aseptically Adding Drug Solution to LVP or SVP

Generally, LVP solutions are used as primary or continuous infusion solutions administered at a slow infusion rate. Drug additives then can be introduced directly into the LVP using a syringe and needle. Drug additives also can be introduced into the LVP at the *y-connection port* in the administration set or by using a minibag as a piggyback on the LVP.

All of these scenarios require a syringe and needle to transfer the drug additive solution into a plastic bag or an administration set injection port. The needle must be at least ½ inch long and not less than 19 gauge to ensure

that the inner diaphragm of the port will be penetrated and that the protective rubber cover will reseal.

To transfer a drug additive to a LVP or SVP container or an administration set with a needle and syringe:

1. Remove the protective covering from the medication port.

2. Assemble the needle and syringe and aseptically withdraw the necessary drug additive volume.

3. Swab the medication port with an alcohol swab.

4. Hold the medication port with one hand and insert the needle into the port with the other hand. Hold the port in such a way that the fingers are out of the way in case the needle punctures the port. Be sure that the medication port is extended fully to minimize the chance of punctures through the port.

5. Inject the drug additive solution.

6. Remove the needle.

7. Mix and inspect the admixture.

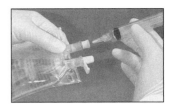

Inspections and End Product Evaluations

The compounded formulation should be inspected for

- container integrity or leaks,

- particulate material, and

- properties such as color, odor, fill volume, consistency, and so on.

Preparations in flexible containers should be squeezed to ensure the absence of unintended holes and slits. Glass bottles should be examined for cracks and leaking stoppers.

Visual inspection will show two of the six characteristics of parenteral solutions: (1) particulate material, and (2) stability if such stability is physically characterized by precipitation or crystallization. The presence (or absence) of particulate material is best determined by holding the parenteral against an illuminated white and black background.[3]

Formulation properties should be known beforehand and documented on the formulation record. The compounded product should be compared to these standards.

The pharmacist also should verify that the product was prepared accurately with respect to

- ingredients (check used vials, ampules, diluents),

- quantities (check syringe volumes used),

- containers (check final solution container), and

- instrumentation (check calibration and settings on repeat or automated dispensing devices).

During compounding, volumes of additives in syringes should be examined to confirm accurate measurement. The volumes of solutions remaining in vials and ampules should be determined to compare to the theoretical volumes required to make the formulation. A mass balance of materials should be evident. Also, additive containers and syringes should be available (not discarded in the trash) until the formulation checks have been completed.

Formulations should be subjected to quality control tests as outlined in the formulation record. These generally are the physical tests that can be conducted within the pharmacy and may involve weight variation, specific gravity, pH, filtration membrane integrity, and the like.

Formulations that are not distributed promptly should be inspected again before leaving the pharmacy. The purpose of the predistribution inspection is to check for defects such as precipitation, cloudiness, and leakage that may have developed during storage.

Special Solutions

Three types of special solutions are irrigation solutions, peritoneal dialysis solutions, and parenteral nutrition solutions.

Irrigation Solutions

Irrigation solutions are sterile solutions, but they are not administered into the venous system. They are packaged in containers larger than 1,000 ml capacity and are designed to empty rapidly. Surgical irrigating solutions (splash solutions) are used to bathe and moisten body tissues, to moisten dressings, or as a washing solution for instruments. They typically are Sodium Chloride for Irrigation or Sterile Water for Irrigation.

Urological irrigation solutions are used during surgery to maintain tissue integrity, and to remove blood to maintain a clear field of vision. Glycine Irrigation 1.5% and Sorbitol Irrigation 3% solutions are used commonly because they are non-hemolytic.

Peritoneal Dialysis Solutions

Dialysis refers to the passage of small particles through membranes. This is the action in which drug molecules in a solution of a higher concentration will move through a permeable membrane into a solution of a lower concentration. This principle is the basis for *peritoneal dialysis* solutions.

Peritoneal dialysis solutions are administered to patients who have compromised kidney function. The solution is administered directly into the peritoneal cavity to remove toxic substances, excessive body wastes, and serum electrolytes by dialysis. These solutions are made hypertonic to plasma so water will not move into the intravascular system but toxic components will move

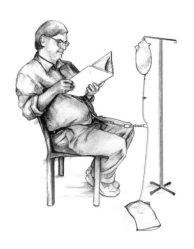

into the dialysis solution.

Peritoneal dialysis solutions are administered several times a day. The solution is permitted to flow into the abdominal cavity and remains in the cavity for 30 to 90 minutes. Then it is drained by a siphon tube into discharge bottles. This procedure may use up to 50 liters of solution per day. For this reason, peritoneal dialysis solutions are supplied in containers larger than 1,000 ml capacity.

Parenteral Nutrition Solutions

Parenteral nutrition solutions are complex admixtures used to provide nutritional support to patients who are unable to take in adequate nutrients via the gastrointestinal tract (enteral nutrition solutions). These admixtures are composed of dextrose, fat, protein, electrolytes, vitamins, and trace elements, and are hypertonic solutions. The two types of parenteral nutrition solutions are administered at different sites depending on the desired patient outcome.

1. *Peripheral parenteral nutrition (PPN)* solutions are most appropriate to prevent malnutrition rather than to correct nutritional problems. PPN solutions are administered into peripheral veins using short, midline, or PICC catheters for periods of less than 2 weeks. PPN solutions do not exceed dextrose concentrations of 12.5% (10% is ideal) and do not exceed amino acid concentrations of 3%–5%. PPN solutions are the preferred formulation for infants and children.

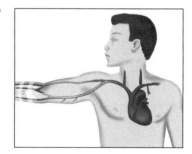

2. *Total parenteral nutrition (TPN)* solutions are given to patients who typically are malnourished or who have conditions that interfere with gastrointestinal nutrient absorption. TPN formulations are administered through central

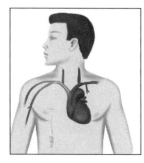

venous catheters and provide all the essential nutrients that promote weight gain, wound healing, and anabolism. All TPN solutions combine seven essential nutrients: water, protein, carbohydrates, fat, electrolytes, vitamins, and trace elements. It is recommended that dextrose concentrations be less than 37% and that amino acid concentrations be less than 7.5%.

Base parenteral nutrition solutions contain amino acids (a source of protein) and dextrose (a source of carbohydrate calories) and are available in 2,000 and 3,000 ml sizes. These solutions, sometimes referred to as *macronutrients,* make up most of the volume of a parenteral nutrition solution. Several electrolytes, trace elements, and multiple vitamins (referred to collectively as *micronutrients)* may be added to the base solution to meet individual patient requirements. Common electrolyte additives are sodium chloride (or acetate), potassium chloride (or acetate), calcium gluconate, magnesium sulfate, and sodium (or potassium) phosphate. Multiple vitamin preparations containing both water soluble and fat soluble vitamins usually are added daily. A trace element product containing zinc, copper, manganese, selenium, and chromium may be added to provide these elements in the TPN.

Intravenous fat (lipid) emulsion (10%–20%) is required as a source of essential fatty acids. It also is used as a concentrated source of calories. Fat provides 9 calories/g compared to 3.4 calories/g provided by dextrose. Intravenous fat emulsions may be admixed into the TPN solution or piggybacked into the TPN line. When intravenous fat emulsion is admixed with the base solution, the resulting solution is referred to as a *total nutrient admixture (TNA)* or three-in-one admixture.

To assure their accurate delivery, nutrition solutions almost always are administered with an intravenous infusion pump. The solutions commonly are administered through an in-line filter in the administration set positioned as close to the patient as possible. But intravenous fat emulsions, either alone or as part of a TNA solution, can be administered through an air-eliminating filter 1.2 micron pore size. An alternative is to piggyback the intravenous fat emulsion into the primary line below the in-line filter.

Foremost of the many things that must be considered regarding parenteral nutrition solutions are the following.

1. The patient's basal energy, total caloric, fluid, caloric sources (carbohydrates, fats, protein), electrolyte, and additive requirements. These needs will be determined as part of an initial assessment and ongoing monitoring of the patient. General information about many of these needs is available in standard resources.

2. The parenteral nutrition formulation itself.

   - Parenteral nutrition formulations are hypertonic solutions. If they are to be administered through a peripheral line, the osmolarity must not exceed 900 mOsmol/Liter. When osmolarities have exceeded this upper limit, irritation, phlebitis, and loss of the line have occurred.

   - The lipid emulsion in TNA solutions is known to extract the plasticizer di-2-ethylhexl phthalate (DEHP) from polyvinyl chloride containers; DEHP is a known carcinogen. TNA solutions, therefore, must be dispensed in a container (such as such as ethylene-vinyl acetate) that does not contain DEHP.

   - Calcium phosphate can precipitate in parenteral nutrition solutions. The precipitate can lead to pulmonary emboli. This precipitate may not be seen in parenteral nutrition solutions. The eye cannot detect particles smaller than 50 microns in size, but particles as small as 6 microns can block the pulmonary vasculature. TNA solutions cannot be inspected visually because of the opacity caused by the lipid emulsions. Therefore, it is recommended that the solution be filtered with a 1.2 micron in-line filter. Calcium and phosphate insolubility can be reduced by understanding the following:[4]

     ○ The final solution pH approximates the pH of the amino acid product used. Calcium and phosphate are more soluble in lower pHs. Parenteral nutrition solutions, however, are less stable at acidic pHs.

     ○ Calcium and phosphate solubility increases as the amino acid concentration increases. If the concentration is too high, however, lipid emulsions may crack.

     ○ Calcium and phosphate solubility is greater if the phosphate source is added early in the order of mixing.

     ○ Calcium and phosphate are less soluble as the temperature of the solution increases.

3. A quality assessment procedure must be performed for compounded parenteral nutrition solutions. Variables such as pH, specific gravity, color, and globular size, as well as sterility and pyrogenicity, should be evaluated. A sample SOP for such a quality assessment has been published.[5]

Biotechnology Drugs: Special Therapeutic Agents

The term *biotechnology* encompasses any technique that uses living organisms for the production or modification of pharmaceutical products. Historically, the word was associated with proteins obtained from recombinant DNA technology. But now, tissue cultures, living cells, and cell enzymes are utilized to make pharmaceutically relevant drugs, so the term has a much broader meaning and involves research achievements from molecular biology, genetics, and immunology.

The development of biotechnology drugs began with the production of proteins such as insulin and human growth hormone. Vaccines were developed to provide immunization protection. Drawing on the understanding of antibody production in the immunization process, therapeutic monoclonal antibodies were developed. Advances in genetics led to the discovery of antisense oligonucleotides as yet another biotechnological agent with therapeutic usefulness.

Today, biotechnological drugs include clotting factors, hematopoietic factors, hormones, interferons, interleukins, monoclonal antibodies, tissue growth factors, vaccines, and cytokines. And as new technologies or techniques are developed (e.g., bi-specific antibodies, super antigens), the armament will continue to increase.

Recombinant DNA and Therapeutic Proteins

The use of proteins to replace or supplement endogenous proteins is a long established treatment for diseases such as diabetes, growth hormone deficiency, and hemophilia. These treatments often are limited by undesired responses to the heterologous protein molecules or contaminants derived from natural sources, as well as the difficulty and expense of obtaining useful quantities from human and animal origin. For example, insulin originally was derived from bovine or porcine sources, so undesired immunological responses to the animal protein were common. Human growth hormone was derived from cadaver pituitary glands, and approximately 50 such glands were required to treat a single child for one year. The product was withdrawn from the market when deaths from Creutzfeldt-Jabok disease were linked to a viral contaminant in the preparation. Another example of the risks associated with using proteins isolated from natural sources was the initial consequence of treating hemophiliacs with clotting factors derived from AIDS- or hepatitis-inflected blood.

Certainly, one technique for creating homologous proteins would be to determine the composition and sequence of amino acids that make up the protein and then synthesize it in a laboratory setting. This might be a viable option for small protein molecules but clearly would be more difficult if dealing with an extremely large protein. Proteins range in size from those containing approximately 50 amino acids to those having more than 3,000 amino acids. But *recombinant DNA technology* made it possible to produce homologous proteins

of varying sizes with a desired structural purity and in quantities sufficient for therapeutic purposes.

Recombinant DNA technology involves isolating the cellular DNA fragments that code for the protein of therapeutic interest, the rapid and specific replication of the protein, and the final purification of the product. The human DNA fragment that produces the protein is identified and isolated. The DNA fragment then is inserted into a circular DNA vector, which can be replicated quickly in host cells such as *E coli*, a common bacterium. Other host cells that might be used include yeast or mammalian cells. The rapid replication process results in large quantities of the human protein that can be recovered from the host's culture media. The proteins produced are highly homologous, which reduces undesired immunogenicity.

Recombinant proteins represent almost all of the approved biotechnology drugs. It is not surprising that the development time for these agents is considerably less than for other conventional drugs because the recombinant protein most often mimics the human endogenous protein. The probability of regulatory success (i.e., achieving FDA approval) with recombinant proteins is about 40% compared to other conventional drugs, which is about 10%.

Problems With Delivery

Recombinant proteins are not without their difficulties. One of the major problems is delivery—i.e., maintaining a therapeutic concentration at a desired target for a desired time. Many routes of administration are being investigated for the delivery of proteins, including nasal, buccal, rectal, vaginal, transdermal, ocular, oral, and pulmonary. Oral administration still proves to be of limited utility in protein delivery, while the nasal and pulmonary routes seem to have the greatest promise.

The nasal route has more permeability and less enzymatic activity than the oral route. Several protein nasal products now are available, including desmopressin, oxytocin, and calcitonin. The route has not been used successfully with proteins of molecular weights greater than 10 kDa. The pulmonary route has been used successfully for leuprolide, insulin, and human growth hormone, with bioavailabilities between 10% and 25%. With both routes, however, questions remain about the long-term safety of administration, optimization of formulations, and molecular size limitations.

Some high clearance proteins require extended biological half lives to increase their effectiveness. Biological half life can be extended by chemically modifying the protein to inhibit its clearance or by controlling the rate at which the protein is administered. Polyethylene glycol (PEG) modification of some proteins increases the half life by inhibiting the glomerular filtration as a result of the larger molecular size. The presence of the PEG modification also interferes with the uptake of the molecule into metabolic pathways. PEG modified adenosine deaminase was the first such modified protein to gain FDA approval.

Modified release delivery methodology has been achieved with biodegradable microspheres. Biodegradable lactic–glycolic acid copolymer based microspheres have been useful for the delivery of several polypeptides and proteins. The first FDA-approved product was a formulation of leuprolide acetate using a poly–lactide–coglycolide) microsphere formulation.[6,7] This formulation provides release of the peptide over 30 days and is used for the treatment of prostate cancer.

Problems With Stability

Proteins become chemically unstable through hydrolysis, oxidation, racemization, adsorption, etc.—the same processes that influence the stability of conventional drugs. A unique stability consideration for proteins, however, is the tertiary or quaternary structure of the molecule. The primary protein structure is defined as the sequence of amino acids and the presence of disulfide bonds, but the tertiary structure of a protein is its overall three-dimensional architecture if only one amino acid chain is involved. If multiple amino acid chains are involved, it is referred to as the protein's quaternary structure. Maintaining this unique structure during all the manufacturing and production processes can be as time-consuming and expensive as making the protein initially.

Problems With Immunogenicity

Although undesirable immunogenicity is reduced with recombinant proteins, it is not eliminated. Antibodies to several recombinant drugs now are known. Some of these antibodies neutralize the pharmacological activity of the drug, and in some cases they decrease the systemic clearance. There is evidence that the immunogenicity of a certain protein may depend on the route of administration. Protein aggregation subsequent to subcutaneous or intramuscular injection leads to a greater antigenic response than soluble protein.

Immunoglobulins: Endogenous Therapeutic Proteins

The body's specific defense response to invading antigens is mediated through the *immune system*. Human immunity is either natural or acquired. *Natural* (sometimes called innate or native) *immunity* depends on the factors that are inborn. Some of these immunity factors are species-specific, race-specific, and individual-specific. In contrast, acquired immunity is conferred to an individual. *Acquired immunity* can result from natural causes (e.g., by infection), in which case it is termed *naturally acquired active immunity*, or it may be developed in response to the administration of a specific *vaccine*, in which case it

is termed *artificially acquired active immunity*. A third type of immunity is termed *acquired passive immunity*, in which immunoglobulins from one individual are introduced into another individual.

Naturally Acquired Active Immunity

Normally, when an antigen invades the body, phagocytes mount a generalized attack response. Indiscriminately, they engulf cellular debris as well as anything recognized as "foreign" or "not self." Occasionally this response is not adequate to protect the individual, and then white cells such as macrophages, T lymphocytes, and B lymphocytes become involved in the response.

- Macrophages are phagocytic cells that alert helper T-cells to the presence of the antigen.
- Helper T-cells stimulate the rapid production of both killer T lymphocytes and B lymphocytes.
- Killer T lymphocytes directly destroy cells that have been infected with the antigen.
- B lymphocytes differentiate into plasma cells that are capable of producing *antibodies* specific to the invading antigen. These antibodies, which are immunoglobulins, attach to the antigen and cause its destruction by phagocytes and the *complement system*.

It has long been known that different antibodies are produced in each individual as part of that person's particular immunological response to antigens. Each B lymphocyte produces only one antibody, but because thousands of B lymphocytes are produced in response to an antigenic attack, they create an in vivo "library" of antibodies that interact with the antigen at many different determinants (i.e., epitopes). Some determinants are more immunogenic than others.

All antibodies have the same basic "Y" protein structure. The protein consists of two heavy and two light polypeptide chains interconnected by disulfide bonds. The heavy and light chains are divided into a *variable region* and a *constant domain*. The constant domain is relatively conserved between the different classes of immunoglobulins (e.g., IgG, IgM). The variable region is heterogenous between the different antibodies and gives the antibody its antigen binding specificity and affinity.

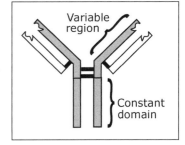

Artificially Acquired Active Immunity

One part of the immunological response is to produce antibodies that are immunoglobulin proteins. Another unique feature of the immune system is that T and B lymphocytes demonstrate "memory," which allows them to recognize and respond to a second exposure of the antigen in a much greater magnitude than after the initial exposure. From the therapeutic standpoint, the ability of T and B lymphocytes to demonstrate memory means that individuals can be more resistant to an antigen on an exposure subsequent to the initial exposure. Thus, individuals are immunized with vaccines and *toxoids* to provide an initial exposure to the antigen. This intentional use of a biological agent to confer immunity to an individual is known as *immunization.*

Vaccines are suspensions of attenuated (i.e., live) or inactivated (i.e., killed) microorganisms or fractions of the microorganisms. *Attenuated vaccines* contain live but significantly weakened microorganisms. *Inactivated vaccines* are composed of killed whole bacteria or viruses or substructures of these organisms. Both of these types of vaccines are capable of producing immunity, but attenuated vaccines typically have more antigenicity and thus are more likely to confer permanent immunity. To maintain adequate antibody titers, inactivated vaccines must be readministered over time.

Vaccines are given to increase the response of individuals to a wide variety of antigens such as hepatitis B, diphtheria, tetanus, pertussis, influenza, measles, rabies, rubella, smallpox, and polio. More recently, vaccines have been developed to assist in treating cancer, AIDS, rheumatoid arthritis, rotavirus gastroenteritis in children, and multiple sclerosis. Vaccines can be monovalent (containing a single immunogen) or can be polyvalent (containing multiple immunogens). Polyvalent vaccines would provide a broader immunity against the immunogen. Vaccines also can be mixed vaccines. For example, the measles, mumps, and rubella vaccine (MMR) is a single product with three different immunogens for three different viral disease states. A mixed biological also can contain a vaccine and a toxoid in the same product (e.g., Diphtheria and Tetanus Toxoids and Pertussis Vaccine Adsorbed for Pediatric Use).

Cancer vaccines are developed to increase the immune system's recognition of cancer cells. These products have to stimulate the production of T lymphocytes, *lymphokine activated killer cells,* and *natural killer cells* because these cell types have antitumor activity. Another application of cancer vaccines is to prevent cancer in patients having a high risk for developing cancer because of family history.

Several methods are used to manufacture vaccines. One method is to grow the microorganism in an appropriate medium under a controlled environment until a desired growth stage is achieved. Microoorganisms can be inactivated with phenol, formaldehyde, heat, or acetone. The microorganism is separated from the medium, resuspended, and further purified with dialysis or centrifugation. One method used to make an attenuated vaccine is to alter the microorganism genetically so it will survive and multiply but not produce the disease.

Subunit vaccines are made using recombinant DNA technology. First, the genes that code for the antigen are introduced into nonpathogenic organisms. This limits the amount of genetic material in the organisms and ensures that the organisms will not become pathogenic. Enough genetic material is present, however, to cause the B lymphocytes to make antibodies.

Toxoids are bacterial toxins modified and detoxified by the use of moderate heat and chemical treatment so the antigenic properties remain while the toxin is rendered nontoxic. Here, antibodies are produced to protect the individual from the disease caused by the naturally occurring toxin. The major problem with toxoids is that they produce inadequate immunological responses when administered alone. Thus, they often are combined with adjuvants (e.g., alum, aluminum phosphate, aluminum hydroxide, aluminum sulfate) to enhance their antigenicity. The combined toxoids and adjuvants are insoluble and remain in tissues for longer periods, thereby creating a prolonged immunological response.

Marketed products may contain a single toxoid (e.g., Tetanus Toxoid), or multiple toxoids, or can be mixed with vaccines (e.g., Diphtheria and Tetanus Toxoids and Pertussis Vaccine Adsorbed for Pediatric Use). The latter example has one vaccine and two toxoids adsorbed on an adjuvant. The advantage of such a mixed product is to provide broad immunization coverage with a minimum number of injections. The strength of a toxoid is in flocculating (Lf) units (e.g., Tetanus Toxoid is 4 to 5 Lf units/0.5 ml dose). A flocculating unit is the smallest amount of toxin that will most rapidly flocculate one unit of antitoxin.

Acquired Passive Immunity

Acquired passive immunity is conferred on individuals when they receive immunoglobulins produced in another human individual or an animal. Acquired passive immunity can be either *natural* or *artificial.* Naturally acquired passive immunity occurs by placental transmission of immunoglobulin G from the mother to the fetus. Because of this transfer, infants may have passive immunity to diphtheria, tetanus, measles, mumps, and other infections for the first 4 to 6 months of life.

Artificially acquired passive immunity is conferred to an individual who receives immunoglobulins for temporary prophylaxis in an epidemic or as an immediate treatment for infections and toxicities. Examples of the latter scenario are the antivenins used to treat bites from poisonous snakes (e.g., North American Coral Snake Antivenin) and spiders (e.g., Black Widow Spider Antivenin). This acquired passive immunity is not long lasting, usually ranging from 1 to 2 weeks, but the function is to protect the susceptible patient during a critical period of exposure.

Products used to confer artificially acquired passive immunity are isolated from human immune sera (homologous sera) or animal immune sera (heterologous sera). Human immune sera is obtained from pooled plasma of adults from the general population (labeled "Immune Globulin") or from hyperimmunized adults who have had the specific disease or who have been immunized against it (labeled "[specific disease] Immune Globulin"). The processed plasma generally contains not less than 15% and not more than 18% protein. An exception is Varicella-zoster Immune Globulin, which contains not less than 10% protein. Most of these preparations are for intramuscular injection; however, two immune globulins (i.e., Immune Globulin Intravenous and Cytomegalo-virus Immune Globulin) are administered intravenously.

Most animal immune sera is prepared from plasma from horses that have been immunized against the specific immunogen. The immunoglobulin fraction of the plasma is harvested and treated with pepsin to remove the complement activating component and render it less immunogenic. Horses also are used to make antitoxins and antivenins. Antitoxins are produced by inoculating horses with increasing doses of the toxins over a period of weeks or months. Antivenins are produced in the same manner, using the venom of selected species of snakes (e.g., pit vipers) and the black widow spider.

Monoclonal Antibodies

As mentioned above, an immune response is initiated when an antigen enters the body. Part of this response is the in vivo "library" of antibodies produced by B lymphocytes. The most efficient response would be to have B lymphocytes produce only the antibodies that completely neutralize the antigen. This would require that only the B lymphocytes that produced those specific antibodies be propagated throughout the response.

An important milestone in such a selective approach came in 1975 when Kohler and Milstein devised a method of growing large numbers of antibody-producing cells from a single B lymphocyte. The B lymphocyte was fused with a myeloma cancer cell to form a hybridoma. The resulting hybridoma retained two main features of its two parent cells: It could grow indefinitely like the cancer cell, and it could produce antibodies such as the B lymphocyte. Consequently, all the antibodies (i.e., immuno-globulins) produced by the hybridoma cells are genetically identical and monospecific and are called *monoclonal antibodies* (MAbs).[8]

Originally, hybridoma cells were developed by immunizing mice with the antigen of interest. The clinical use of these monoclonal antibodies, however, caused humans to produce anti-mouse antibodies that shorted the biological half life of the monoclonal antibody. Newer methods have been derived to circumvent or minimize these problems. Using recombinant DNA technology, other rodent–human monoclonal antibodies have been produced with human constant domains (typically the most immunogenic part of an antibody) and rodent variable regions. Another approach has been to develop *primatized antibodies* by combining cynomolgus monkey variable regions with human constant domain fragments. Antibodies also can be made using *bacteriophage particles* instead of animals.

Other areas of research with monoclonal antibodies have shown that in some cases the entire antibody is not necessary to attain the desired therapeutic activity. A distinct physicochemical advantage can be obtained by using a portion of the antibody. An example of the latter is *human tissue plasminogen activator* (i.e., alteplase, tPA), which is used for thrombolytic therapy following myocardial infarction. The tPA must be administered in relatively high concentrations because of its rapid plasma clearance ($t_{1/2}$ = 5 minutes), which results in part from tPA's poor solubility. A portion of the tPA antibody was found to be more clinically useful (i.e., reteplase, recombinant plasminogen activator) because it possessed superior solubility and had the additional advantage of being produced by *E coli*.

Parts of antibodies are made by treating antibodies with *proteolytic enzymes*. When the enzyme *papain* is used, two identical variable region fragments (Fab; antigen binding) are separated from the constant domain (Fc). If the enzyme *pepsin* is used, one F(ab')₂ fragment (consisting of two covalently linked F(ab') fragments) is separated from a subdivided constant domain (sFc). The smaller fragments tend to be less immunogenic and have demonstrated greater tumor penetration ability than the corresponding intact immunoglobulin.

In diagnostic applications, the smaller fragments have demonstrated greater renal, biliary, and colonic uptake at 24 hours compared to the corresponding intact immunoglobulin, because they undergo more renal filtration and biliary excretion as a result of their smaller size. They also have been more successful at detecting smaller lesions (i.e., < 2 cm) not seen on a CT scan.

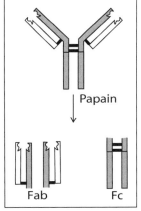
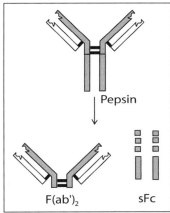

The sFc fragments have been used as an attachment point for toxins (e.g., ricin), cytokines, radiolabeled isotopes (e.g., alpha emitters), and genes, thereby broadening their utility as delivery vehicles in cancer therapy. Theoretically, therapeutic agents attached to a monoclonal antibody should target the desired tumor cells with great precision, but the reality is that the majority of monoclonal antibodies do not reach their targets; less than 0.1% reach the desired cells. The reason for this difference between theory and utility is the extensive barriers within tumors that impede antibody distribution. These include a torturous vasculature, increased hydrostatic pressure, and heterogeneity of antigen distribution within tumors.

Monoclonal antibodies also have been the basis for many "in home" diagnostic test kits. Other kits are restricted to use by physicians and include products for infectious disease processes such as AIDS, chlamydia trachomatis, and streptococcal throat infections. The use of pregnancy tests kits has been widespread for years. One product is available to help prevent pregnancy by predicting ovulation and allowing the woman to know when to avoid intercourse. Monoclonal antibody test kits also will be available to analyze blood or plasma concentrations for a number of drugs (e.g., digoxin, phenytoin, theophylline).

Antisense Technology

Recombinant DNA technology, immunizations, and monoclonal antibodies all increase the expression of some type of protein. Antisense technology has the opposite outcome in that it inhibits protein expression.

The sequence of a nucleotide chain that contains the information for protein synthesis is called the *sense sequence*, which is a specific mRNA responsible for making a protein. The nucleotide chain that is complementary to this sense sequence is called the *antisense sequence*, a short *oligonucleotide* of 10 to 20 base pairs. When the oligonucleotide binds to the mRNA, protein synthesis is inhibited because the bound mRNA cannot be translated by ribosomal function. In addition, the bound mRNA recruits RNase H, which degrades the mRNA itself. So if the protein is implicated in causing a disease state, preventing its expression would be of therapeutic value.

Several antisense molecules have progressed to clinical trials for viral diseases (e.g., herpes simplex, HIV) and cancer. The antisense molecules in these trials all have a modified phosphodiester backbone in which one of the non-bridging oxygens on the phosphate has been replaced with a sulfur atom. It also is suggested that these antisense molecules produce favorable therapeutic results by increasing the production of immunoglobulins and interferons, and by activating natural killer cells.[9]

Other technologies under investigation are adaptations of the antisense mode of action. *Ribozymes* are RNA molecules that possess enzymatic RNA degrading activity. The ribozymes are directed to the sense sequence of the protein implicated in the disease state. One ribozyme molecule can be involved in the destruction of thousands of target RNA molecules because of its enzymatic activity, and in some cases has a greater specificity than an antisense molecule.

Compounding Biotechnology Drugs

Biotechnology drugs are inherently unstable molecules, and their degradation profiles can be complex. These drugs can be lost in several ways when they are being manipulated in a compounding or administration process. Loss can occur as the result of improper pH, storage, filtration, sorption, or inappropriate agitation of the drug.

Two formulation excipients contained in most of the biotechnology formulations are stabilizing agents and buffering agents. *Stabilizing agents* can be surfactants, amino acids, fatty acids, or metal ions. A list of common stabilizing agents has been published.[10] *Buffering agents* are included to control pH because it is a critical factor in maintaining protein stability.

With few exceptions, biotechnology formulations are stored in a refrigerator (2°–8°C, 35°–36°F), to avoid freezing. In many instances, freezing will not harm the biotechnology agent but will damage the container that holds the agent and lose some of the formulation.

Filters used in compounding or administration of biotechnology formulations can result in the loss of drug because many filters will bind protein drugs. Filters that have been shown to minimize protein adsorption are made of polyvinylidene difluoride, polycarbonate, polysulfone, and regenerated cellulose. If a filter is part of a intravenous administration set, the biotechnology drug should be administered at a site distal to the filter.

Protein-like molecules can adsorb to their containers, resulting in loss of drug. This sorption can be minimized by adding albumin (0.1%) to the formulation, or by using siliconized containers. If siliconized containers are to be used, the glassware should be soaked in a silicone solution, then dried at 250°C for 5 to 6 hours.

Agitation of a reconstituted biotechnology drug will cause a froth (i.e., foam) to form in the container. Frothing is caused by the physical decomposition of the protein's quaternary struc- 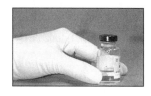 ture and can affect the potency of the formulation. To avoid frothing, the formulation can be mixed by rolling the vial in the hands or gently swirling it.

Before compounding any biotechnology formulation, the product information always should be consulted, as many instructions for the proper manipulation and use of the product are product-specific. Examples of specific instructions include:

- use in the presence of heparin
- how to store the product
- how to store the diluent
- how to reconstitute the vial
- whether or not to shake the vial
- administration schedule
- dilution instructions with other parenterals
- adsorption to tubing
- availability of patient use brochures
- whether an in-line filter is to be used
- compatibility with other products for dilution or co-administration.

The Future of Biotechnology Drugs

Many research and development efforts are under way in the field of biotechnology drugs. A few of these are discussed next.

Physical Approaches

Experimentation into "manmade" monoclonal antibodies (e.g., rodent–human and monkey–human) is just the beginning of modifying immunoglobulins. Targeting or transporting therapeutic molecules attached to monoclonal antibodies will be an important area of therapeutics because this will increase specificity to the desired target and reduce delivery to undesired sites.

Research also is continuing on new delivery methods for proteins. Interest is directed to delivering proteins via transdermal, nasal, pulmonary, and parenteral routes of administration. A *microsphere based injection* system (Prolease®) delivers proteins over days to months.

Liposomes are being considered as a means of delivering regulatory proteins (e.g., insulin, growth hormone) to tissues without metabolic degradation. *Liposomes* are vesicular structures composed of several phospholipid layers (e.g., phosphatidylcholine, cholesterol, phosphatidylglycerol) surrounding an aqueous core, and with the outer shell capable of providing direction to specific target cells.

Typically, liposomes are taken up preferentially by the reticuloendothelial system (RES) and circulate for a short time (i.e., minutes to hours) depending on their size, charge, and phospholipid layer constituents and rigidity. But "stealth" liposomes, which have been formulated using polyethylene glycol (PEG), seem to avoid the body's rapid clearance mechanisms. As mentioned, an adenosine deaminase formulation has been approved for patients with severe combined immunodeficiency disease (SCID).[11]

Gene Therapy

The goal of *gene therapy* is to deliver a segment of DNA (i.e., a gene) inside a cell's nuclear material. The first gene therapy experiments began in 1990. Yet, after years of experimentation, it has not become a viable therapeutic option.

Currently, gene therapy is restricted largely to diseases caused by a single gene and to treatment in only one person. This therapy may not be available for years in diseases caused by multiple genes. And the question of treating one individual and having the treatment extend to the individual's offspring is raising enormous ethical and scientific questions (e.g., genetic discrimination, preempting adult-onset disorders). If gene therapy involves the germ line cells (i.e., sperm and eggs), the new gene will be expressed in the individual's offspring. If the gene therapy is carried out in somatic cells (e.g., bone marrow cells or other specific body organ cells), however, the alteration is not extended and expression of the gene will end with that individual.

The principle of gene therapy is simple, but the major difficulty is to deliver the gene to the proper place and have it available at the proper time. Several steps are involved in this process: The gene has to be directed to the appropriate cells in the body; it has to arrive at the cellular nucleus; it has to occupy a safe place in the chromosomes without disrupting the surrounding genes; and it has to be controlled so the gene will be utilized only when needed.

Several different techniques have been used to carry out the gene delivery process. In general, they might be divided into two strategies. One strategy is to remove the appropriate cell population from the body, modify the cellular DNA, and then place the treated cells back in the body. This technique has several limitations. First, it is expensive, requiring special laboratory equipment and time. Second, the procedure must be repeated because the modified cells generally do not propagate for long periods. Third, this procedure can be used to treat only certain tissue cells; tissues that must remain in the body at all times cannot be treated.

A second delivery strategy is to place the gene directly into a specific tissue in the body or to deliver the material to that tissue through systemic circulation. But the fundamental requirement is that the gene be delivered inside the appropriate cell. One of the most common approaches is to deliver the gene in a vector such as a retrovirus, a lentivirus, an adenovirus, or an adeno-associated virus. *Viruses* are organisms that contain genetic material encased in protein coats that effectively inject their genetic material into their target host cells. To use them as vectors, the viral genetic material is removed (so the host cell will not be disrupted when the viral DNA is integrated into the host genome) and replaced with the desired human gene. As the virus propagates, it is injecting the human gene of interest and not the viral DNA.

Viruses have several limitations as delivery vectors, one of the most limiting is that vectors still elicit immune responses even though much of their material has been removed. Some genes are simply too large for a single virus to carry, and other vectors will not infect nondividing cells. In addition, these vectors are highly selective and do not infect every cell type. This can be both a positive and a negative attribute. If the desire is to deliver a gene to only one cell type and a virus is known that infects that cell type, specific delivery can be obtained. If no virus infects the desired cell type, however, delivery with any virus to that cell type will be problematic.

Liposomes containing the DNA segment have been investigated as a delivery vehicle. The technique has been effective only in delivering genetic material to a small percentage of cells and is significantly less effective than viral delivery. One advantage might be that these liposomal complexes can be lyophilized, which enhances the stability of the preparations.

NOTES

1. <797> Pharmaceutical Compounding—Sterile Preparations: The United States Pharmacopeia 29/National Formulary 24. The United States Pharmacopeial Convention, Inc., Rockville, MD, 2005, pp. 2735–2751.

2. Allen, L. V., Jr. Standard Operating Procedure for General Aseptic Procedures Carried Out at a Laminar Airflow Workbench. *International Journal of Pharmaceutical Compounding* 2:242–278, 1998.

3. Allen, L. V., Jr. Standard Operating Procedure for Particulate Testing for Sterile Products. *International Journal of Pharmaceutical Compounding* 2:78, 1998.

4. Lima, H. A. Drug Stability and Compatibility: Special Considerations for Home Health Care. *International Journal of Pharmaceutical Compounding* 1:301–305, 1997.

5. Tran, T., Kupiec, T. C., and Trissel, L. A. Quality-Control Analytical Methods: Particulate Matter in Injections: What Is It and What Are the Concerns? *International Journal of Pharmaceutical Compounding* 10:202–204, 2006.

6. Sharifi, R. and Soloway, M. Clinical Study of Leuprolide Depot Formulation in the Treatment of Advanced Prostate Cancer. *Journal of Urology* 143:68–71, 1990.

7. Okada, H., Heya, T., Ogawa, Y., Toguchi, H., and Shimamoto, T. Sustained Pharmacological Activities in Rats Following Single and Repeated Administration of Once-a-Month Injectable Microspheres of Lleuprolide Acetate. *Pharmaceutical Research* 8:584–587, 1991.

8. Köhler, G. C., and Milstein, C. Continuous Cultures of Fused Cells Secreting Antibody of Predefined Specificity. *Nature* 256:495–497, 1975.

9. Anderson, W. F. Gene Therapy: The Best of Times, The Worst of Times. *Science.* 288:627–629, 2000.

10. Allen, L. V., Jr. Biotechnology Preparations (chapter 23). In *The Art, Science, and Technology of Pharmaceutical Compounding*, 2nd edition. American Pharmaceutical Association, Washington, DC, 2002, pp. 393–400.

11. Cavazzana-Calvo, M., Hacein-Bey, S., de Saint Basile, G., Gross, F., Yvon, E., Nusbaum, P., Selz F., Hue, C., Certain, S., Casanova, J. L., Bousso, P., Deist, F. L., and Fischer, A. Gene Therapy of Human Severe Combined Immunodeficiency (SCID)-X1 Disease. *Science* 288:669–672, 2000.

CHAPTER TWENTY-SEVEN

Home Infusion Care

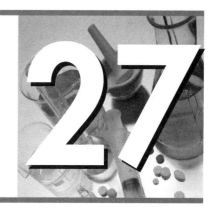

WHAT STARTED THE HOME HEALTH CARE (SOME-times called alternate-site health care) movement is subject to debate. Some believe it began in the 1970s, when *total parenteral nutrition (TPN)* solutions were being provided on an outpatient basis. Others claim that advances in infusion device technology, such as the *patient controlled administration (PCA)* devices in the 1980s, were responsible for its beginning. These infusion control devices allowed patients to regulate their own analgesic therapy (within certain restrictions) and demonstrated that patients and caregivers could provide successful therapy with a minimum of professional help.

Regardless of the initial impetus, home health care is the fastest growing segment of the health care system. Today, home infusion care includes nutrition, antibiotic and antiviral, chemotherapy, pain management, chelation, inhalation, intravenous immune globulin, steroids, cardiac agents, human growth hormone, blood products/transfusions, colony-stimulating factors, and hydration therapies. Projections of the continued growth of the home infusion care industry are based on several factors, the most prominent of which are[1,2]

- availability of improved infusion devices (programming for continuous, intermittent, tapering, and circadian administration),
- therapies that are cost-effective, and
- a larger percentage of the aging population that will require this type of care.

Guidelines

Home health care presents unique challenges to patients and health care professionals alike. The home care of a patient must be coordinated with the patient, family members (caregivers), the pharmacist, and other health care professionals. ASHP has set forth guidelines and standards for the role of the pharmacist and pharmacy in home health care.[3,4] Both of these documents identify the pharmacist as the primary provider of pharmaceutical care in the home. This care is to include products and monitoring of the patient's infusion therapy, oral medications, home hospice services (if appropriate), and parenteral and enteral nutrition.

The ASHP *Pharmacist's Role in Home Care* outlines many of the pharmacist's areas of responsibility, some of which are as follows:

- Conduct an initial patient assessment to
  - ensure that each patient referred for home care is assessed based on a predetermined admission criterion, and
  - develop a complete patient home care record database.
- Provide patient and caregiver education, training, and counseling including
  - proper and correct techniques for administration of drugs
  - equipment use and maintenance
  - potential adverse effects, drug–drug interactions, etc., and their management
  - proper storage, handling, and disposal of drug, supplies, and biomedical waste
  - emergency procedures.
- Select proper infusion devices, ancillary drugs, and ancillary supplies including
  - selection of emergency medications and supplies.
- Develop a pharmaceutical care plan covering
  - potential drug therapy problems and their proposed solutions
  - desired outcomes of drug therapy
  - a monitoring plan.
- Provide ongoing clinical monitoring to
  - ensure that relevant information is obtained from the patient and given to the other health care providers.
- Communicate effectively with patient, caregiver, and other health care providers.
- Take responsibility for proper acquisition, compounding, dispensing, storage, delivery, and administration of all medications and related equipment supplies.

The ASHP *Minimum Standards for Home Care Pharmacies* adds details and more explanation concerning the responsibility areas listed above. In addition, that document sets out requirements for leadership and management of the pharmacy involved in home care, as well as the necessary physical facilities. These standards also address issues of sterile compounding for the home care setting as follows:

- Medications must be aseptically compounded, often in quantities sufficient for multiple day use.

- Extended beyond use dates are required so a multiple day supply of medications can be dispensed and delivered.

- Products must be packaged for transit from the pharmacy to the home site in light of the expected environmental conditions.

- Medication must be delivered under conditions that will ensure maintenance of product potency and purity.

- Vascular access should be maintained for the intended duration of therapy, which may range from days to years.

- Administration devices should be selected and maintained to administer drugs accurately and safely in a variety of therapeutic regimens.

The USP/NF chapter <797> regulates sterile products prepared in a pharmacy but intended for administration in settings other than a health care facility.[5] Sections of that chapter dictate that pharmacists are responsible for ensuring that the quality and integrity of the compounded sterile preparation (CSP) are maintained during transit and use in its final location. It guides the use of appropriate packaging that is capable of maintaining proper temperature and conditions during shipment via common carriers (FedEx, UPS, USPS). The chapter goes on to require a formal training program to instruct the patient or caregiver in how to store, administer, and dispose of the CSP. It also requires that the pharmacist clinically monitor patients receiving CSPs.

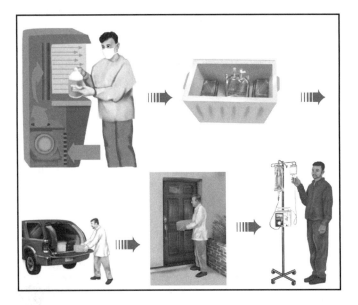

Administration and Equipment

In the context of the standards, guidelines, and regulations above, compounding takes on an expanded connotation beyond just mixing ingredients together to produce an acceptable formulation. These new or expanded opportunities might be summarized as

- formulating sterile products to retain stability and sterility during transport and long-term storage in the patient's home,

- providing products that require multiple manipulations and special handling or storage conditions in the patient's home,

- administering one product over a long time (e.g., longer than 24 hours),

- establishing and maintaining vascular access, and

- providing new infusion delivery systems.

Several of these areas have been addressed elsewhere in this book concerning sterile compounding. Nevertheless, vascular access must be established and maintained in patients receiving moderate to long-term IV therapy at home.

Types of Catheters

Most infusions conducted in the home setting will access the patient's vascular system through a catheter. Catheters are placed in two primary locations: close to the surface (*peripheral venous catheters*) and deeper in the body (*central venous catheters*).

Peripheral Venous Catheters (PVC)

PVCs are inserted into veins close to the surface and are used for up to 72 hours. Peripheral catheters are easy to insert, and most nurses can do this at a patient's bedside. PVCs usually are inserted in veins on the arms, hands, feet, or scalp.

For 20%–50% of patients, PVCs likely will cause problems such as pain and irritation. Some drugs cause vein irritation because of the drug's pH or osmolarity, and longer contact times with the blood vessels because the blood flow in peripheral veins is slow. Another problem is *infiltration*—breakdown of a vein that allows the drug to leak into tissues surrounding the catheter site, causing edema and/or tissue damage.

A *midline catheter* is a longer peripheral catheter that goes from the insertion site to a deep vein. These catheters are intended to stay in place for a week or longer. A *PICC* (peripheral inserted central catheter) is a very fine catheter that is threaded through the

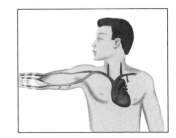

peripheral vein into the subclavian vein. A PICC has the same characteristics as a *central venous catheter*, but a skilled nurse can insert it at the bedside.

Central Venous Catheters (CVC)

CVCs are placed deeper in the body, are more complicated to place, and should be placed by a physician. Central catheters are used for therapy with a duration of 1 to 2 weeks. Common sites of insertion are the subclavian vein (which lies below the clavicle) and the jugular vein in the neck. The femoral vein (in the groin area) also is used, but this is the least desirable site because of the risk of infection. A subclavian catheter is placed deeper in the vein so the end enters the superior vena cava close to the heart, where the blood flow is the greatest. A larger blood flow will dilute a more concentrated solution such as total parenteral nutrition, chemotherapy, or phenytoin. Problems with subclavian catheters are the possibility of lacerating the subclavian vein (i.e., missing the vein and puncturing a lung) and a higher risk for infection, as the procedure is more invasive.

Multiple Lumen Catheters

In some instances several incompatible drugs must be given simultaneously and multiple lumen catheters are used. Because each lumen exits the catheter at a different location, the drugs are not allowed to mix before being diluted in the bloodstream. Multiple lumen catheters are available with one, two, three, or four lumens.

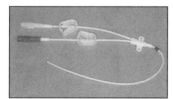 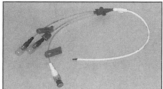

Implantable Infusion Devices

Some patients have home infusion care for months or even years, requiring frequent or continuous drug administration as with total parenteral nutrition, chemotherapy, or the coagulation factors in severe hemophilia. For these patients, infusion devices are implanted surgically to provide long-term vascular access and reduce the risk of infection. Implantable infusion devices include external *tunnel catheters* (Hickman or Broviac) and an internal port such as the Port-a-Cath®.

Tunnel Catheters

In using tunnel catheters, a surgeon inserts the catheter below the breast and moves it under the skin into the subclavian vein. At the exit through the skin, the catheter has a cuff to which the body's connective tissue attaches and seals off bacterial entry into the surgical area. Tunnel

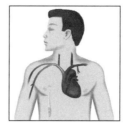

catheters allow the patient to provide self-care, and the catheters can be placed discretely under clothing. Table 27.1 gives examples of the different types of tunnel catheters and their advantages and disadvantages.

TABLE 27.1: EXAMPLES OF TUNNEL CATHETERS

Hickman	Leonard
Long-term central access *Advantages:* • Dacron cuff provides point of attachment • Clamp eliminates need for Valsalva maneuver • Provides single or multiple lumen *Disadvantages:* • Requires surgical insertion • Usually removed by a physician	Double lumen catheter (otherwise, same as Hickman) *Advantages:* • Same as Hickman *Disadvantages:* • Is double lumen only • Requires surgical insertion • Usually must be removed by a physician
Broviac	**Groshong**
Identical to Hickman, but smaller inner lumen (for pediatric patients and patients with small central vessels) *Advantages:* • Small lumen is appropriate for pediatric patients *Disadvantages:* • Provides single lumen only • Requires surgical insertion • Usually must be removed by a physician	1. Provides single or double lumen with pressure-sensitive two-way valve (opens inward with aspiration and opens outward with infusion) 2. Is used with patients with heparin allergy or if heparin is contraindicated *Advantages:* • Two-way valve eliminates need for heparin flushing • Dacron cuff provides point of attachment • Two-way valve decreases chance of air embolism • Two-way valve eliminates need for clamp on catheter *Disadvantages:* • Same as Hickman

Port-a-Cath

A Port-a-Cath is a small device made of stainless steel, titanium, or plastic, about the diameter of a 25-cent coin. The port has a reservoir for instilling fluids, and the reservoir is covered by a silicone rubber septum. The port is implanted subcutaneously in the chest wall, and a catheter connects the port to a vein.

Huber point needles with a 90° bend are used when accessing the port. The special design of the needle

 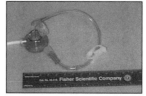 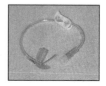

moves the silicone rubber in the port's septa around the needle and prevents coring. A Port-a-Cath septum lasts up to 2,000 punctures with a 22-gauge Huber point needle.

Catheter Recommendations

The pharmacist will be called upon to make recommendations about which catheter should be used in a home care setting. Table 27.2 presents a guide to the different types of catheters and their advantages and disadvantages.

Vascular Access

Patient vascular access occludes or becomes sluggish through catheters as a result of mechanical factors, fibrin build up or thrombosis, drug precipitates, or lipid deposits. Catheter occlusion can interrupt the infusion of medications, nutrients, and fluids. Sluggish flow of solution can reduce the dosage administered in a defined period of time and can prevent the catheter from being used to obtain blood specimens. Uncorrected catheter occlusion can lead to venous thrombosis, septicemia, permanent obstruction, chronic venous insufficiency, and pulmonary embolism.[6]

Mechanical occlusion—the easiest malfunction to observe—typically is caused by twisted or kinked tubing in the administration set, a clogged in-line filter, a suture securing the vascular access device that is too tight, or the catheter not being positioned correctly. This last problem can be suspected if the occlusion is corrected or improved by changing the patient's position.

Thrombotic occlusion occurs when fibrin deposits within or around the vascular access device. One test for a thrombotic occlusion is the ability to infuse fluids but not withdraw blood through the same device. Each home care provider will require a detailed procedure for clearing thrombotic occlusions with a hemolytic drug. In the past, urokinase and streptokinase have been used to clear occlusions, but urokinase has been removed from the market and the manufacturer of streptokinase has reminded practitioners repeatedly that its product is not indicated to restore patency to intravenous catheters. Alteplase and reteplase are newer fibrin specific thrombolytic agents.

The most common precipitate involved in vascular access occlusion is calcium

TABLE 27.2: TYPES OF CATHETERS AND THEIR ADVANTAGES AND DISADVANTAGES

Catheter Type	Advantages and Disadvantages
Short peripheral catheters (inserted directly in hand or arm)	*Advantages* • Immediate access • Short-term therapies of 7 or fewer days • Patients with good venous access • Nonirritating therapies (such as isoosmotic, near isoosmotic, or ≤10% dextrose) *Disadvantages* • Frequent site change needed (48–72 hours) • Higher incidence of phlebitis
Midline peripheral catheters (inserted above or below elbow; tip remains in proximal end of extremity)	*Advantages* • Therapies of 2 to 4 weeks • Insertion is easier than with PICC catheters • Can use with peripheral therapies requiring greater hemodilution • Nonirritating therapies (such as isoosmotic, near isoosmotic, or ≤10% dextrose) • No X-ray verification *Disadvantages* • Greater rates of phlebitis than PICC lines • Frequent site changes (48–72 hours) • Greater discomfort and restriction than with PICC lines
PICC catheters (inserted above elbow; tip can be stopped in the axillary, subclavian, or brachiocephalic vein or in the superior vena cava)	*Advantages* • Therapies up to 1 month • Easily inserted by skilled personnel • Increased comfort and less arm restriction • For hypertonic and highly irritating therapies • Generally fewer complications with insertion and access *Disadvantages* • Patients with sclerotic veins may not be candidates for placement • Superior vena cava placement must be verified by X-ray
Midclavicular catheters (tip can be stopped in axillary, subclavian, or brachiocephalic vein)	*Advantages* • Therapies up to 3 months (depending on tip location) • Reduce risk of complications (insertion and dwell) • Nonirritating therapies (such as isoosmotic, near isoosmotic, or ≤10% dextrose) *Disadvantages* • High incidence of incorrect positioning and thrombosis
Subclavian (untunneled) catheters (tip remains in superior vena cava)	*Advantages* • For multiple access needs in acute-care settings • For diagnostic/therapies access needs • Hypertonic solutions that require rapid dilution • Long-term therapies (TPN, antibiotics, chemotherapy) *Disadvantage* • Higher risk of complications with insertion and access
Surgically placed tunnel catheters (tip remains in superior vena cava)	*Advantages* • For longer-term therapies • For regular or recurring therapies • For patient or physician preference • Hypertonic solutions that require rapid dilution *Disadvantages* • Requires surgical insertion • Usually must be removed by a physician • Higher risk of complications with insertion and access
Surgically implanted Port-a-Cath (tip remains in superior vena cava)	*Advantages* • For intermittent longer-term therapies • For regular or reoccurring therapies • For patient or physician preference • No external apparatus when not in use *Disadvantages* • Requires surgical insertion • Possibility of missing septum with Huber needle and injecting subcutaneously • Requirement and expense of a Huber needle

phosphate. Calcium phosphate is the result of a chemical incompatibility that forms when calcium and phosphate are in the same formulation. This is particularly true of total parenteral nutrition solutions. The best way to avoid this type of occlusion is to prevent it from happening in the first place.

In TPN solutions, choose components (amino acid products, cysteine HCl, calcium salts) that will reduce the pH. Calcium and phosphate are more soluble at low pH. Using lower pH solutions, however, is not recommended for TNA solutions. Therefore, mix the phosphate prior to the calcium, and mix the solution very well between additions. If the solution is not for immediate use, store it in the refrigerator. Calcium and phosphate are more soluble at lower temperatures. If possible, avoid warm ambient temperatures during administration. If an occlusion does occur, use 0.1N HCl to attempt to open the access device; the acid converts the insoluble dibasic calcium phosphate to the more soluble monobasic calcium phosphate.

Drug precipitates also occlude devices. One of the most important (and most incorrectly done) steps to help prevent these precipitates is to flush the administration line with saline *before* introducing heparin into the line. Many drugs are incompatible with heparin and will precipitate. If a drug has precipitated in the line, use 0.1N HCl for drugs that are soluble in acid and 1M sodium bicarbonate for those soluble in a base.

When catheters are manufactured, a waxy lipid remains within the catheter. If this waxy material collects inside the catheter to the point at which the catheter is occluded, a 70% alcohol solution can be used to dissolve it and open the catheter.

In all of these manipulations, use a 10 ml syringe to execute the procedures. Small syringes such as 1 ml or 3 ml cause too much pressure in the plastic catheter, which can damage it.

Pumps

Pumps are used in many situations related to home health care. Pharmacists use automated compounding pumps that simultaneously dispense multiple components to make parenteral nutrition solutions. Examples of such devices include Nutrimix®, MicroMacro®, Hyper-Former®, Automix®, and Micromix®. These devices help meet the demand for increased complexity in parenteral nutrition solutions, yet optimize personnel preparation time. They are housed inside of laminar flow hoods, which greatly reduces the space available for other operations. Each model generally requires personnel to receive training about its operation. The different models are unique, and training on one pump generally does not translate to other pumps.[7]

In the home care setting pumps are used as infusion systems. The two categories or types of infusion pumps

SOME FACTORS TO CONSIDER WHEN SELECTING AN INFUSION SYSTEM
• Ease of operation
• Ease of training end user (patient or caregiver)
• Alarm features
• Ambulatory status
• Number of therapies
• Whether a caregiver will be in the home
• Cost of the system
• Reliability of the system
• Availability of the system
• Ability of system to minimize waste
• Storage space needed at home
• Repair costs

are stationary and ambulatory. In selecting an infusion system, many factors must be considered. The pharmacist will make a recommendation for an infusion system.

Stationary infusion pumps ensure delivery accuracy and offer portability and a wide range of capabilities and features. Some systems can use generic IV administration sets instead of a proprietary set. They are used extensively in institutional settings. In home use they can be too large or too heavy or lack the desired portability, but they are important delivery systems for many patients.

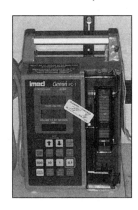

The small *ambulatory pump* may be the preferred system if the patient is nearly or fully ambulatory, but this is not always the best system to use. Consideration

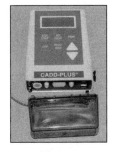

must be given to the type of therapy being given, length of the infusion cycle, and the patient's desire to wear and use such a device. These devices offer a lower up-front acquisition cost and use less expensive disposable administration sets.

Some of these pumps are therapy specific—meaning that they are

SOME STATIONARY INFUSION PUMPS	
Gemini PC-1	Alaris Medical Systems
IVAC 7000	Alaris Medical Systems
Flo-Gard 6201	Baxter Healthcare
280RT	Graseby Medical, Inc.
HomeFusion RT	McGaw, Inc.
Sigma 8000	McGaw, Inc.

SOME AMBULATORY INFUSION DEVICES

Provider One	Abbott Laboratories
microSTAR	Alaris Medical Systems
Multifuse System	AmerMed Corporation
VIVUS 2000	I-Flow Corporation
Genie	Invacare Infusion Systems
Stratus	McGaw, Inc.
Model TPN	Microject, Inc.
CADD-Prizm VIP	SIMS Deltec
CADD-PLUS	SIMS Deltec
Dual Rate Syringe Infuser	Baxa Corporation

designed to meet the delivery protocol of a single therapy. Many pumps have multiple therapy capabilities. These can be used for a variety of delivery protocols such as TPN, antibiotics, pain management, and chemotherapy.

Beyond Use Dates in Home Care Settings

Within an institutional environment, assigning beyond use dates usually is not a problem because sterile formulations are prepared and administered within 24 hours. Assigning beyond use dates to sterile formulations intended for home care, however, can be problematic because preparation and administration times are much longer and factors such as uncontrolled and unmonitored temperature and storage conditions must be considered.

The first source of information about assigning a beyond use date would be the manufacturer's package insert or approved labeling. If the formulation is compounded in accordance with the conditions stated in the labeling, the manufacturer's date is the appropriate beyond use date to use. The same is true if the formulation compounded is an official USP/NF compounded formulation. If the compounding deviates from conditions in the approved labeling of manufactured products, however, the pharmacist should first consult the manufacturer for advice about a beyond use date. When requesting stability information, the pharmacist should communicate to the manufacturer the deviations from the package insert. Pharmacists should obtain a letter from the manufacturer certifying the beyond use dating period provided.

If a beyond use date cannot be obtained from the manufacturer, the pharmacist should refer to relevant publications to obtain information about stability, compatibility, and degradation. Direct extrapolation of the information to the specific compounded formulation requires that the scientific study data utilized the same drug source, the same drug concentration and the same

compounding procedures, stored the formulation in the same container, and subjected the formulation to the same anticipated environmental variables. Classic references such as Trissel's *The Handbook of Injectable Drugs* and King's *Guide to Parenteral Admixtures* do not include extended stability information.

Beyond use dates described in the USP/NF chapter <795> are to be assigned to CSPs that lack justification from either the manufacturer or literature sources or by direct testing evidence.[8] The USP/NF also recommends that the pharmacy establish and follow written policies and procedures governing determination of the beyond use dates for all of its compounded products. These manuals could contain detailed descriptions and forms about beyond use dates assigned to each product and also include

- copies of product specific stability studies based on a stability indicating analytical procedure
- copies of letters from manufacturers certifying the beyond use dating
- predictive materials such as publications, charts, tables
- in-house quality control data collected for compounded formulations.

It should be remembered that each compounded formulation could have a beyond use date that is different from those contained in the policies and procedures manual if there is a difference in any of its components or the home care environment.

> The degree of error or inaccuracy would be dependent upon the extent of differences between the CSP's characteristics (such as composition, concentration of ingredients, fill volume, container type and material) and the characteristics of the products from which stability data or information are to be extrapolated. Thus, the greater the doubt of the accuracy of theoretically predicted beyond use dating, the greater the need to determine dating periods experimentally.

NOTES

1. Lima, H. A. Compounded Nutritional Solutions—A Market Overview. *International Journal of Pharmaceutical Compounding* 2:334–337, 1998.

2. Lima, H. A. Home Infusion and Alternate-Site Health Care: The Big Picture. *International Journal of Pharmaceutical Compounding* 1:294–297, 1997.

3. American Society of Hospital Pharmacists. ASHP Guidelines on the Pharmacist's Role in Home Care. *American Journal of Hospital Pharmacy* 50:1940–1944, 1993.

4. American Society of Health-System Pharmacists. ASHP Guidelines: Minimum Standards for Home Care Pharmacies. *American Journal of Health-System Pharmacy* 56:629–638, 1999.

5. <797> Pharmaceutical Compounding—Sterile Preparations: The United States Pharmacopeia 29/National Formulary 24, The United States Pharmacopeial Convention, Inc., Rockville, MD, 2005, pp. 2735–2751.

6. McKinnon, B., Lima, H. A. Catheter Occlusion: Causes and Solutions. *International Journal of Pharmaceutical Compounding* 2: 342–346, 1998.

7. Bertch, K. E. Parenteral Nutrition Equipment and Devices. *International Journal of Pharmaceutical Compounding* 2:338–341, 1998.

8. <795> Pharmaceutical Compounding—Nonsterile Preparations: The United States Pharmacopeia 29/National Formulary 24, The United States Pharmacopeial Convention, Inc., Rockville, MD, 2005, pp. 2731–2735.

ADDITIONAL READING

McElhiney, L. F. Educating the Caregiver and Community Pharmacist to Facilitate Provision of Consistent Compounded Medication From the Inpatient to Ambulatory Setting. *International Journal of Pharmaceutical Compounding* 7:394–398, 2003.

CHAPTER TWENTY-EIGHT

Ophthalmic Formulations

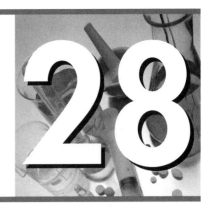

D RUGS ARE ADMINISTERED TO THE EYES IN A WIDE variety of dosage forms. Because of the importance of the eyes in daily living, ophthalmic formulations are compounded using the same standards as intravenous formulations. Unique features, however, apply to formulations used in the eye.

Physiology of the Eye

When looking at the exterior of the eye, several structures are evident:

- the *eyelids,*
- the *sclera*—the "white" portion of the eye,
- the *iris*—the "color" portion of the eye, and
- the *pupil*—black opening into the eye.

The *eyelids* protect the entire eye structure, but the *conjunctiva* lines the back of the eyelids and attaches to the outer surface of the sclera. In most places the conjunctival attachment is loose and therefore allows freedom of movement for the eye. The *conjunctival sac or cul-de-sac* is the space between the eyeball and the eyelids where tear fluid flows. It has a maximum capacity of about 30 microliters. Figure 28.1 shows the structures of the eye.

The *sclera*—the white portion of the eye—forms a relatively tough covering for the internal ocular structures. Along with the *cornea*, it constitutes the external protective covering of the eye. The sclera contains the microcirculation, which partly nourishes the cornea. The cornea actually has several layers. The order of the prominent layers from the external to the internal surface of the cornea is as follows:

1. *Epithelium*: five or six layers of cells with a basement membrane about 60–65 nm (nanometers) thick.

2. *Bowman's layer*: fibrils that run parallel to the external surface of the cornea; the layer is about 12 microns thick.

3. *Stroma*: layers of collagen fibril bundles loosely interlaced with each other; the stroma accounts for about 90% of the cornea.

4. *Descemet's membrane*: formed by secretions from the underlying endothelial cells about 10 microns thick.

5. *Endothelium*: a single layer lining Descemet's membrane.

The cornea has no blood supply within itself, so blood is supplied by the sclera and the conjunctiva. Many nerve fibers in the structure, however, account for its sensitivity. Figure 28.2 shows some of the corneal structures.

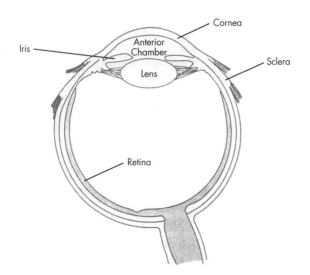

FIGURE 28.1: ANATOMICAL STRUCTURES OF THE EYE

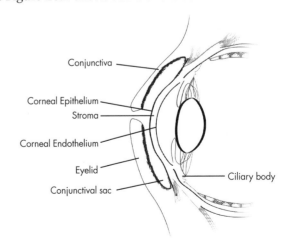

FIGURE 28.2: STRUCTURES OF THE CORNEA

The *iris* is a colored, circular membrane suspended behind the cornea. The iris is connected to the *ciliary body* and forms the boundary between the *anterior and posterior chambers* of the eye. The iris controls the size of the pupil, which determines the amount of light that enters the eye. The *pupil* is the variable aperture in the middle of the iris; its size is controlled by contractions and relaxations of the iris.

The *lens*, positioned behind the iris, refracts the light entering through the pupil onto the *retina*. The lens is avascular but receives its sustenance from the *aqueous humor* and the *vitreous humor*. The *zonules* are thin, delicate filaments that suspend and maintain the lens in position. They are bundles of fibrils 80–120 Å wide (1 angstrom = 1.0×10^{-10} meters) and contain collagen-like glycoprotein and acidic mucopolysaccharides. The *retina* is the innermost surface of the eye. It contains the light-sensitive nerve elements necessary for sight.

The three intraocular fluids of the eye are the *precorneal film*, the *aqueous humor*, and the *vitreous humor*. The precorneal film covers the corneal and conjunctival surfaces. Commonly called tears, the precorneal film includes tears, but two other layers surround the tear layer as well. The film is secreted by the conjunctival and lacrimal glands and is a clear, watery fluid containing numerous salts, glucose, and the enzyme lysozyme. It serves to lubricate and cleanse the surface of the eye. The structure of the precorneal film has three layers consisting of:

1. an outer lipid layer—about 0.1 microns thick

2. a middle aqueous layer, the tear fluid—about 7 microns thick

3. an inner mucoid layer—about 0.02 to 0.05 microns thick.

The isotonic film is produced at a rate of about 1.2 μl/min and has an average pH of 7.4 (range = 7.3 to 7.7). A pH below 4 or above 9 causes the film to lose its consistency; however, the film can maintain its structure when substantially hypertonic solutions (e.g., 2% sodium chloride solution) are added. Spontaneous blinking replenishes the precorneal film by pushing a thin layer of film ahead of the eyelid margins as they come together. The excess fluid is directed into two small tubes, called the *lacrimal canalicula*, that lead into the lacrimal sac. The film enters the lacrimal canalicula aided by capillary attraction and contraction of eyelid muscle.

The *aqueous humor* (about 300 μl in volume) is an ultrafiltrate of the blood formed by the ciliary body. It is secreted by the ciliary processes into the posterior chamber, moves to the anterior chamber, and flows out of the anterior chamber at a turnover rate of approximately 1%/min. Most of the drainage is through the *Canal of Schlemm* in the *trabecular meshwork* (1.8–2.5 μl/minute),

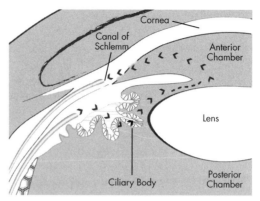

FIGURE 28.3: AQUEOUS HUMOR FLOW IN THE EYE

but a small portion drains through the anterior face of the ciliary body (0.2–0.5 μl/minute). The aqueous humor has a viscosity of about 1.03 relative to water and is slightly hyperosmotic to plasma by 3 to 5 mOsmol/L. It also carries nutrients, substrates, and metabolites to the avascular tissues of the eye. Figure 28.3 illustrates the origin of and flow patterns of aqueous humor in the eye.

The *intraocular pressure* of the eye results from the resistance produced by aqueous humor as it passes into the Canal of Schlemm. In humans, the normal intraocular pressure is about 12–20 mm Hg. Sustained elevated intraocular pressures (i.e., glaucoma) of 25–30 mm Hg can compress the retinal artery, causing reduced nutrition to the retina, atrophy of the retina, or even blindness. Patients can have chronic *open angle glaucoma* when the drainage efficiency of the trabecular meshwork is reduced. *Angle closure glaucoma* is caused when the iris mechanically blocks the outflow of aqueous humor from the trabecular meshwork. If this condition is not corrected surgically, blindness may result in a few days.

The *vitreous humor* (sometimes called the vitreous body) is a clear mass, filling the posterior cavity of the eye. The total weight is about 3.9 g, and the volume is about 3.9 ml. It is a gelatinous mass with a fine fibrillar network composed primarily of large proteoglycan molecules. Materials can diffuse slowly through the vitreous humor, but there is little flow of the humor itself. The pH is 7.5 with a viscosity of 4.2 relative to water.

Physiological Considerations for Drug Delivery

The unique anatomy and physiology of the eye has profound consequences on effective drug delivery. Following ophthalmic administration, a significant portion of an administered dose can be lost via three mechanisms:

1. *Immediate loss from spillage.* The normal volume of the precorneal film is estimated to be 7–10 μl. The

estimated maximum volume of the conjunctival cul-de-sac is about 30 µl. The normal commercial eye-dropper dispenses 50–75 µl of solution; thus, more than half of the dose will be lost from the eye by overflow. The ideal volume of drug solution to administer would be 5–10 µl; however, microliter dosing eyedroppers generally are not available to patients.

2. *Lacrimal drainage.* The precorneal film washes the eyeball as it flows from the lacrimal gland across the eye and drains into the lacrimal canalicula. The canalicula terminate in the lacrimal sac, which directs the drainage toward the opening in the nose via the nasolacrimal duct. In humans, the entire precorneal film volume turns over every 2–3 minutes. This rapid washing and turnover account for loss of an ophthalmic dose in a relatively short time.

3. *Absorption through the conjunctiva.* The conjunctiva has substantial blood flow, and absorbed drugs can enter the systemic circulation via this route.

The unique structure of the eye also allows systemic absorption of a drug through several sites. One is through the conjunctiva, because it has a good blood supply and thin membranes. Another site is via the lacrimal drainage system through the nose directly into the gastrointestinal system, or the drainage may be aspirated into the lungs, where absorption can occur again. A third site is through the cornea and into the aqueous humor; the aqueous humor leaves the eye via the Canal of Schlemm directly into the systemic circulation.

A drug also can be administered systemically to produce an ophthalmic effect. Two mechanisms are possible for this "reverse" effect:

1. The drug is secreted into the lacrimal gland and becomes part of the precorneal film.

2. The drug enters the interior of the eye via the aqueous humor.

Even though the volumes involved in both the precorneal film and the aqueous humor are small, some drugs do produce an ophthalmic effect when administered systemically. An example is orally administered tetrahydrocannibol to treat glaucoma.

Administered drugs whose therapeutic activity is directed at any of the interior structures of the eye (iris, pupil, ciliary body, etc.) must be absorbed through the cornea. The corneal structure poses three potential barriers to drug permeation:

1. entrance into the cornea through the epithelium,

2. transport through the stroma, and

3. entrance into the anterior chamber through the endothelium.

In assessing these potential barriers, drug permeability in excised rabbit corneal preparations was studied for a number of drugs.[1] For hydrophilic drugs the epithelium appears to contribute significantly to penetration resistance, whereas the stroma and endothelium offer little resistance. As drugs become more lipophilic, the stroma and endothelium contribute more significantly to barrier resistance. For most lipophilic drugs, the epithelium contributes minimally, but the stroma and endothelium become significant barriers. Table 28.1 shows the percentage of barrier resistance for each class of drug.

The epithelium is composed of flat, tightly fitting squamous cells. The layer resists penetration partly because it is selective for lipophilic compounds but mostly because it has low porosity and high tortuosity. The stroma, which accounts for 90% of the total corneal thickness, consists of 78% water interspersed with collagen fibrils. The stroma allows relatively free diffusion of dissociated (i.e., ionized) molecules through its matrix because of its large aqueous environment, low tortuosity, and high porosity. The endothelium is selective for lipophilic compounds (i.e., undissociated or unionized).

Most ophthalmic drugs are formulated as aqueous solutions of their salts. The salt form generally is used to ensure good solubility in the precorneal film. When the

TABLE 28.1: PERCENTAGE CONTRIBUTION OF EACH CORNEAL BARRIER TO DRUG PERMEABILITY

Drugs	Percentage Resistance of Corneal Barrier			Log PC*
	Epithelium	Stroma	Endothelium	
Lipophilic				
Bevantolol	7	44	49	2.19
Bufurolol	18	50	32	2.31
Penbutolol	1	46	53	2.53
Propranolol	7	45	48	1.62
Slightly Lipophilic				
Cyclophosphamide	72	10	13	0.38
Levobunolol	58	15	27	0.72
Metoprolol	48	18	34	0.28
Oxprenolol	45	21	34	0.69
Timolol	68	9	23	0.34
Hydrophilic				
Acebutolol	91	1	8	0.20
Atenolol	97	1	2	−1.52
Nadolol	95	1	4	−0.82
Phenylephrine	95	1	4	−1.00
Sotalol	95	1	4	−1.25
Tobramycin	95	1	4	<−2.00

*octanol/buffer (pH 7.65) partition coefficient

solution is administered, the neutralizing action of the precorneal film will bring the pH of the solution to the physiological pH range of the eye. At this point the drug will assume its characteristic unionized:ionized ratio and the unionized moiety will penetrate the cornea. Once the drug passes the epithelium, the undissociated free base will dissociate to a degree. The dissociated moiety will move through the stroma because of its water soluble nature. At the junction of the stroma and endothelium, some of the dissociated moiety will exist as the undissociated species, and this undissociated species is what passes through the endothelium into the aqueous humor. Again, the equilibrium between the undissociated and dissociated species exists, and the dissociated form readily diffuses through the aqueous humor to the iris and the ciliary body.

Therefore, corneal drug absorption occurs because of the equilibrium between undissociated and dissociated moieties of the drug, and once the drug arrives in the aqueous humor, it can be removed from the eye into the systemic circulation, creating "sink" conditions. Thus, drug absorption through the cornea is a "microcosmic" representation of the general phenomena responsible for most drug movement through biological membranes throughout the body. Transcorneal transport (drug penetration into the eye), however, is not effective, as only an estimated one-tenth of a dose penetrates the eye.

Types of Ophthalmic Formulations

The roles of ophthalmic formulations are to protect and heal the eye. To fulfill these roles, ophthalmic formulations are prepared with the same standards as parenteral products with respect to sterility, particulate matter, isotonicity, buffers, preservatives, and so on. The primary requirement for an ophthalmic formulation is its sterility. The eye can accommodate variations in particulate matter, isotonicity, and the like, but not variations in sterility. Every ophthalmic product must be sterile in its final container. Preservatives are added to ophthalmic formulations to prevent microbial contamination of the formulation after the package is opened.

The ASHP has prepared a Technical Assistance Bulletin on Pharmacy-Prepared Ophthalmic Products.[2] This bulletin outlines the many considerations inherent in compounding ophthalmic formulations. The bulletin stresses the need for established policies and procedures. It states that all ophthalmic compounding must be performed in a laminar flow hood and gives some general information about how to filter sterilize solutions. Ophthalmic suspensions and ointments cannot be filtration sterilized and must either be sterilized as a finished product or have each component sterilized separately and then combined using aseptic techniques. Many of

the topics mentioned in the bulletin superficially will be discussed in much more detail in this chapter.

Ophthalmic formulations include aqueous solutions, aqueous suspensions, gels, ointments, and inserts. Most drugs administered in ophthalmic formulations are intended for local activity. The formulation delivers the drug on the eye, into the eye, or onto the conjunctiva, where local activity occurs. Drugs are administered to the eye for local effects such as miosis, mydriasis, and anesthesia, or to reduce intraocular pressure in treating glaucoma. Some drugs are used to aid in eye examinations and surgery. Many of the categories of drugs applied to the eye are given in Table 28.2.

TABLE 28.2: OPHTHALMIC DRUGS BY THERAPEUTIC CATEGORY

Category of Drug	Therapeutic Use	Examples
Anesthetics	Pain relief preoperatively and postoperatively	Tetracaine, proparacaine
Anti-infective agents	Systemic and local application for ophthalmic infection	Bacitracin, tetracycline, trimethoprim, gentamicin, norfloxacin
Antifungal agents	Fungal endophthalmitis and fungal keratitis	Amphotericin B, natamycin, flucytosine
Antihistamines	Relief of itching caused by pollen, ragweed, and animal dander	Peniramine
Anti-inflammatory agents (corticosteroids and NSAIDs)	Allergic conjunctivitis, non-specific, superficial keratitis, herpes zoster keratitis, cyclitis	Prednisolone, dexamethasone, loteprednol (steroids) diclofenac, flurbiprofen, ketorolac (NSAIDs)
Antiviral agents	Herpes simplex virus, cytomegalovirus retinitis	Trifluridine, idoxuridine, vidarabine, foscarnet
Astringents	Conjunctivitis	Zinc sulfate
β-Adrenergic blocking agents	Elevated intraocular pressure, chronic open angle glaucoma	Betaxolol, timolol
Miotics	Glaucoma, accommodative esotropia, myasthenia gravis	Pilocarpine, echothiophate, demecarium, latanoprost
Mydriatics and cycloplegics	Dilation of the pupil	Atropine, homatropine, cyclopentolate, phenylephrine, tropicamide
Protectants/artificial tears	Lubrication of surface of the eye	Carboxymethylcellulose, methylcellulose, hydroxypropylmethyl cellulose, polyvinyl alcohol
Vasoconstrictors	Soothing, refreshing, and removing redness caused by minor eye irritation	Naphazoline, oxymetazoline, tetrahydrozoline

Solutions

Ophthalmic solutions are the most commonly used ophthalmic formulation. They interfere minimally with vision, but because they wash out quickly from the cul-de-sac, they may require frequent application. Ophthalmic solutions are sterile, free from foreign particles, and specially prepared for instillation in the eye. Most ophthalmic solutions are dispensed in eyedropper bottles or plastic containers called *droptainers*. Patients should be shown how to instill the drops properly in their eyes, and every effort should be made to emphasize the need for instilling only one drop per administration, not two or three drops. When more than one drop is to be administered, at least 5 minutes should elapse between administrations. Immediately after instilling a drop on the eye, pressure should be placed on the lacrimal sac for 1 or 2 minutes. This reduces the rate of drug loss through this pathway.

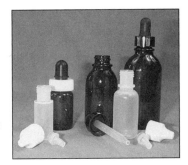

Suspensions

Ophthalmic suspensions are aqueous formulations that contain solid particles. The solid particles act as a reservoir that increases the contact time and duration of action of a drug as compared to a solution. The solid undissolved particles tend to adhere to the conjunctiva. As the drug is absorbed, these solid particles dissolve to replenish the absorbed drug. The recommended particle size is smaller than 10 microns, to minimize irritation to the eye. The micronized form of the drug can be used to meet this requirement.

For aqueous suspensions, the physicochemical parameters of intrinsic solubility and dissolution rate must be considered. The *intrinsic solubility* determines the amount of drug actually in solution and available for absorption, but as the drug is absorbed, new solid particles must dissolve to replenish the absorbed drug. The requirement here is that the particles have a dissolution rate within the formulation's residence time in the eye that is rapid enough to provide this reservoir effect. If the dissolution rate is too slow, the suspension formulation has no more benefit than a saturated solution of the drug.

Gels

Aqueous gels incorporate agents such as polyvinyl alcohol, poloxamers, Carbopols®, hydroxyethyl cellulose, hydroxypropyl cellulose, or hydroxypropylmethyl cellulose in the formulation. Ophthalmic gels generally require only 5% of the gelling agent, so the gel base is about 95% aqueous. These more viscous formulations have been shown to produce a three-fold to five-fold increase in corneal absorption. Products used to treat open angle glaucoma can be applied at bedtime (e.g., pilocarpine gel, Pilopine HS®) or once a day (e.g., timolol maleate, Timoptic XE®).

The hydroxypropyl cellulose gel base without drug has been used to treat moderate to severe cases of dry eye (i.e., keratoconjunctivitis sicca). Dry eye syndrome usually is the result of a deficiency in precorneal film production, so installation of a formulation such as the Lacrisert® keeps the cornea wetted.

Ointments

Ointments typically are used to maintain longer contact between the drug and the eye. They also may be the required formulation because an appropriate ophthalmic solution could not be produced as a result of difficulties with drug solubility, stability, or other problems. Most ointments blur the patient's vision because they remain viscous and are not easily removed by the tear fluid. Thus, ointments usually are used at night as adjunctive therapy to eyedrops used during the day.

Ophthalmic ointments tend to keep the drug in contact with the eye longer than suspensions do. Most ophthalmic ointment bases are a mixture of mineral oil and white petrolatum and have a melting point close to body temperature. Sometimes anhydrous lanolin is used to take up an ingredient that was dissolved in a small amount of water. The aqueous solution is incorporated into the lanolin, and then the lanolin is mixed with the remaining ointment base ingredients. The micronized form of the ingredients is used because ointments must be nonirritating and free from grittiness. Sterile ointments are prepared by first sterilizing all of the individual ingredients and then combining them under aseptic conditions. Ophthalmic ointments also must contain preservatives.

Typically, ophthalmic ointment tubes are small, holding approximately 3.5 g of ointment, and are fitted with narrow gauge tips that permit the extrusion of narrow bands of ointment. The tubes can sterilized conveniently by autoclaving or by ethylene oxide.

Official compendia provide tests to determine the level of particulate matter in ophthalmic ointments. In these tests, the content of 10 ointment tubes is melted in flat-bottom Petri dishes and then allowed to solidify. The mass is scanned under a low-power microscope fitted with a micrometer eyepiece. In an acceptable test, all 10 tubes do not exceed 50 particles that are 50 microns or larger, and not more than one tube is found to contain 8 such particles.

Inserts

Ocular inserts are not compounded but, instead, must be manufactured. Ocusert® is a nonerodible ocular device designed to release pilocarpine at a controlled rate for 7 days. The Ocusert system is an elliptical membrane that is soft and flexible and consists of three components:

1. The drug reservoir is composed of the active drug (pilocarpine) and alginic acid.

2. The rate controlling membrane is composed of a ethylene-vinyl acetate copolymer that also serves as the housing of the drug reservoir.

3. A border ring containing titanium dioxide, which helps visualize the device.

The device weighs about 20 mg and has the dimensions of 13.4 mm × 5.7 mm × 0.3 mm.

The pilocarpine Ocusert is available as Pilo-20®, which releases 20 µg/hr and Pilo-40®, which releases 40 µg/hr. Thus, the patient is exposed to about one-eighth the amount of pilocarpine that would be delivered with traditional liquid drop therapy. The continuous delivery of pilocarpine provides constant control of intraocular pressure, whereas drop therapy would allow the pressure to peak and valley between administrations. Clinical acceptance of the device has been moderate because the device is uncomfortable for some patients and has a tendency to float on the eyeball, particularly in the morning upon arising. Also, the cost differential is considerable.

Some inserts are designed to dissolve in tear fluid. These inserts are made of dried polymeric solutions that have been fashioned into a film or a rod. An example of this type of insert is Lacrisert®, which is used to treat moderate to severe dry eye syndrome when "artificial tears" solutions do not provide symptomatic relief. The insert is composed of 5 mg hydroxypropyl cellulose in a rod-shaped insert about 1.3 mm in diameter and about 3.5 mm long. The insert is placed in the cul-de-sac between the eyeball and the eyelid, where it imbibes water from the precorneal film and forms a gel-like mass. This mass softens and dissolves slowly, releasing the polymer, which provides additional ocular lubrication and thickens the existing precorneal film.

Formulation Considerations for Ophthalmic Products

Ophthalmic formulations are intended to protect the eye, so they are prepared with the same standards as parenteral products with respect to sterility, particulate matter, isotonicity, pH and buffer capacity, preservatives, and so on.

Sterility

Sterility, defined as the absence of viable microbial contamination, is an absolute requirement of all ophthalmic formulations. Contaminated ophthalmic formulations may result in eye infections that could result in blindness, especially if *Pseudomonas aeruginosa* is the infecting organism. This gram-negative bacillus can cause complete loss of sight in 24 to 48 hours. Therefore, ophthalmic formulations must be prepared in a laminar flow hood using the same aseptic techniques as intravenous formulations. The sterile formulations must be packaged in sterile containers. Suspensions should not be filtered, as the filter will remove the drug. Obviously, ointments cannot be filtered. For these formulations the individual ingredients are sterilized separately, and then they are formulated using aseptic techniques.

A sterile ophthalmic solution in a multiple dose container can be contaminated in a number of ways unless precautions are taken. The tip of the dropper while out of the container can touch the surface of a table if the dropper is laid down, or it can touch the patient's eyelid or eyelash during administration. If a droptainer type of container is used, the dropper tip can touch the eyelid or eyelash during administration, or the patient may touch its edge or cap.

Particulate Matter

Ophthalmic solutions must be free from foreign particles. This clarity normally is achieved by filtration. In many instances, clarity and sterility are achieved in the same filtration step. It is essential that both the solution and the intended container be free of particulate's matter. The container and closure must be sterile, clean, and non-shedding so they will not contribute particles to the solution during prolonged contact.

Solution pH

The physiologic pH of tears is approximately 7.4. From a comfort and safety standpoint, this would be the optimal pH for ophthalmic formulations, but formulating a product at this pH is not always possible because of the drug's solubility, chemical stability, or therapeutic activity. Therefore, some compromise in the formulation pH may be necessary.

When a formulation is administered to the eye, it stimulates the flow of tears. Tear fluid is capable of quickly diluting and buffering small volumes of formulations, so a fairly wide range of formulation pH can be used. Ophthalmic solutions generally are buffered in a pH range from 4.5 to 11.5,[3] but the useful range to prevent corneal damage is 6.5 to 8.5.[4]

Buffers and Buffer Capacity

Once the optimal solution pH for the drug has been determined, buffers are needed to maintain that pH for the expected shelf life of the product. Just as compromises might be required in choosing the optimal solution pH for a formulation, compromises might be required in selecting the optimal buffer capacity of the solution. On the one hand, the buffer capacity must be large enough to maintain the product pH for a reasonably long shelf life. Changes in product pH may result from the interaction of components with one another or with the package (e.g., glass, plastic, rubber closures). On the other hand, the buffer capacity must be low enough to allow rapid readjustment of the formulation's pH to the physiological pH upon administration. Buffer capacities ranging from 0.01 to 0.1 are adequate for most ophthalmic solutions.

The precorneal film contains buffers that maintain pH at the physiologic value of 7.40. The proteins, carbonic acid, and organic acids in tears act as buffer systems in the eye. Solutions instilled in the eye may have a pH that is significantly different from 7.40; these solutions cause minimal discomfort to the patient because of the buffer systems in the eye. Generally, tissue irritation is correlated with differences in the pH between the film and the solution being administered, volume of solution being used relative to the volume of the film, and buffer capacity of the drug solution and the film. The more the precorneal film departs from the drug solution in those parameters, the more discomfort the patient feels. The buffer capacity of the solution instilled in the eye seems to have a greater effect on irritation than the pH does.

Several buffer systems have been developed primarily for ophthalmic solutions.[5] Formulation tables are available based on using two solutions to prepare the buffer: One solution will be the acid or base, and the other solution will contain the appropriate salt form. The solutions are mixed in the ratio shown in the example below for the desired pH. This example is given for Sorenson's modified phosphate buffer. Additional buffer systems are included in the Appendix to this chapter.

EXAMPLE: Preparation of Sorensen's Modified Phosphate Buffer with Specific pH

Acid stock solution (1/15 M sodium biphosphate):
Sodium biphosphate, anhydrous   8.006 g
Purified water   qs   1,000 mL

Alkaline stock solution (1/15 M sodium phosphate):
Sodium phosphate, anhydrous   9.473 g
Purified water   qs   1,000 mL

Required Volume of Stock Solutions

pH	mL of Acid Stock Solution	mL of Alkaline Stock Solution	Grams of Sodium Chloride Required for Tonicity
5.9	90	10	0.52
6.2	80	20	0.51
6.5	70	30	0.50
6.6	60	40	0.49
6.8	50	50	0.48
7.0	40	60	0.46
7.2	30	70	0.45
7.4	20	80	0.44
7.7	10	90	0.43
8.0	5	95	0.42

Isotonic Buffers

Ophthalmic solutions have to be both isotonic and buffered, so each of these elements can be dealt with separately. These separate topics have been presented elsewhere in this book. With ophthalmic solutions, however, another alternative is to use an isotonic buffer that addresses both elements at one time.

Adding any compound to a solution will affect the isotonicity, as isotonicity is a property of the number of particles in solution. Therefore, the osmotic pressure of a solution will be affected not only by the drug but also by any buffer compounds included in the formulation. After these compounds have been added, though, the solution still may not be isotonic. Sodium chloride may have to be added to bring the solution to isotonicity, as shown in the previous example. Two approaches that involve using an isotonic buffer follow.

Approach 1

In the first approach, the drug is dissolved in an appropriate volume of water (V value) to make the solution isotonic. Then the remaining volume needed in the formulation is supplied by an isotonic buffer.

EXAMPLE:

Procaine HCl		2%
Aqua. dist.	q.s. ad	15 ml

The formulation requires 0.3 g of procaine hydrochloride. V value tables can been found in standard references (these have been presented elsewhere in this book) and are tabulated to indicate how many ml of water, when added to 0.3 g of drug, will result in an isotonic solution. For procaine hydrochloride, 7 ml of water added to 0.3 g of drug will make an isotonic solution. Therefore, 0.3 g procaine hydrochloride is dissolved in 7 ml water, and then a sufficiently buffered and isotonic vehicle of appropriate pH is added to make 15 ml.

The pH of an isotonic procaine hydrochloride solution is 5.6. Therefore, an isotonic buffer of approximately the same pH would be used. One commonly used isotonic buffer is the Sorenson's modified phosphate buffer. The closest Sorenson's buffer to pH 5.6 would be pH 5.9, so to complete the formulation, 8 ml of pH 5.9 Sorensen's buffer would be added to the 7 ml of procaine hydrochloride solution. Individual amounts of the Sorenson's buffer to add can be determined as follows:

90 ml/100 ml × 8 ml = 7.2 ml of 0.0667 M NaH_2PO_4

10 ml/100 ml × 8 ml = 0.8 ml of 0.0667 M Na_2HPO_4

0.52 g/100 ml × 8 ml = 0.04 g of NaCl

Therefore, the compounding procedure would be to weigh 0.3 g procaine hydrochloride and 0.04 g NaCl, add 7 ml of H_2O, 7.2 ml of 0.0667 M NaH_2PO_4, and 0.8 ml of 0.0667 M Na_2HPO_4. Finally, the solution is filtration sterilized and packaged in a sterile final container.

The limitation to this approach is that the final formulation pH may be different from the desired pH. The final pH will depend on the two pHs and buffer capacities of the Sorensen's buffer and the aqueous drug solution.

Approach 2

In the second method, Sorensen's buffer is used as the entire solvent of the formulation. In this situation, the sodium chloride equivalent of the active drug is subtracted from the "NaCl required for isotonicity" as shown in the example below. This method has the advantage that the pH of the final solution will be the pH of the selected Sorensen's buffer.

EXAMPLE:

Ampicillin sodium	30 mg/ml
Sodium chloride	q.s.
Make 15 ml of sterile, buffered, isotonic solution	pH 6.6

1. A ratio calculation will show that 0.45 g of ampicillin sodium is needed for this formulation.

$$\frac{30 \text{ mg}}{\text{ml}} \times 15 \text{ ml} = 450 \text{ mg} = 0.45 \text{ g}$$

2. The sodium chloride equivalent for ampicillin sodium is 0.16. Therefore, the drug will contribute osmotic pressure as if it were 0.072 g of sodium chloride.

$$0.45 \text{ g} \times 0.16 = 0.072 \text{ g}$$

3. To have a pH of 6.6, 9.0 ml of monobasic sodium phosphate solution and 6.0 ml of dibasic sodium phosphate solution are needed. Then, to adjust the isotonicity, 0.0735 g of sodium chloride is needed, but the ampicillin sodium equivalent will account for 0.072 g, so 0.0015 g of sodium chloride must be added.

$$0.49 \text{ g}/100 \text{ ml} \times 15 \text{ ml} = 0.0735 \text{ g of NaCl}$$

$$0.0735 \text{ g} \times 0.072 \text{ g} = 0.0015 \text{ g of NaCl}$$

Therefore, the compounding procedure would be to weigh 0.45 g of ampicillin sodium and 0.0015 g of sodium chloride. Finally, 9.0 ml of monobasic sodium phosphate solution and 6.0 ml of dibasic sodium phosphate solution are added and the solution is filtration sterilized and packaged in a sterile final container.

Preservatives

Ophthalmic preparations may be packaged in multiple dose containers. Because of the possibility of inadvertent bacterial contamination with repeated patient use, a preservative should be added. The preservative must prevent the growth of, or destroy, microorganisms introduced accidentally into the preparation during use. Preservatives do not produce sterility immediately and should not be the sole means of sterilizing the formulation.

Preservatives must be evaluated within both the formulation and the packaging. They also must be evaluated for effectiveness when the preparation is first opened, and then for a period of time after that initial opening. This often is done by measuring both chemical stability and the effectiveness of the preservative over a given period of time and under varying conditions.

Preservatives commonly used in ophthalmic formulations are listed in Table 28.3. These concentrations are for formulations that will have direct contact with the eye and not for ocular devices such as contact lens products.

TABLE 28.3: COMMON PRESERVATIVES IN OPHTHALMIC FORMULATIONS

Preservative	Maximum Concentration (%)
Benzalkonium chloride	0.013
Benzethonium chloride	0.01
Chlorobutanol	0.5
Phenylmercuric acetate	0.004
Phenylmercuric nitrate	0.004
Thimerosal	0.01
Methylparaben	0.1–0.2
Propylparaben	0.04

Because preservatives do not produce sterility immediately, they should not be the sole means of sterilizing a product. Patients should be counseled that the product may be easily contaminated by touching it to the eyes. Droptainers are less likely to be contaminated than those that must be opened and the dropper removed. The plastics used to make these, however, are reactive with a number of solutions and may not be as acceptable as glass bottles.[6]

Antioxidants

Some drugs can be chemically degraded by oxidation. If such a drug is present in the formulation, an antioxidant should be added. The common agents and their maximum concentration used in ophthalmic formulations are shown in Table 28.4. Because sulfites can cause allergic type reactions in certain people, patients should be questioned

TABLE 28.4: COMMON ANTIOXIDANT AGENTS AND THEIR MAXIMUM CONCENTRATIONS

Antioxidant	Maximum Concentration (%)
Ethylenediaminetetraacetic acid	0.1
Sodium bisulfite	0.1
Sodium metabisulfite	0.1
Thiourea	0.1

Adapted from "Featured Excipients: Antioxidants," by L. V. Allen, Jr., in International Journal of Pharmaceutical Compounding 3:52–55, 1999.

about this potential reaction before including the antioxidant in the formulation. Ethylenediaminetetraacetic acid (also known as Edetic Acid or EDTA) is not often used in ophthalmic formulations because of its low water solubility. Instead, disodium edetate, the disodium salt of EDTA, is used because of its high solubility in water.

Viscosity

Viscosity measures the resistance of a solution to flow when a stress is applied. The viscosity of a solution is given in *poise* units. The unit *centipoise* (cp or the plural cps) is equal to 0.01 poise and is most often used in pharmaceutical applications. Compounds used to enhance viscosity are available in various grades such as 15 cps, 100 cps, etc. The grade number refers to the viscosity that results when a fixed percentage aqueous solution is made. Generally the solutions are 1% or 2%, and the viscosity is measured at 20°C.

Viscosity enhancers are used in ophthalmic solutions to increase their viscosity. This enables the formulation to remain in the eye longer and allows more time for the drug to exert its therapeutic activity or undergo absorption. Commonly used viscosity enhancers and their maximum concentrations are given in Table 28.5.

The most common viscosity desired in an ophthalmic solution is between 25 and 50 cps. The actual concentration of the enhancer required to produce that viscosity will depend on the grade of the enhancer. For example, if methylcellulose 25 cps is used, a 1% solution will create a viscosity of 25 cps. If methylcellulose 4000 cps is used, a 0.25% solution will provide the desired viscosity. Standard references give tables of viscosities produced by percentage solutions and grades of ingredients.

Packaging

The traditional ophthalmic glass container with accompanying glass dropper (sometimes called medicine dropper) has been supplanted almost completely by the low density polyethylene droptainer. In only a few instances are glass containers still in use, usually because of a stability problem. Droptainers are easier to handle than glass bottles, but the plastic packaging is permeable to a variety of substances including light and air. The plastic package also may contain a variety of extraneous substances used in their manufacturing, such as lubricants, antioxidants, and reaction quenchers. Some of these substances may leach out of the plastic and into the ophthalmic solution over time. Volatile materials also may move from the solution into or through the plastic containers.

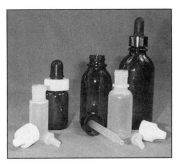

Packaging standards have been proposed to help reduce confusion in labeling and in identifying various topical ocular medications. The standard colors for drug labels and bottle caps are given in Table 28.6.

TABLE 28.6: STANDARD COLORS FOR DRUG LABELS AND BOTTLE CAPS

Therapeutic Class	Color
β-blockers	Yellow, blue, or both
Mydriatics and cycloplegics	Red
Miotics	Green
NSAIDs	Gray
Anti-infectives	Brown, tan

TABLE 28.5: COMMON VISCOSITY ENHANCERS AND THEIR MAXIMUM CONCENTRATIONS

Viscosity Enhancer	Maximum Concentration (%)
Hydroxyethyl cellulose	0.8
Hydroxypropylmethyl cellulose	1.0
Methylcellulose	2.0
Polyvinyl alcohol	1.4
Polyvinylpyrrolidone	1.7

Observing Formulations for Evidence of Instability

The evidence of instability for ophthalmic solutions, suspensions, and ointments is the same as for non-ophthalmic solutions, suspensions, and ointments. Solutions must be free of precipitation; suspensions must be free of caking; and ointments must be free of separation and from the formation of grittiness or granules.[7] In addition, the formulations must be free of microbial contamination as might be evidenced by cloudiness, gas formation, discoloration, or odor.

Because ophthalmic formulations are intended for short-term use, conservative beyond use dates would seem reasonable. The USP/NF chapter <795> recommends beyond use dates not longer than 14 days for water containing formulations (e.g., solutions and suspensions). Ophthalmic ointments are semisolids, and probably will contain some water. Although not specifically stated in the USP, the recommendations for water containing formulations should be applied to the ointments.[8]

Certainly one concern in assigning a beyond use date to a ophthalmic formulation is the potential for contamination once the formulation is used. The addition of preservatives should assure a beyond use date of 14 days. Unpreserved ophthalmic formulations should be dispensed only for immediate use. If their use is delayed, they should be stored in a refrigerator and warmed to room temperature just before use.

NOTES

1. Schoenwald, R. D. Ocular Drug Delivery: Pharmacokinetic Considerations. *Clinical Pharmacokinetics* 18:255–269, 1990.

2. American Society of Hospital Pharmacists. ASHP Technical Assistance Bulletin on Pharmacy-Prepared Ophthalmic Products. *American Journal of Hospital Pharmacy* 50:1462–1463, 1993.

3. Allen, L.V., Jr. Compounding Ophthalmic Preparations. *International Journal of Pharmaceutical Compounding* 2:184–188, 1998.

4. Thompson, J. E. Ophthalmic Solutions (chapter 27). In *A Practical Guide to Contemporary Pharmacy Practice*, 2nd edition. Lippincott Williams & Wilkins, Baltimore, MD, 2004, pp. 27.1–27.5.

5. Allen, L.V., Jr. Buffer Solutions for Ophthalmic Preparations. *International Journal of Pharmaceutical Compounding* 2:190–191, 1998.

6. Allen, L.V., Jr. Preservation, Sterilization, and Sterility: Testing of Ophthalmic Preparations. *International Journal of Pharmaceutical Compounding* 2:192–195, 1998.

7. <1191> Stability Considerations in Dispensing Practice: The United States Pharmacopeia 29/National Formulary 24. The United States Pharmacopeial Convention, Inc., Rockville, MD, 2005, pp. 3029–3031.

8. <795> Pharmacy Compounding—Nonsterile Preparations: The United States Pharmacopeia 29/National Formulary 24. The United States Pharmacopeial Convention, Inc., Rockville, MD, 2005, pp. 2731–2735.

APPENDIX TO CHAPTER 28
Buffers and Buffer Solutions

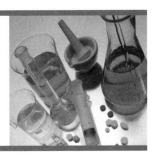

Boric Acid Buffer (pH 5)

Boric acid		19 g
Purified water	qs	1,000 mL

Boric Acid-Sodium Borate Buffer

Boric acid		0.43 g
Sodium borate		4.2 g
Purified water	qs	1,000 mL

Sorensen's Modified Phosphate Buffer

Acid stock solution (1/15 M sodium biphosphate):

Sodium biphosphate, anhydrous		8.006 g
Purified water	qs	1,000 mL

Alkaline stock solution (1/15 M sodium phosphate):

Sodium phosphate, anhydrous		9.473 g
Purified water	qs	1,000 mL

Preparation of Sorensen's Modified Phosphate Buffer with Specific pH

	Required Volume of Stock Solutions		
pH	mL of Acid Stock Solution	mL of Alkaline Stock Solution	Grams of Sodium Chloride Required for Tonicity
5.9	90	10	0.52
6.2	80	20	0.51
6.5	70	30	0.50
6.6	60	40	0.49
6.8	50	50	0.48
7.0	40	60	0.46
7.2	30	70	0.45
7.4	20	80	0.44
7.7	10	90	0.43
8.0	5	95	0.42

Gilford Buffer

Acid stock solution:

Boric acid		12.4 g
Potassium chloride		7.4 g
Purified water	qs	1,000 mL

Alkaline stock solution:

Sodium carbonate, monohydrate		24.8 g
Purified water	qs	1,000 mL

Preparation of Gilford Buffer with Specific pH

	Required Volume of Stock Solutions	
pH	mL of Acid Stock Solution	mL of Alkaline Stock Solution
6.0	30	0.05
6.2	30	0.1
6.6	30	0.2
6.8	30	0.3
6.9	30	0.5
7.0	30	0.6
7.2	30	1.0
7.4	30	1.5
7.6	30	2.0
7.8	30	3.0
8.0	30	4.0
8.5	30	8.0

Palitzsch Buffer

Acid stock solution:

Boric acid		12.404 g
Purified water	qs	1,000 mL

Alkaline stock solution:

Sodium borate, decahydrate		19.108 g
Purified water	qs	1,000 mL

Preparation of Palitzsch Buffer with Specific pH

	Required Volume of Stock Solutions	
pH	mL of Acid Stock Solution	mL of Alkaline Stock Solution
6.8	97	3
7.1	94	6
7.4	90	10
7.6	85	15
7.8	80	20
7.9	75	25
8.1	70	30
8.2	65	35
8.4	55	45
8.6	45	55
8.7	40	60
8.8	30	70
9.0	20	80
9.1	10	90

Sodium Acetate-Boric Acid Buffer

Acid stock solution (pH 7.6):

Boric acid		19 g
Purified water	qs	1,000 mL

Alkaline stock solution (pH approx. 5):

Sodium acetate, trihydrate		20 g
Purified water	qs	1,000 mL

Preparation of Sodium Acetate-Boric Acid Buffer with Specific pH

	Required Volume of Stock Solutions	
pH	mL of Acid Stock Solution	mL of Alkaline Stock Solution
5.0	100	–
5.7	95	5
6.05	90	10
6.3	80	20
6.5	70	30
6.65	60	40
6.75	50	50
6.85	40	60
6.95	30	70
7.1	20	80
7.25	10	90
7.4	5	100
7.6	0	100

Atkins and Pantin Buffer

Acid stock solution (0.2 M boric acid solution):

Boric acid		12.405 g
Sodium chloride		7.5 g
Purified water	qs	1,000 mL

Alkaline stock solution (0.2 M sodium carbonate solution):

Sodium carbonate, anhydrous		21.2 g
Purified water	qs	1,000 mL

Preparation of Atkins and Pantin Buffer with Specific pH

	Required Volume of Stock Solutions	
pH	mL of Acid Stock Solution	mL of Alkaline Stock Solution
7.6	93.8	6.2
7.8	91.7	8.3
8.0	88.8	11.2
8.2	85.0	15.0
8.4	80.7	19.3
8.6	75.7	24.3
8.8	69.5	30.5
9.0	63.0	37.0
9.2	56.4	43.6
9.4	49.7	50.3
9.6	42.9	57.1
9.8	36.0	64.0
10.0	29.1	70.9
10.2	22.1	77.9
10.4	15.4	84.6
10.6	9.8	90.2
10.8	5.7	94.3
11.0	3.5	96.5

Feldman Buffer

Acid stock solution:

Boric acid		12.368 g
Sodium chloride		2.925 g
Purified water	qs	1,000 mL

Alkaline stock solution:

Sodium borate, decahydrate		19.07g
Purified water	qs	1,000 mL

Preparation of Feldman Buffer with Specific pH

	Required Volume of Stock Solutions	
pH	mL of Acid Stock Solution	mL of Alkaline Stock Solution
5.0	100	0
6.0	100	0.4
7.0	95	5
7.1	94	6
7.2	93	7
7.3	91	9
7.4	89	11
7.5	87	13
7.6	85	15
7.7	82	18
7.8	80	20
7.9	76	24
8.0	73	27
8.1	69	31
8.2	65	35

CHAPTER TWENTY-NINE

Otic Formulations

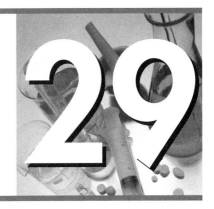

E AR DISORDERS ARE QUITE COMMON AND CAN INVOLVE any or all three anatomical sections of the ear. Problems of the outer ear, however, are the ones most often treated by compounded formulations. Typically, formulations such as solutions, suspension, or gels are used. Compounded ointments can be used to treat dermatological conditions on the ear lobe.

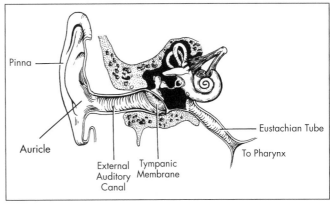

"Human Ear" by Hans F. E. Wachtmeister and L. J. Scott, Chapter 31 in General Biology Laboratory Manual: Encounters with Life, 7th edition (Denver, CO: Morton Publishing Company, 2006), p. 288.

Physiology of the Ear

The ear can be divided anatomically into three sections: the outer (or external) ear, the middle ear, and the inner (or internal) ear. The external ear consists of three structures: the *pinna* (part of the ear lobe), the *auricle,* and the *external auditory canal.* The purpose of these structures is to collect and transmit sound waves to the middle ear.

The auricle is the opening to the ear and is surrounded by the *ear lobe.* The auricle consists of a thin layer of highly vascular skin that is firmly attached to cartilage but has no fatty tissue or subcutaneous tissue. The skin that covers the auricle is especially susceptible to bleeding when scratched, because of a lack of flexibility and a large blood supply to the area. The skin also is highly innervated, causing disproportionate ear pain when inflammation is present.[1,2]

The external auditory canal starts at the auricle and ends at the tympanic membrane. The external auditory canal of adults tends to be "S"-shaped, and that of children tends to be shorter and straighter. As the external auditory canal proceeds toward the tympanic membrane, the skin becomes thicker and contains both apocrine and exocrine glands along with hair follicles.

Cerumen is the waxy material commonly called *ear wax.* It is formed when the oily secretions from the exocrine glands mix with the fatty fluid from the apocrine glands in the external auditory canal. The cerumen serves to lubricate the canal and entrap dust and foreign materials. It also provides a waxy, waterproof barrier to pathogens. Cerumen normally moves outward toward the auricle as the jaw moves when talking or chewing, so the external auditory canal is self-cleaning. Under normal conditions, bacterial growth is inhibited because the cerumen contains *lysozymes* and an acidic pH.[3]

Uses of Otic Formulations

Formulations to treat the most common ear disorders are outlined below.

Bacterial Growth in External Auditory Canal

The external auditory canal provides an ideal environment for bacterial growth, as it is both warm and moist. The skin in this region can be damaged by objects inserted into the ear, such as cotton-tipped swabs or hairpins, or from improperly fitting hearing aids, or from ear piercing. Once the integrity of the skin is lost, a bacterial infection can be introduced.

Otic solutions and suspensions are used to treat infections in the external auditory canal. The solvents typically are glycerin, propylene glycol, vegetable oils (e.g., olive oil), mineral oils, or low molecular weight polyethylene glycols (PEG 300), because they adhere to the canal wall better than water or alcohol. Suspensions are expected to provide a longer drug effect, or they may be required because of insolubility of the drug. Fine powders (talc or lactose) used as insufflations might be considered to further extend the contact time, but these can form a powder–wax buildup in the canal and, therefore, are not used often.

Ear Wax Impaction in External Auditory Canal

Up to about 6% of the general population experiences ear wax impaction.[4] Excess ear wax can form particularly in individuals who have a narrow or misshapen ear canal or excessive hair in the canal. It also can form in individuals with overactive apocrine and exocrine glands. It can also occur in those who wear hearing aids or ear plugs because the cerumen is prevented from its natural outward flow from the canal. Another way by which cerumen can become impacted in the canal is if cotton-tipped swabs used in the ear push the cerumen deeper into the canal.

The cerumen remaining in the ear will become dry and difficult to remove from the canal. A typical treatment is to use a formulation containing carbamide peroxide, glycerin, hydrogen peroxide, and olive oil. The carbamide peroxide and hydrogen peroxide contribute a mechanical "bubbling" action that softens and breaks up the dried cerumen. These also have anti-infective properties. Glycerin is hygroscopic and absorbs moisture, which helps soften the cerumen. The olive oil also serves as a softening agent and retains the formulation in the ear longer because of its viscosity.

An ear irrigation solution is used following the treatment with the carbamide peroxide formulation. The ear is flushed gently with the irrigation solution, using a soft rubber ear syringe. These solutions use water and alcohol (ethanol and isopropyl) because they have low viscosity and flow out of the canal easily. It is important for water to leave the canal because it could support bacterial growth if it were left in the canal. Alcohol, which can be used at full strength, will not support bacterial growth. Irrigation solutions also may contain surfactants to enhance the spreading of the solution, and weak boric acid (0.5%–1%) or aluminum acetate solutions to lower the pH in the canal.

Swimmer's Ear

In the condition called swimmer's ear (otitis externa), water becomes lodged between a cerumen impaction and the tympanic membrane. This is most common in people who spend a lot of time in water, such as swimmers, but also can result from excessive sweating in humid environments. Trapped water can encourage bacterial growth, leading to inflammation and infection of the external auditory canal. Also, some loss of hearing may occur gradually.

Formulations used to treat swimmer's ear include isopropyl alcohol, glycerin, boric acid, hydrocortisone, ethyl alcohol, and acetic acid. If infection is present, aminoglycoside antibiotics and corticosteroids also can be added. The alcohol helps to reduce the surface tension of the water, which aids in its removal from the canal. Glycerin absorbs the water, and acetic acid reduces the

pH in the canal, thereby minimizing bacterial growth. A combination of acetic acid (2%) in aluminum acetate solution and boric acid (2%–5%) in isopropyl alcohol can be used to both re-acidify and dry the canal.

Skin Disorders of the Ear

The outer ear is a skin-covered structure and is susceptible to the same dermatologic conditions as other parts of the body. Skin conditions are treated using a variety of topical dermatological preparations. *Contact dermatitis* may result from either an allergy or an irritant and usually is treated with a 2.5% aluminum acetate solution that possesses antipruritic and anti-inflammatory properties. This solution also has antibacterial properties because it lowers the pH at the area of application.

Seborrhea, or *psoriasis,* can affect the ear, so treatment of the primary condition involves routine medications. The itching associated with these conditions, however, can be treated with topical hydrocortisone, triamcinolone, or dexamethasone formulations. Otic gels and ointments are appropriate for these formulations and are applied directly to the skin of the ear. Otic ointments typically use petrolatum as the base and contain antibacterial, antifungal, and corticosteroid ingredients.

Boils form in the ear skin when a localized infection of the hair follicles develops into a superficial pustule with a core of pus. Boils generally are self-limiting and can be treated with warm compresses and topical antibiotics. Ear pain, however, may be exaggerated, as mentioned previously. Topical analgesics, along with systemic analgesics, may be needed to minimize the pain. Antipyrine, the most common topical analgesic, is formulated in a vehicle of propylene glycol or anhydrous glycerin. The hygroscopic vehicles reduce swelling of the ear tissue (and thus some pain) and retard bacterial growth by drawing moisture from the swollen tissues into the vehicle.

How to Use Otic Drops

Before beginning a course of treatment, the patient needs to know several aspects involved in administering eardrops. First, the patient should be made aware of the purpose of the formulation. For example, if the formulation is to remove impacted cerumen, the drops are to be instilled and then removed with an irrigation solution. If the drops are to treat an infection or inflammation, they are to be instilled and left in the ear.

Second, patients should understand the length of time they are to use the formulation. For antibiotic eardrops, the content of the entire bottle does not have to be used. Patients should continue using the drops for 3 days beyond the time the ear symptoms disappear. Products for swimmer's ear or otitis externa may require up to 7 to 10 days to demonstrate symptomatic relief.

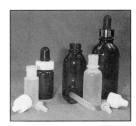

HOW TO USE EARDROPS

1. Wash your hands with soap and warm water.

2. Warm the dropper bottle in your hands. If a suspension, shake well prior to withdrawing medication.

3. Draw up a small amount of medication into the medicine dropper.

4. Lie on your side so the affected ear points toward the ceiling.

5. Position the tip of the medicine dropper just inside the affected ear canal. Avoid touching the dropper against the ear or anything else. For adults, hold the ear lobe up and back; for children, hold the earlobe down and back.

6. Squeeze the directed number of drops into the ear canal and allow the drops to run into the ear.

7. Remain lying down for 3 to 5 minutes so the medication has a chance to spread throughout the ear canal; gently massage the area around ear to aid the spreading and distribution of the eardrops in the canal.

8. Place a clean cotton pledget just inside ear to prevent leakage of the solution when the head is held in an upright position.

9. Replace the cap tightly on the bottle.

TIPS

- Do not use eardrops if your eardrum has been damaged.

- Avoid using very hot or very cold eardrops. The medication should be at room temperature or slightly warmer. If necessary, warm the drops by holding the bottle in your hand for a few minutes.

- Have someone else instill eardrops if this is easier for you.

without needles, as appropriate for the method of administration. Otic ointments can be packaged in an ophthalmic tube because this allows a small amount of ointment to be placed in the ear canal with a minimum of waste.

Observing Formulations for Evidence of Instability

Many otic preparations are self-preserving because of the high concentration of glycerin, propylene glycol, or alcohol. If these agents are not present, a preservative should be added to minimize bacterial growth. When preservation is required, agents such as chlorobutanol (0.5%), thimerosal (0.01%), or methylparaben and propylparaben combinations are commonly used.

NOTES

1. Allen, L. V., Jr. Compounding for Otic Disorders. *Secundum Artem* 13:1–6, 2005.

2. Krypel, L. Otic Disorders (chapter 30). In *Handbook of Nonprescription Drugs,* 14th edition, edited by R. R. Berardi. American Pharmacists Association, Washington, DC, 2004, pp. 723–738.

3. Hughes, E., Lee, J. H. Otitis externa. *Pediatric Review* 22:191–197, 2001.

4. Jabor, M. A. Cerumen Impaction. *Journal Louisiana State Medical Society* 149:358–362, 1997.

ADDITIONAL READING

Allen, L.V., Jr. Basics of Compounding for Disorders of the External Ear. *International Journal of Pharmaceutical Compounding* 8:46–48, 2004.

Third, if a patient is prone to develop ear infections as a result of swimming or showering, a physician might be consulted about prophylactic medication, or the patient might consider using form-fitting ear plugs that would keep water from entering the ear. Also, a hair blow dryer on a low setting could be used to dry out the ear.

Packaging

Solutions and suspensions should be packaged in small (5 to 15 ml) dropper bottles, droptainers, or syringes

CHAPTER THIRTY

Radiopharmaceuticals

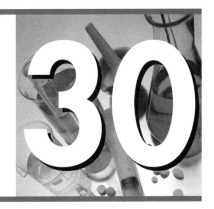

RADIOPHARMACEUTICALS ARE DRUGS THAT CONTAIN a *radionuclide* component and a *drug molecule* component. A radionuclide is an individual atom that exhibits radioactivity, and the drug molecule is the carrier of the radioactive atom. The radionuclide spontaneously transforms into another nuclide with the emission of energy most often in the form of particulate or electromagnetic radiation. This spontaneous transformation (decay) occurs because of an unstable configuration of protons and neutrons in the atomic nucleus. The process changes the configuration of protons and neutrons each time it occurs and ultimately will lead to a stable nucleus. The emitted radiation has medicinal application and is used for the in vivo diagnosis and treatment of disease.

Most radionuclides emit radiation that can be externally (i.e., outside the body) monitored or measured. But radioactive drugs, when compared to traditional drugs, generally lack any pharmacological activity because they are administered in *tracer* (i.e., very small) quantities. For example, the largest dosage of radionuclide administered in nuclear medicine is 200 mCi of I–131. This is equivalent to 1.6 µg of iodine, which is only 0.5% of the average daily intake of iodine in the diet. Tracer amounts of radiopharmaceuticals are given so the physiological parameter can be observed or measured but not perturbed.

Radiopharmaceuticals are formulated in a variety of dosage forms. Although some radiopharmaceuticals are manufactured in their final product form, most radiopharmaceutics must be prepared either on-site or in a near-by facility. Injection dosage forms include intravenous solutions, colloids, suspensions, and intrathecal solutions. Oral administration may involve a solution or a capsule. Gases and aerosols are used for inhalation administration.

Preparing radiopharmaceuticals can be a simple compounding task (e.g., reconstituting reagent kits with Tc–99m sodium pertechnetate). A majority of radiopharmaceuticals are administered parenterally, so aseptic techniques are used in their preparation. Some radiopharmaceutical compounding, however, can be quite complex (e.g., operating a cyclotron). These types of radiopharmaceutical preparations require a knowledge of the chemical reactions used to label the drug molecule component with a radionuclide (e.g., covalent bonding, transchelation, coordination complexation). Another type of specialized knowledge involves infection control procedures when formulating radiolabeling blood cells from patients who are affected with blood borne pathogens (e.g., HIV, hepatitis).

Physical Characteristics

The spontaneous decay of a radionuclide releases energy most often in the form of alpha, beta, or gamma radiation.[1] These types of radiation have different physical properties which dictate how the radionuclide can be used therapeutically. Other modes of decay are neutron radiation, positron emission, electron capture, and isomeric transition.

Types of Radiation

Alpha radiation particles consist of two protons and two neutrons. Of the three most common types of radiation, the alpha particle has the largest mass and charge and is identical to the helium nucleus, i.e., the helium atom less two electrons. As an alpha particle loses energy, its velocity decreases and it will attract two electrons into its K-shell and become an ordinary helium atom. The range of alpha particles in air is about 5 cm, and the range is less than 100 microns in tissue. These particles are unable to pierce the outer layers of skin or penetrate a thin sheet of paper. Because of the charge, however, they can cause damage to an immediate cellular area.

Beta radiation exists in two types because there are two kinds of electrons—negative electrons (negatrons) and positive electrons (positrons). The positron is identical to the negatron in all aspects except that its charge is +1 instead of −1. Therefore, when electrons are emitted from radioactive nuclei as beta particles, they will be either β− and β+. Beta particles may have a range of more than three meters in air and up to 1 mm in tissue, depending on the specific energy of the beta particle.

Alpha and beta particles release large amounts of energy over a short distance, and so are locally destructive to tissue. As a result, radionuclides that emit these particles are useful as therapeutic agents if they are deposited internally or in strategic proximity to the lesions. Beta emitting radionuclides are used more commonly than alpha emitters because beta particles are not as destructive as alpha particles.

The third type of radiation is not a particle, so it is fundamentally different from alpha and beta particles. Gamma rays are electromagnetic vibrations radiated as photons at a velocity of 3.0×10^{12} m/sec. Thus, they are comparable to light but have a much shorter wavelength. Because of the short wavelength and high energy, they are highly penetrating.

Activity and Half Life

Radioactivity is expressed as the number of nuclear transformations per unit time. As the transformation proceeds, fewer atoms are left to decay so the overall radioactivity decreases over time. All of the atoms of a radionuclide do not decay at the same instant, but the fraction of atoms decaying does remain constant. The combination of the decreasing radioactivity and the constant fraction decaying provides a decay equation that allows activity to be predicted at any point in time. This relationship is:

$$A_e = A_0 e^{-\lambda t}$$

where

A_e = specific activity at time t

A_0 = initial activity

λ = decay constant

t = time

Decay tables are available that have the $e^{-\lambda t}$ portion of the equation tabulated for many hours. Thus, when using such a table, the equation above becomes:

$$A_e = A_0 \times \text{(fraction remaining)}$$

Such a table for the pertechnetate ion ($^{99m}TcO_4^-$) is shown as Table 30.1.

EXAMPLE: The activity and time of a $^{99m}TcO_4^-$ sample obtained from a radionuclide generator was 25 µCi at 9:00 a.m. What is the activity of the sample at 2:30 p.m.?

The time between 9:00 a.m. and 2:30 p.m. is 5.5 hours. The decay factor for 5 hours is 0.562, and the factor for 0.5 hours is 0.944. Therefore, the expected activity can be calculated as:

25 µCi × 0.562 × 0.944 = 13.3 µCi

The time required for a radionuclide to decay to 50% of its original activity is its half life ($t_{1/2}$). The half

TABLE 30.1: PREDICTED DECAY FRACTION OF THE PERTECHNETATE ION

Hours	Fraction Remaining	Hours	Fraction Remaining
0	1.000	6	0.501
5 minutes	0.990	7	0.447
10 minutes	0.981	8	0.398
0.25	0.971	9	0.355
0.5	0.944	10	0.316
1	0.891	11	0.282
2	0.794	12	0.251
3	0.708	18	0.126
4	0.631	24	0.063
5	0.562		

"Radiopharmaceuticals," by Robert P. Shrewsbury, in Pharmaceutics Laboratory. http://pharmlabs.unc.edu/radiopharm/pretext.htm. Last accessed August 09, 2007.

lives of radionuclides vary widely. For example, carbon-14 has a half life of 5,730 years, whereas sodium-24 has only a 15 hour half life. Some radionuclides have half lives that are just minutes. The relationship between a radionuclide's decay constant and half life is inverse; the faster the decay process, the shorter is the half life. The following equation gives the mathematical relationship:

$$t_{1/2} = \frac{0.693}{\lambda}$$

Table 30.2 lists some common radionuclides and their physical characteristics.

TABLE 30.2: COMMON RADIONUCLIDES AND THEIR PHYSICAL CHARACTERISTICS

Radionuclide	Half Life	Decay Radiation*	Energy (keV)
O–15	2.0 minutes	β+	511
N–13	10.0 minutes	β+	511
C–11	20.4 minutes	β+	511
F–18	110.0 minutes	β+	511
Tc–99m	6.0 hours	IT	140
I–123	13.2 hours	EC	159
Mo–99	66.0 hours	β–	740
In–111	67.3 hours	EC	173, 247
Tl–201	73.0 hours	EC	69–81
Ga–67	78.3 hours	EC	90, 190, 298
Xe–133	5.3 days	β–	83
I–131	8.1 days	β–	361

*method of decay: IT = isomeric transition; EC = electron capture

Uses of Radiopharmaceuticals

Nuclear medicine is a subspecialty of radiology dealing with the diagnosis and therapy of diseases. The use of radiopharmaceuticals in nuclear medicine provides radiographic images related to the biochemical and physiological properties of tissues or organs. Other radiological imaging modalities such as X-ray, computerized tomography (CT), magnetic resonance, and ultrasound imaging also are used to detect altered physical and anatomical properties of tissues and organs.[2]

Diagnosis

Many radiopharmaceuticals are used to perform in vivo organ function tests and diagnostic imaging. Radiopharmaceuticals help to diagnose the presence of disease, observe the progression of the disease following specific therapy interventions, and evaluate drug induced toxicity. For example, some radiopharmaceuticals are used to evaluate myocardial and cerebral perfusion. Tc–99m labeled macroaggregated albumin particles can detect pulmonary embolism before and after thrombolytic therapy. Drug induced toxicity can be illustrated with doxorubicin therapy. Tc–99m labeled radiopharmaceuticals are used to monitor the left ventricular ejection fraction to assess a patient's risk of developing doxorubicin induced heart failure.

The criteria for an ideal diagnostic agent include

- easy detection and quantification,
- localization in the tissue of interest,
- appropriate radioactive and physical half life,
- chemical stability during preparation and in vivo application, and
- availability at a cost effective price.

Any radiopharmaceutical used in a diagnostic study must provide adequate energy (i.e., gamma radiation) for imaging without perturbing the tissue and without producing any biological effect. As mentioned previously, tracer amounts of radiopharmaceuticals are used to achieve these requirements. The small quantities of administered drug used in diagnostic studies will produce blood concentrations far below the minimum effective concentration.

One of the most important requirements of the radiopharmaceutical is that it preferentially distributes to the organ or part of the body that is being diagnostically imaged. This *targeting* is achieved through a combination of many factors including the dosage form administered, the route of administration, the properties of the drug molecule component of the radiopharmaceutical, and the nature of the radionuclide itself.

For example, if the radionuclide is an ion, a salt, or an ion complex and is all or essentially all of the radiopharmaceutical, the radionuclide portion of the radiopharmaceutical will determine the site of localization. In other instances the drug molecule portion of the radiopharmaceutical will determine the localization. For example, I–131 as the iodide anion naturally localizes in the thyroid gland. But I–131 orthoiodohippurate is secreted actively into the urine in the kidney. Greater specificity now is available with newer radiopharmaceuticals that are radiolabeled monoclonal antibodies and peptides; for example, I–131 radiolabeled IgG anti-B1 murine monoclonal antibody, In-111 imciromab pendetide, and In-111 labeled pentetreotide.

The ideal characteristics of radiopharmaceuticals with respect to their localization properties should be that they

- localize rapidly and exclusively in the organ of interest,
- localize more in pathological tissue than normal tissue,
- be metabolically inert unless metabolism determines targeting,
- clear rapidly from background tissues, and
- are excreted rapidly after the study is completed.

Some examples of radiopharmaceuticals, their tissue or organ of localization, and the mechanisms involved in the localization are given in Table 30.3. They are assigned into two general mechanistic categories:

1. *Function* indicates that localization is governed more by the biological processes and properties of the body.
2. *Mechanical* implies that the physical property of the radiopharmaceutical is more important in determining the localization profile.

To be of any diagnostic value, the radiopharmaceutical has to emit gamma radiation so its location can be monitored externally with a gamma camera. Camera images are compared to control images, and the presence of "cold spots" or "hot spots" are used when making diagnostic decisions. For example, a normal image of a radioactive drug phagocytized by the liver will appear as a random uniform distribution of radiation throughout the liver. If a hepatic tumor is present, a space or void (i.e., a cold spot) will be seen in the distribution of radiation because the tumor takes up less radionuclide. Hot spots are created when an area of the tissue takes up more radioactive drug.

The emission energy must be high enough so it escapes the body without being attenuated but low enough to undergo a satisfactory photoelectric interaction in the camera's photon detecting crystal. Gamma cameras are set up conventionally to detect radiation in the 60 to 400 keV range, but some applications require that the range be extended to allow detection of 511 keV photons.

TABLE 30.3: LOCALIZATION MECHANISMS OF DIAGNOSTIC RADIOPHARMACEUTICALS

Function Mechanisms			
Radiopharmaceutical	Drug Molecule Component	Tissue or Organ Location or Use	Mechanism
Tc–99m DTPA	Diethylenetriaminepentaacetic acid	Kidney (glomerular filtration)	Passive diffusion
I-123		Thyroid	Active transport
Tc–99m DISIDA	Diisopropylacetanilidoiminodiacetic acid	Liver	Active transport
F-18 FDG	Fluorodeoxyglucose	Heart	Metabolic trapping
In-111 pentetreotide	Octreotide-D-Phe-DTPA	Somatostatin receptor	Receptor binding
Tc–99m arcitumomab	IgG murine monoclonal IMMU-4 Fab	Colorectal disease	Antibody binding
In-111 satumomab pendetide	IgG1 murine monoclonal B72.3 conjugated with DTPA	Extrahepatic malignant disease	Antibody binding
Mechanical Mechanisms			
Tc–99m MAA	Macroaggregated albumin	Lung perfusion	Capillary blockage
Tc–99m SC	Sulfur colloid	Liver and spleen scan	Phagocytosis
Tc–99m RBC	Red blood cells	Spleen	Sequestration
In-111 DTPA	Diethylenetriaminepentaacetic acid	CSF flow	Localization in compartment space
Tc–99m RBC	Red blood cells	Cardiac function studies	Localization in compartment space
Xe-133		Pulmonary ventilation scan	Localization in compartment space
Tc–99m IDA	Iminodiacetic acid	Bile leaks	Abnormal extravasation
Tc–99m RBC	Red blood cells	GI bleeding	Abnormal extravasation

The diagnostic studies conducted with radiopharmaceuticals can be termed *static* or *dynamic*. Static imaging studies can provide morphological information such as blood flow patterns, organ size, shape, or position, and the presence of space occupying lesions. Dynamic studies provide information by collecting data throughout the rate of accumulation and removal of the radionuclide from a specific organ. As mentioned before, I–131 orthoiodohippurate is secreted actively into the urine. Measuring the time course of radioactivity in the kidney from the time the drug is administered through the time it is all secreted in the urine will give a measure of kidney function. This example of a dynamic study is a *renogram*, which is used to assess renal function in patients with transplanted kidneys.

Liver Imaging

Tc–99m disofenin (diisopropylacetanilidoiminodiacetic acid, DISIDA) is a lipophilic complex that is taken up by hepatic hepatocytes via active transport. Following intravenous administration, the radiopharmaceutical is distributed in the liver, bile ducts, and gallbladder, and ultimately is excreted into the intestinal tract. When evaluating acute cholecystitis, activity is distributed normally except that no activity is seen in the gallbladder. Uptake of Tc–99m DISIDA into the gallbladder is delayed in the presence of chronic cholecystitis. Gallstones in the common bile duct that block bile flow will be seen as an absence of excretion activity into the intestinal tract.

Bone Imaging

Bone imaging is helpful in identifying metastatic lesions in bone secondary to breast cancer and prostate cancer. Bone imaging is also used to differentiate cellulitis (soft tissue infection) from osteomyelitis (bone infection). Tc–99m medronate (methylene diphosphonate) is used for such imaging and shows a uniform uptake in normal bone as the radiopharmaceutical is chemisorbed to hydroxyapatite crystals in the tissue. Metastatic lesions are seen as hot spots due to a greater concentration of amorphous calcium phosphate compared to hydroxyapatite.

Heart Imaging

Myocardial perfusion imaging with thallous chloride (Tl-201) is used for many purposes but most commonly with exercise stress testing to differentiate ischemic and infarcted tissue. A typical exercise stress test involves a stress period and a rest period. In the stress period the patient is exercised on a treadmill until the heart blood flow is increased two to three times, the Tl-201 is injected intravenously, and the imaging is done between 15 and 40 minutes after injection. During the rest period that follows, the patient is allowed to rest for 4 hours, and then the imaging is repeated.

Tl-201 distributes in the heart tissue in proportion to blood flow. During the stress period, then, normally perfused tissue will take up radioactivity and appear "hot," whereas poorly perfused (i.e., ischemic) or non-perfused (i.e., infarcted) tissue will appear "cold." During the rest period, Tl-201 leaves normal areas more quickly than ischemic areas. Thus, during this 4 hour period, the ischemic tissue will appear to be "filling in" with activity while there is no "filling in" seen in infarcted areas.

Lung Imaging

Blood perfusion in the lung can be detected with Tc–99m macroaggregated albumin (MAA). The Tc–99m MAA is a suspension of particles ranging in size from 10 to 90 microns. These particles are large enough to become trapped in the lung capillaries, which are only 6 to 10 microns in size. Normal lung tissue shows a uniform distribution of radioactivity in the scan. When a pulmonary embolism is present, the Tc–99m MAA particles cannot distribute beyond the blockage, and portions of the lung will appear "cold."

Airway ventilation scans often are done in conjunction with a lung perfusion study. In a typical scenario, a positive lung perfusion scan is found and it must be determined if the obstruction is caused by an embolism or is caused by vasoconstriction secondary to poor ventilation. During the "wash in" phase of the ventilation study, the patient breathes Xe-133 gas until a constant amount of radioactivity is present in the lungs. During this "equilibrium phase," Xe-133 diffuses into poorly ventilated tissues. The patient then breathes in room air and exhales the radioactive Xe-133 into a trap (the "wash out" phase). In the poorly ventilated segments, wash out is much slower than in normal lung tissue.

Therefore, if the perfusion study is positive and the airway ventilation study is also positive, there is a high probability that poor ventilation is caused by chronic obstructive pulmonary disease (COPD) or asthma. If the lung ventilation scan is normal, however, the diagnosis of the positive perfusion study will be a pulmonary embolism.

Therapy

Radiopharmaceutical therapy has significant advantages over chemotherapy and external beam irradiation.

- Radiopharmaceuticals allow the therapeutic effect to be accomplished without causing any pharmacological effect, which minimizes side effects.

- Radiopharmaceutical therapy exposes neighboring cells to lethal irradiation even if the radionuclide is not taken up in the cells.

- Radiopharmaceutical therapy allows for selective therapy in terms of localization of target and in energy emissions.

The choice of the radiopharmaceutical for a given therapy is based on the type of radiation and energy required for treatment, and tissue localization preferences, and the tissue areas that must be affected. Larger tissue areas to be treated require that the radionuclide cover more *tissue range*. The range of beta particles is in millimeters and alpha particles in micrometers.

Therapeutic dosages of radiopharmaceuticals are much higher than doses given for diagnostic purposes. For example, the therapeutic dosages of I–131 used to treat hyperthyroidism and thyroid cancer are 5 to 10,000 times greater than the diagnostic dose. The amount of radioactivity administered to a patient is measured in units of *microcuries* (μCi or 10^{-6} Ci) and *millicuries* (mCi or 10^{-3} Ci). The Curie (Ci) is equal to 3.7×10^{10} disintegrations (atoms decaying) per second (dpm) and is the traditional measure of radioactivity used in the United States. The international unit of radioactivity is the *Becquerel* (Bq), which is equal to one disintegration per second. Thus, 1 mCi = 3.7×10^7 Bq. The amount of radiation absorbed by a body tissue is termed the *radiation dose* and is measured in units of *rads*. One rad (radiation absorbed dose) is equal to 100 ergs of energy absorbed in 1 g of tissue. The international unit of absorbed dose is the *Gray*, which equals 100 rads.

The optimum therapeutic dosage of a radiopharmaceutical is the dose that provides the desired outcome with the least exposure to the patient. Radiopharmaceuticals with shorter half lives allow higher doses while limiting patient exposure. The half life, however, must be long enough to allow for the drug to be prepared and administered, and to complete the treatment. Common radiopharmaceuticals used in therapeutics are shown in Table 30.4.

TABLE 30.4: THERAPEUTIC BETA EMITTING RADIONUCLIDES

Radionuclide	Half Life (Days)	Energy (keV) mean/max	Tissue Range (mm) mean/max
I–131	8.1	190/606	0.95/2.4
Sr–89	50.5	583/1,470	2.92/8.0
P–32	14.3	694/1,709	3.47/8.7
Sm–153	1.9	233/804	1.16/3.0
Rh–186	3.8	766/2,116	1.75/5.0

Positron Emission Tomography

Positron emission tomography (PET) is a type of emission computerized tomography that produces tomographic images, i.e., slices or planes through a patient in which each slice is displayed without the confusing data from above or below that slice. PET allows cross-sectional imaging, which can be quantitated to measure regional physiological function and chemical reactions within various organs of the body. Applications of PET have been used to map regional blood flow and blood volume, to quantitate the rates of metabolism, and to examine specific receptor binding.

Tracers used in PET imaging are natural biochemicals labeled with radionuclides of carbon, nitrogen, oxygen, and fluorine. This allows physiological and biochemical analysis at a specificity beyond that possible with traditional nuclear imaging. Moment-to-moment changes in tracer concentration in the blood or tissue can be determined in absolute units. PET also has the advantage of detecting chemical changes that often occur prior to anatomic changes in most disease states. This allows earlier diagnoses and interventions.

Historically, PET evolved with its main focus on studies of the brain and heart. PET also is a valued diagnostic tool for the diagnosis and treatment monitoring of patients with lymphoma, as a means of assessing estrogen receptors and primary and metastatic breast cancers, and for better identifying the recurrence of resectable colorectal tumors. In another application, PET is used to study glucose metabolism in tumor cells. Glycolysis is accelerated in tumors and F–18 fluorodeoxyglucose is used to trace this metabolism rate. Table 30.5 lists common positron emitting radiopharmaceuticals and their typical applications.

Positron emission tomography uses radiopharmaceuticals in which the radionuclide decays by emitting a positron. When the positron is emitted, it travels a short distance (i.e., 1 to 4 mm) in body tissues before expending its 511 keV energy and combining with an electron. When the positron and electron combine, they simultaneously release two photons, each having a specific energy and emitted at a 180° angle from each other. By detecting the two photons, a low background, high resolution, and highly specific radionuclide specific imaging can be obtained.

Radionuclides used in PET have short half lives, which allow large doses of radioactivity to be administered without undue radiation exposure to the patient. The high doses allow the collection of statistically significant images in a short time interval. The short half lives also permit the procedure to be repeated within a brief

TABLE 30.6: POSITRON EMITTING RADIONUCLIDES

Radionuclide	Half Life (min)	Maximum Positron Energy (keV)	Maximum Tissue Range (mm)
F–18	109.7	0.6	2.4
C–11	20.3	1.0	5.0
N–13	10.0	1.2	5.4
O–15	2.0	1.7	8.2
Ga–68	68.3	1.9	9.1
Rb–82	1.3	3.1	16.0

period without confounding background activity from the previous administration. Table 30.6 shows properties of positron emitting radionuclides.

It is desirable to use a radionuclide with the shortest possible half life to complete the physiological study being conducted. The consequence, however, is that the production facilities for the radionuclide must be close to the site where the imaging occurs. Therefore, most PET radionuclides are produced in cyclotrons that are on-site, which effectively restricts PET facilities to large medical centers. As alternatives to cyclotrons, parent/daughter generator systems are being investigated as possible production methods for PET radionuclides. Such systems would liberate the dependence on the hospital cyclotrons and would make PET a viable diagnostic tool away from the large medical center.

Preparation and Quality Assurance of Radiopharmaceuticals

The radionuclides used in medicine and pharmacy are produced artificially in reactors or cyclotrons. Most are produced by bombarding a stable nucleus with subatomic particles such as neutrons and protons that have been produced in a reactor or particle accelerator. Radionuclides therefore are (1) byproducts of a nuclear fission reaction, (2) products of activation or transmutation neutron reactions, or (3) products of an accelerator such as a cyclotron.[3,4]

Fission Byproducts

Fission is a process in which a relatively heavy nucleus splits into two new nuclei of nearly equal size with the simultaneous emission of two or three neutrons. The fission reaction usually is initiated by bombarding a stable nucleus (e.g., enriched uranium) with a neutron. For each neutron that bombards the target, an average of 2.5 new neutrons is produced. These intermediate neutrons are very active and immediately cause fission reactions with other nuclei, thereby perpetuating the reaction. This continuous fission reaction is called a *chain*

TABLE 30.5: POSITRON EMITTING RADIOPHARMACEUTICALS USED IN PET IMAGING PROCEDURES

Radiopharmaceutical	Application
O–15 oxygen	Cerebral oxygen extraction and metabolism
O–15 carbon monoxide	Cerebral and myocardial blood volume
O–15 water	Cerebral and myocardial blood volume
N–13 ammonia	Myocardial blood flow
C–11 acetate	Myocardial metabolism
F–18 fluorodeoxyglucose	Cerebral, myocardial and tumor glucose metabolism

reaction. Many different types of radionuclides are produced in one such fission reaction, varying in atomic masses between 70 and 170 and having mass numbers that peak at 90 and 140. The radionuclide of interest must be separated chemically from the others before use. This process is the major source of Xe–133, I–131, and Mo–99.

Neutron Reactions

Some radionuclides are prepared by *neutron activation* or *transmutation* reactions by bombarding a stable nucleus with neutrons. Activation reactions use low energy neutrons to bombard the target which results in low specific activity radionuclides that decay by emitting a *negatron*, although some also emit gamma radiation. The resulting radionuclide has the same chemical properties as the target nucleus, so chemical separation generally is not possible. Activation reactions are used with higher atomic weight elements and result in the production of low specific activity radionuclides.

Transmutation reactions use neutrons of higher energy that allow a proton to escape from the nucleus and produce an isobar. Chemical separation is possible here. Transmutation reactions are used with lower atomic weight elements and result in high specific activity radionuclides.

Cyclotrons

Cyclotrons are used only with charged particles such as electrons, protons, or alpha particles. The principle is to accelerate the particles almost to the velocity of light and then bombard a target. The charged particles move toward an oppositely charged electrode. Electrodes in a cyclotron are semicircular devices called "Dees," and two Dees are placed in an evacuated chamber enclosed in an electromagnetic field. The polarity of each Dee is changed rapidly back-and-forth (~10^7 times per second), so the particles increase in speed, and the semicircular path of the two Dees causes the particles to move in a circular orbit. Once the required particle energy is reached, the particles exit and are directed onto the target. Radionuclides produced by this method include I–123, Ga–67, In–111, Tl–201, F–18, O–15, N–13, and C–11.

Radionuclide Generators

Generators have been developed to produce a short half life daughter radionuclide from a long half life parent radionuclide. The daughter nuclide is separated from the parent within the generator system. The molybdenum–99/Tc–99m generator system is the most readily available generator system.[5,6] The system consists of an alumina (Al_2O_3) column on which Mo–99 is adsorbed as ammonium molybdate. Radioactivity decay of Mo–99 produces Tc–99m that is eluted from the column with sterile, pyrogen free normal saline. Molybdenum–99 has a half life of 67 hours, so the generator can generate Tc–99m over a period of 1 to 2 weeks.

The technetium eluted from the column is in the form of sodium pertechnetate in the +7 oxidation state. As such, it is not very reactive and must be reduced to a lower value to become chemically reactive. This reduction typically is done using the stannous ion. The reduction reaction is accomplished most frequently using a reagent kit. The kit contains a sterile dosing vial that has a measured amount of the drug molecule component (e.g., sodium thiosulfate) that will be labeled with the radionuclide (Tc–99m), as well as other components (e.g., stannous chloride) needed to accomplish the labeling procedure. The sodium pertechnetate from the generator is added to the dosing vial, then acid is added, the vial is heated, and the sodium pertechnetate is reduced and undergoes reaction to form Tc–99m–drug in the sterile vial. Table 30.7 gives examples of radionuclide generators.

TABLE 30.7: EXAMPLES OF GENERATOR SYSTEMS

Parent	Parent Half Life	Daughter	Daughter Half Life
Ge–68	271 days	Ga–68	68 minutes
Rb–81	4.7 hours	Kr–81m	13 seconds
Mo–99	67 hours	Tc–99m	6.0 hours
Xe–122	20 hours	I–122	3.6 minutes
Cd–109	453 days	Ag–109m	39.2 seconds
Sn–113	118 days	In–113m	1.7 hours

Quality Assurance

All radiopharmaceuticals are legend drugs and are subject to all the regulations that apply from state medical and pharmacy practice acts and FDA regulations. Because they are radioactive, they also are regulated by state boards of radiological health. If they are produced as fission byproducts covered by the Atomic Energy Act (1954), they also are regulated by the Nuclear Regulatory Commission. The USP also has two chapters governing the use of radiopharmaceuticals.[7,8] A preamble to these chapters was published in the Nuclear Pharmacy Compounding Guidelines (2001) by the American Pharmaceutical Association (APhA-APPM).[9]

Each radiopharmaceutical has a USP/NF monograph that states the chemical, physical, and biological standards required before using the radiopharmaceutical. These requirements include radionuclide purity, radiochemical purity, chemical purity, pH, particle size, sterility, pyrogenicity, and specific activity. When the radiopharmaceutical has been prepared commercially, the manufacturer assures these requirements. If the radiopharmaceutical has to be prepared or compounded before administration, however, nuclear pharmacists have the responsibility for assuring that the product complies with the requirements.

Radionuclide purity is the portion of the desired radionuclide present in the total radioactivity measured. Common examples of radionuclide impurity are Au–198 contaminated with Au–199 and Tc–99m contaminated with Mo–99. Radionuclide purity can be measured by gamma ray spectroscopy, half life measurement, or other physical measurements that detect the presence of extraneous nuclides.

Radiochemical purity is the fraction of the stated radionuclide present in the stated chemical form. This measures the presence of nonradioactive contaminants. For example, when Tc–99m is eluted from the generator column, aluminum is leached from the column and appears as a chemical impurity in the eluate. This form of purity typically is determined with thin layer or column chromatography. The acceptable purity percentage depends on the radionuclide, as shown in Table 30.8 for a few representative radiopharmaceuticals.

TABLE 30.8: USP/NF REQUIREMENTS FOR RADIOCHEMICAL PURITY OF RADIOPHARMACEUTICALS

Radio-pharmaceutical	Drug Molecule Component	Radiochemical Purity (%)
Pertechnetate		95%
Sulfur Colloid		92%
MAA	Macroaggregated albumin	90%
GH	Growth hormone	90%
MDP	Methylene diphosphonic acid	90%
HDP	Hydroxymethylene diphosphonate	90%
DTPA	Diethylenetriaminepentaacetic acid	90%
PYP	Stannous pyrophosphate	90%
MIBI	Hexakis-2-methoxyisobutylisonitrile	90%
IDA	Iminodiacetic acid	90%
MAG3	Mercaptoacetyltriglycine	90%
DMSA	Dimercaptosuccinic acid	85%
HMPAO	Hexamethyl propylene amine oxime	80%

NOTES

1. Onofre, T. D. Physics of Radioactive Decay (chapter 21). In *Textbook of Nuclear Medicine*, edited by M. A. Wilson, Lippincott Raven Publishers, Philadelphia, PA, 1998, pp. 371–384.

2. Wilson, M. A., Hammes, R. J. Radiopharmaceuticals (chapter 22). In *Textbook of Nuclear Medicine*, edited by M. A. Wilson, Lippincott Raven Publishers, Philadelphia, PA, 1998, pp. 385–414.

3. Mills, S. L. Physical Requirements for a Nuclear Pharmacy. *International Journal of Pharmaceutical Compounding* 2:426 (1998).

4. Hilliard, N. Nuclear Pharmacists Training and Certification. *International Journal of Pharmaceutical Compounding* 2:427 (1998).

5. Shaw, S. M. Introduction to Nuclear Pharmacy. *International Journal of Pharmaceutical Compounding* 2:424–425 (1998).

6. Basmadjian, N. Prescription Preparation in a Nuclear Pharmacy: Three Case Studies. *International Journal of Pharmaceutical Compounding* 2:429–431 (1998).

7. <821> Radioactivity: The United States Pharmacopeia 29/National Formulary 24. The United States Pharmacopeial Convention, Inc., Rockville, MD, 2005 pp. 2755–2762.

8. <823> Radiopharmaceuticals for Positron Emission Tomography—Compounding: The United States Pharmacopeia 29/National Formulary 24. The United States Pharmacopeial Convention, Inc., Rockville, MD, 2005 pp. 2763–2766.

9. Nuclear Pharmacy Compounding Guidelines. Prepared by Nuclear Pharmacy Compounding Practice Committee, Section on Nuclear Pharmacy Practice, Academy of Pharmacy Practice and Management (APPM), American Pharmaceutical Association (APhA), Washington DC, 2001.

Index

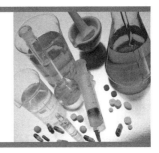